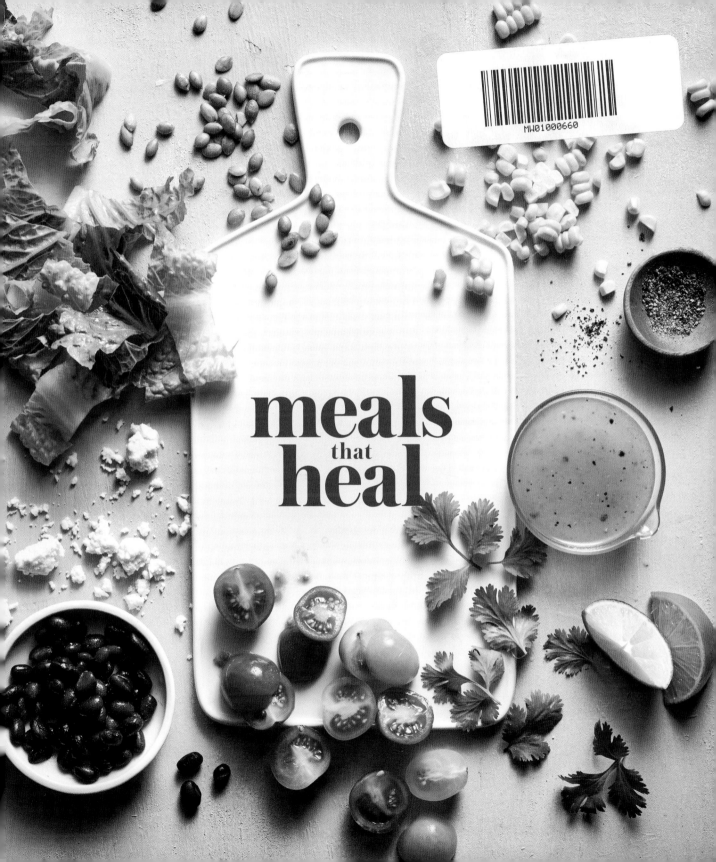

meals
that
heal

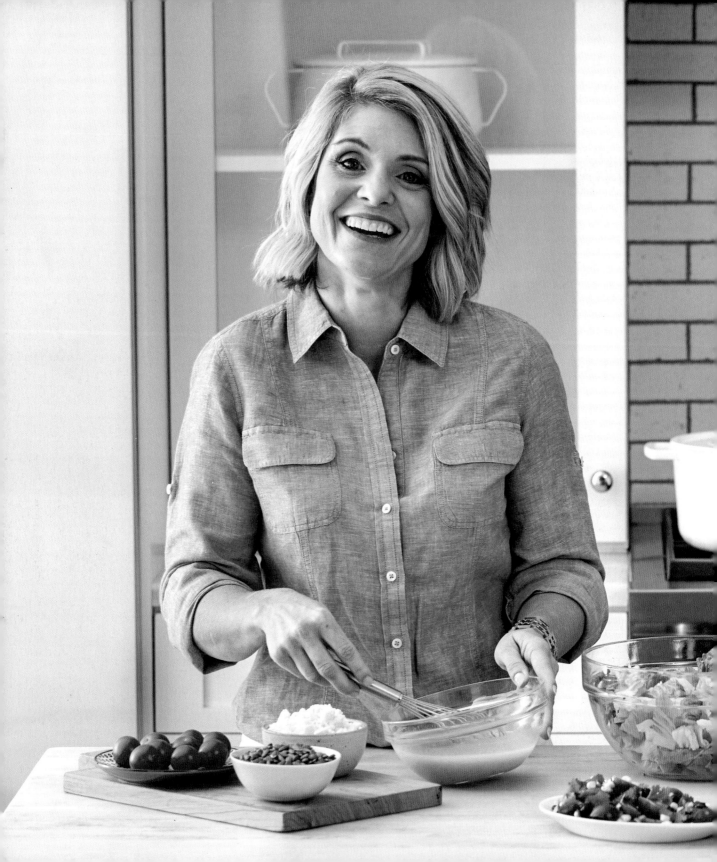

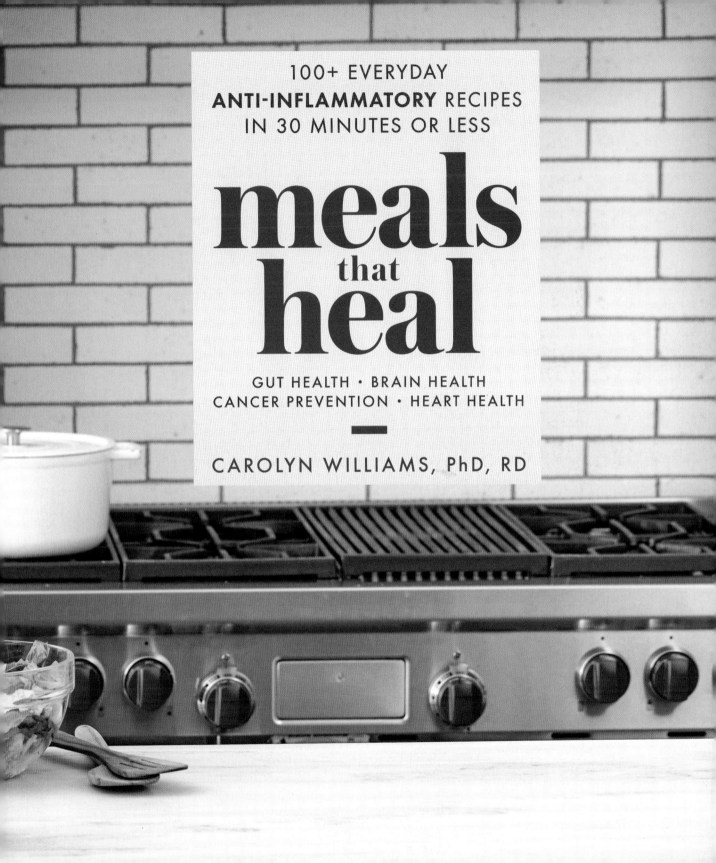

100+ EVERYDAY
ANTI-INFLAMMATORY RECIPES
IN 30 MINUTES OR LESS

meals
that
heal

GUT HEALTH · BRAIN HEALTH
CANCER PREVENTION · HEART HEALTH

———

CAROLYN WILLIAMS, PhD, RD

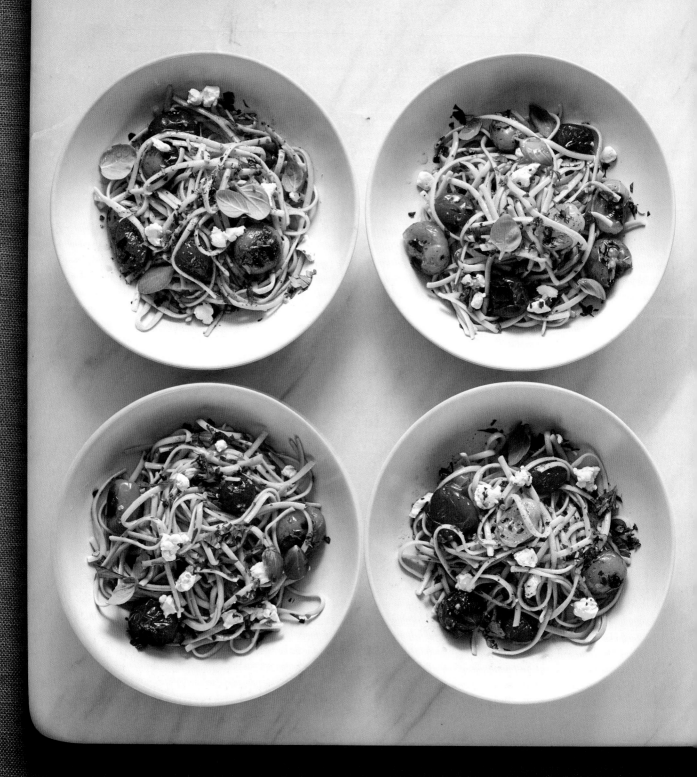

contents

This publication contains the opinions and ideas of its author. It is intended
to provide helpful and informative material on the subjects addressed in the
publication. It is sold with the understanding that the author and publisher are not
engaged in rendering medical, health, or any other kind of personal, professional
services in the book. The reader should consult his or her medical, health, or other
competent professional before adopting any of the suggestions in this book or
drawing inferences from it.

The author and publisher specifically disclaim all responsibility for any liability,
loss or risk, personal or otherwise, which is incurred as a consequence, directly or
indirectly, of the use and application of any of the contents of this book.

TILLER
P R E S S

An Imprint of Simon & Schuster, Inc.
1230 Avenue of the Americas
New York, NY 10020

Photographers: Alison Miksch, Jen Causey, Antonis Achilleos, Caitlin Bensel
Prop Stylists: Kay Clarke, Cindy Barr, Audrey Davis, Lindsey Lower,
   Missie Crawford
Food Stylists: Margaret Dickey, Mary Claire Britton, Tina Stamos,
   Emily Nabors Hall, Karen Rankin

First Tiller Press trade paperback edition June 2019

TILLER PRESS and colophon are trademarks of Simon & Schuster, Inc.

For information about special discounts for bulk purchases,
please contact Simon & Schuster Special Sales at
1-866-506-1949 or business@simonandschuster.com.

The Simon & Schuster Speakers Bureau can bring authors to your live event.
For more information or to book an event, contact the Simon & Schuster Speakers
Bureau at 1-866-248-3049 or visit our website at www.simonspeakers.com.

Interior design by AnnaMaria Jacob

Manufactured in the United States of America

10 9 8 7 6 5 4 3 2

Library of Congress Cataloging-in-Publication Data is available.

ISBN 978-1-9821-3078-7
ISBN 978-1-9821-3079-4 (ebook)

This book is dedicated to my children, Madeline and Griffin, and to my grandmother Norma Sikes, who was the quintessential role model for how to gracefully accomplish anything you set your mind to.

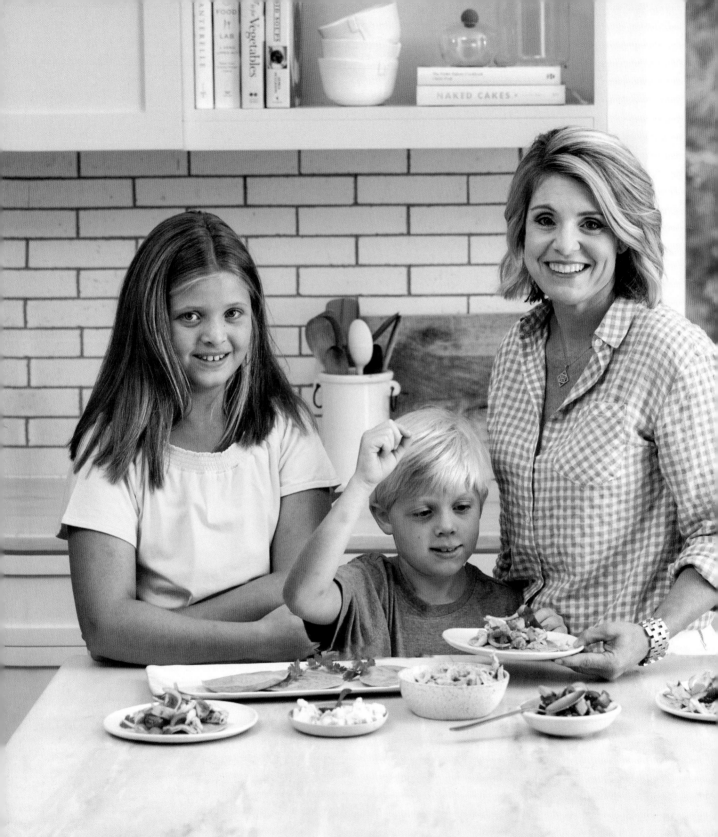

welcome

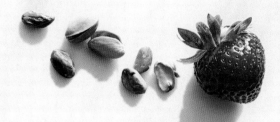

WHAT IF I TOLD YOU that the root of most ailments, from skin irritations to the onset of autoimmune diseases, was caused by one primary underlying condition called inflammation? A few years ago, I probably would have rolled my eyes and put this cookbook back on the shelf for being too hippie health nut. So how did I become convinced more than ever that an anti-inflammatory lifestyle is almost as important as wearing sunscreen or buckling your seat belt? And then end up actually writing an anti-inflammatory cookbook?

It started when I was asked to collaborate on an article for *Cooking Light* in 2016, reviewing emerging research on the role foods play in preventing dementia and brain diseases like Alzheimer's. Study results were significant, pointing toward the importance of an anti-inflammatory diet that included antioxidants. And while I was intrigued by the results, anti-inflammatory eating wasn't the nutrition direction I wanted to take—or so I thought!

Over the next few months, life dropped numerous writing assignments in my lap, all on food's relationship with various health conditions: multiple sclerosis, gut health, cancer, irritable bowel, diabetes, and obesity. It wasn't until the end of all those assignments, after digging through piles of research, that I noticed something: *every* condition that I'd just reported on was caused by chronic inflammation. The *real key* to eating healthy—for all ages—was reducing inflammatory foods and increasing certain nutrients.

My challenge then became how to make anti-inflammatory foods easy, quick, and most importantly, taste good. Was this even possible? I'm a busy mom, so I needed realistic recipes, not 8-hour bone broth or homemade almond milk! While the concepts may be complicated, I was determined that the solution didn't have to be. And I figured that if I could get my family to adopt a more anti-inflammatory way of eating, then I had something.

Fast-forward 18 months and that "something" is *Meals That Heal*, a family-friendly cookbook with recipes that you can tailor to any health condition. It is my sincere hope that this book becomes a staple in your home.

Here's to health and healing! Let's eat!

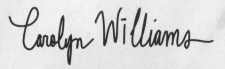

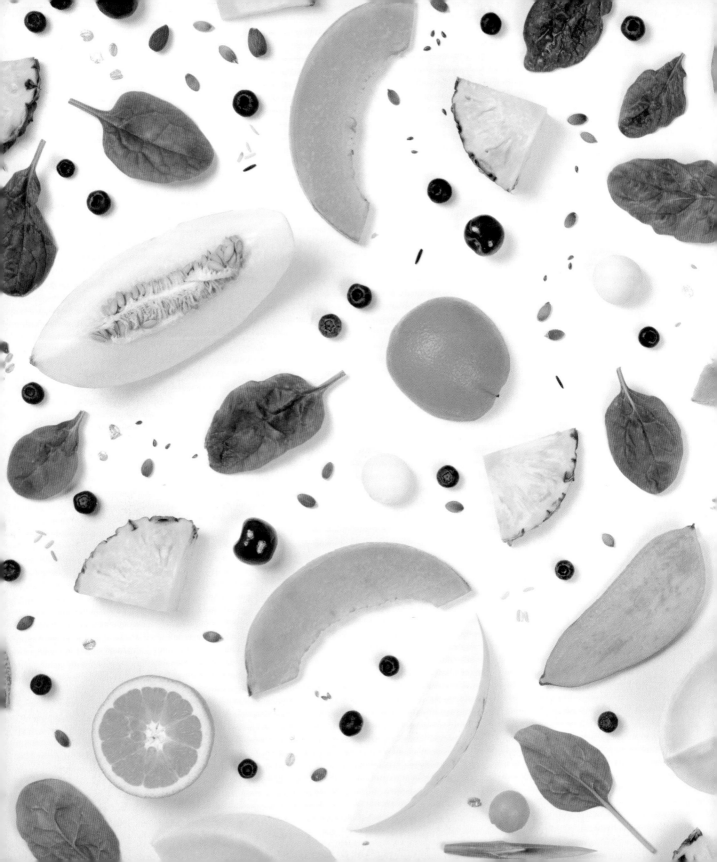

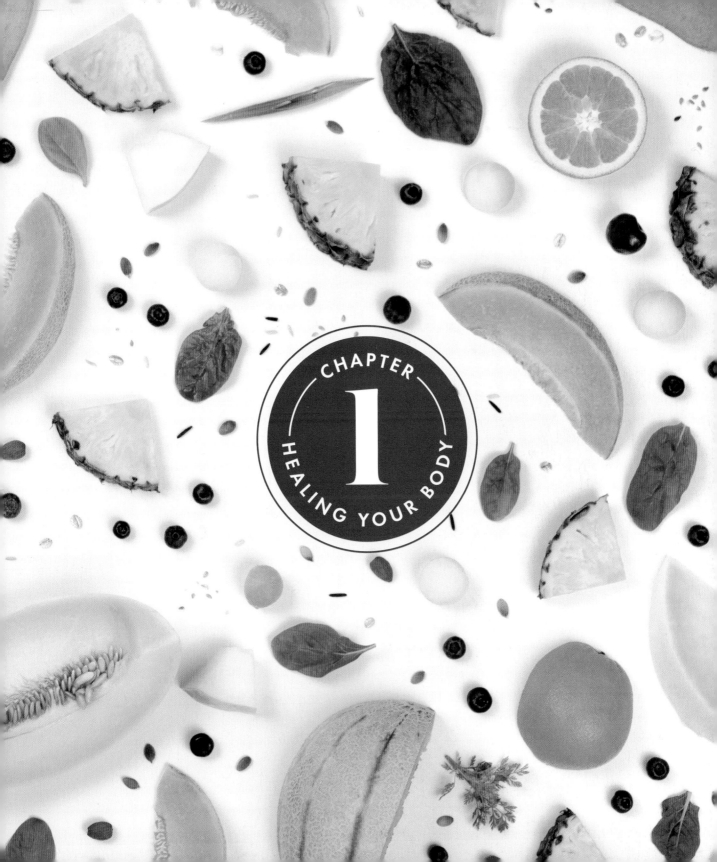

CHAPTER

1

HEALING YOUR BODY

Low energy

Joint pain

Bloating

Allergies and food sensitivities

Digestion issues

Inability to concentrate or focus

Aging faster than expected

Headaches

Itching and eczema

Memory loss

High blood pressure

Any of these sound familiar?

THE MAJORITY OF THE POPULATION in the United States suffers from at least one, if not several, of these conditions, and chronic inflammation is at the root of them all. Though its symptoms often seem vague and nonspecific, this type of inflammation is like a small fire burning inside the body that, over time, gets stoked and encouraged by other irritants, taking a gradual toll on the body by damaging cells, overworking the immune system, and creating imbalances that can lead to long-term health issues. In fact, low levels of ongoing inflammation have been blamed for increasing rates of heart disease, diabetes, cancer, autoimmune diseases, arthritis, depression, and Alzheimer's and Parkinson's diseases.

Chronic inflammation is difficult to understand and difficult to recognize because it has no overt symptoms—making it even harder to diagnose and treat. And there's still a lot we don't know about it. But one thing that research does confirm is that you can prevent future diseases—as well as heal or improve most existing conditions—through food choices. Anti-inflammatory eating involves only a few small changes, and *Meals That Heal* will show you how delicious—not to mention easy and quick—this new healthy approach can be!

inflammation: the good and the bad

Inflammation is a natural healing response by the body, but there are two types: acute and chronic. Acute inflammation is a short-term, healthy response by the immune system that initiates healing or fighting off a pathogen like harmful bacteria. While a little bothersome, acute inflammation slowly goes away over a few days as healing occurs. Chronic inflammation, on the other hand, is not so healthy, and unlike acute inflammation, it doesn't subside. Instead, it continues long-term for months or even years.

Chronic inflammation is also insidious, meaning it develops quietly with few noticeable symptoms (and often those symptoms could be related to many things), and it continues, often slowly increasing in intensity. The effects are that aging occurs at a faster rate and the body is pushed closer, and more quickly, to diseases and conditions like diabetes, cancer, dementia, heart disease, autoimmune issues, Alzheimer's, and other inflammatory-related conditions (see page 17).

Here's a quick snapshot of how acute and chronic inflammation differ:

	ACUTE OR "GOOD" INFLAMMATION	CHRONIC OR "BAD" INFLAMMATION
WHAT IS IT?	Healthy short-term immune system response to a stimulus	Ongoing, low-level immune system response to an unresolved stimulus or continuous irritant
CAUSES (STIMULUS OR IRRITANT)	Harmful bacteria, toxin, cut, bruise, sprain, injury, burn, allergic reaction	An acute inflammation or infection not being completely resolved, foreign bodies (chemicals, allergens, additives, etc.), or continuous irritants (stress, diet, lack of sleep, sedentary lifestyle, autoimmune reaction)
IMMUNE RESPONSE	Immediate, minutes to hours	Delayed
SIGNS	Swelling, redness, pain, pus	No overt symptoms, only subtle ones that could be attributed to a variety of things; symptoms typically increase in severity as inflammation builds.
HEALTH IMPACT	Inflammation slowly subsides with healing or resolution of initial cause, usually within a few days to weeks. The body returns to its normal healthy state.	Until it is resolved, inflammation continues and may be encouraged or exacerbated by other foreign bodies or irritants to initiate damage or disease at a higher rate than normal.

signs and symptoms of chronic inflammation

High blood pressure	Atherosclerosis	Insulin resistance
High LDL, low HDL cholesterol levels	Weight gain	Inability to lose weight
Memory loss	Depression	Joint pain
Stiffness	Bloating and gas	Constipation
Accelerated aging	Abnormal changes or mutations in healthy cells	New sensitivities to foods, beauty products, or environmental stimuli
Lack of energy		

chronic inflammation–associated diseases or ailments

CARDIOVASCULAR AND METABOLIC

Hypertension
Atherosclerosis
Heart attack or stroke
Heart disease
Obesity

Metabolic syndrome
Type 2 diabetes
Nonalcoholic fatty liver disease

NEUROLOGICAL

Depression
Dementia
Degenerative brain diseases
(Alzheimer's, Parkinson's)

BONE AND JOINT

Joint deterioration
Osteoarthritis

AUTOIMMUNE

Lupus
Multiple sclerosis
Crohn's disease
Rheumatoid arthritis
Type 1 diabetes

DIGESTIVE

Irritable bowel syndrome
Colitis
Crohn's disease

OTHERS

Cancer development
Cancer growth
Asthma
Hay fever
Skin conditions
(like rashes or eczema)
COPD
(chronic obstructive pulmonary disease)

what causes chronic inflammation?

While there is still a lot we don't know about the initiation and development of chronic inflammation, we do know that lifestyle habits—particularly food choices—play a key role in both encouraging and calming inflammation. And it likely won't come as a surprise to learn that the typical American diet includes too many of those top inflammatory foods and not nearly enough foods that calm inflammation.

TOP FOOD INFLAMERS:

- Refined, low-fiber starches that create a high glycemic response
- Added sugars
- Fried foods
- Trans and saturated fats
- Excessive omega-6 intake relative to omega-3
- Processed foods
- Artificial sweeteners
- High-fat meats and processed meats
- Excessive alcohol or caffeine
- Excessive calorie intake
- Excessive carbohydrate intake
- Chemicals and compounds used on and in food—artificial colors, flavorings, preservatives, pesticides, and others used in the raising and/or manufacturing of food

OTHER LIFESTYLE INFLAMERS:

- Stress and emotional health
- Inactivity
- Gut permeability and dysbiosis (see page 18)
- Ongoing lack of sleep
- Excess body weight
- Environmental pollutants and toxins

why haven't I heard about chronic inflammation?

"Inflammation" wasn't a word that grabbed my attention until just a few years ago. I realized that every disease or condition I researched was, at its root, the result of some type of inflammation. There are several reasons why it's relatively unknown or spoken about—even in doctors' offices.

- Inflammation is difficult to diagnose or measure; initial signs are subtle and attributable to a variety of things. When you can't see it, feel it, or put your finger on an exact problem (or if there even is a problem), it's hard to wrap your head around inflammation being a true issue.
- While inflammation is a fundamental concept in all aspects of medicine and health, most medical training focuses on treatment, not prevention, and doctors receive very little training on how to effectively talk to patients about behavior and lifestyle changes. It's understandable why a lot of physicians are more comfortable treating the issue with a prescription to the pharmacy, rather than a prescription to healthy cooking classes or for daily meditation.

WHY NOT JUST TAKE ASPIRIN?

Often, people take prescription and over-the-counter anti-inflammatory medications like aspirin, ibuprofen, and naproxen sodium to ease acute inflammation symptoms such as swelling, headaches, and pain. So why can't taking a few of these put an end to chronic inflammation?

- **MANY ANTI-INFLAMMATORY MEDICATIONS** work by halting production of the compounds in the body that trigger inflammation, so while you may get temporary easing of symptoms, nothing is being done to stop the irritant that's causing inflammation.
- **CHRONIC INFLAMMATION** doesn't usually present specific and immediate symptoms like a sprained ankle or fever might, so we aren't usually cued to think about taking medication.
- **MOST ANTI-INFLAMMATORIES** are designed to alleviate acute inflammation that lasts a few days—not several months or years. Long-term intake of these drugs can increase risk of heart attack and stroke, as well as cause GI issues.

how inflammatory diseases develop

In case you're more of a visual person like me, relating the concept of chronic inflammation to something that I could picture—albeit very simplistic compared to the true process—helped me to understand it more fully.

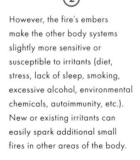

① Chronic inflammation starts as a small, contained fire in the body. Initially, it's not a big problem (few if any noticeable symptoms) since the fire is localized.

REAL-LIFE SCENARIO: Eating a higher-carb diet and drinking soda routinely triggers increased blood glucose and insulin levels, and body weight, as well as low-level chronic inflammation.

② However, the fire's embers make the other body systems slightly more sensitive or susceptible to irritants (diet, stress, lack of sleep, smoking, excessive alcohol, environmental chemicals, autoimmunity, etc.). New or existing irritants can easily spark additional small fires in other areas of the body.

REAL-LIFE SCENARIO: Stress at work and a sedentary lifestyle trigger high blood pressure, insulin resistance, and abnormal cholesterol values.

③ The overall effect of having more small fires burning may make symptoms become more noticeable or serious. Unless the fires are put out, this pattern continues.

REAL-LIFE SCENARIO: Routinely not getting enough sleep, combined with the continuation of previous lifestyle habits, triggers prediabetes.

④ Eventually the small fires combine to become a larger fire (diagnosis of condition or disease).

REAL-LIFE SCENARIO: The smaller "fires" turn into a diagnosis of type 2 diabetes, a heart attack, and/or increased rate of aging and accelerated onset of dementia.

gut health and inflammation

Health buzzwords like "gut health" and "good bacteria" are thrown around all the time now, and for many, they often walk the line between seeming a little "out there" and overwhelming—a combination that can make you want to turn the page. But there's legitimacy to maintaining a healthy gut, because it has a direct relationship to inflammation.

the role of a healthy gut

Without sliding down a dark hole of complex microbe-gut talk, let me share the basics of the relationship. During digestion, foods are gradually broken down as they make their way through the gastrointestinal (GI) tract, with the goal being to dismantle the food into single nutrients or components small enough to be absorbed through the intestinal walls and into the body. It's the variety of good bacteria that largely determine gut permeability—the level to which the nutrients in foods, as well as foreign bodies and irritants, can enter or "leak" into the bloodstream.

HEALTHY GUT:

- An intestinal tract with a variety of plentiful good bacteria provides a strong, fairly impermeable barrier in the lining of the intestines.
- The strong microbe barrier allows digested nutrients to pass through, but prevents—or greatly limits—foreign compounds (toxins, chemicals, bad bacteria, etc.) and waste products from escaping into the rest of the body.

NOT-SO-HEALTHY GUTS:

- An intestinal tract where the good bacteria have been reduced or the balance disrupted (a state called dysbiosis) provides a weakened, much more permeable barrier with holes or gaps in the intestinal lining.
- The weaker, fairly permeable microbe barrier allows digested nutrition to pass through, but also allows foreign bodies and waste components to cross the intestinal walls into the rest of the body as well.
- Research suggests that it's "leaking" of foreign bodies and waste from the gut into the body that augments or encourages inflammation and initiates or worsens symptoms and diseases.

the influence of diet on gut health

While there are still many unknowns, research suggests that there are key components in the typical American diet—too many added sugars, saturated fats, and processed foods, and too little fiber—that are largely responsible for disrupting gut health. What appears to restore or maintain the gut is a diet consisting of less-processed, whole foods with plenty of fiber-rich fruits and vegetables, as well as foods that either contain "good" bacteria or support their growth.

super gut-promoters: probiotics and prebiotics

Probiotic and prebiotic foods are those that offer additional support to maintain a healthy gut microbiome, and each plays a unique role:

- **Probiotics** actually contain live strains of good bacteria, and regular intake helps to re-inoculate the intestinal lining with microbes that may have been killed or significantly reduced in number. Probiotic foods include dairy foods such as yogurt and kefir labeled as having "live cultures," as well as some aged cheese, and nondairy cultured yogurts. Fermented foods like sauerkraut, miso, tempeh, and kombucha are other probiotic sources.
- **Prebiotics** are nondigestible food components that serve as nourishment to the gut's good bacteria and help them to thrive. Most fruits, vegetables, legumes, and whole grains contain some prebiotics, but specific foods rich in them include onions, garlic, leeks, asparagus, barley, oats, bananas, apples, and whole wheat foods.

food's direct relationship to inflammation

① Food/toxins are eaten, digested, and absorbed into the body's intestinal wall.

② Diet and environment can weaken and make holes in the intestinal wall, allowing food particles and toxins to leak out into the bloodstream.

③ Systemic inflammation begins to develop, starting with mild, nondescript symptoms. (See page 15 for a general list.)

④ Symptoms exacerbate and perpetuate each other, leading to larger effects on specific organs or body systems.

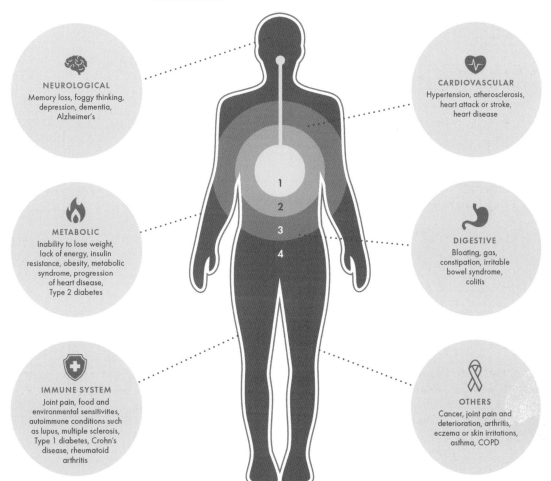

NEUROLOGICAL
Memory loss, foggy thinking, depression, dementia, Alzheimer's

METABOLIC
Inability to lose weight, lack of energy, insulin resistance, obesity, metabolic syndrome, progression of heart disease, Type 2 diabetes

IMMUNE SYSTEM
Joint pain, food and environmental sensitivities, autoimmune conditions such as lupus, multiple sclerosis, Type 1 diabetes, Crohn's disease, rheumatoid arthritis

CARDIOVASCULAR
Hypertension, atherosclerosis, heart attack or stroke, heart disease

DIGESTIVE
Bloating, gas, constipation, irritable bowel syndrome, colitis

OTHERS
Cancer, joint pain and deterioration, arthritis, eczema or skin irritations, asthma, COPD

If you're a little overwhelmed, then let me share some good news:

———

Adopting a less inflammatory lifestyle and diet can not only *heal* your body and *improve* current symptoms, but it can also *prevent* future diseases and *slow* aging.

Even more encouraging is that it only takes a few changes—not a drastic overnight overhaul—to move toward more anti-inflammatory eating. To reduce inflammation and heal the body, research points to these three steps:

INCREASE ANTI-INFLAMMATORY FOODS: Add and increase your intake of foods that ease inflammation as well as nourish and protect the body from further damage. All the *Meals That Heal* recipes are based on this most important guideline and these foods.

REDUCE INFLAMMATORY FOODS: Slowly reduce and eliminate those irritants that you regularly consume.

RESTORE AND NOURISH GUT HEALTH: As you increase foods that heal and protect, incorporate those that also nourish gut health to rebuild and maintain your microbiome of good bacteria.

what's most important?

Increasing anti-inflammatory foods appears to be the most important aspect by far. The reasoning? Many of the key anti-inflammatory foods—vegetables, fruits, legumes, whole grains, nuts, herbs, and spices—actually provide a double boost to your body since most contain phytochemicals and antioxidants. So, in addition to soothing inflammation, these foods' antioxidants and bioactive compounds also prevent or slow oxidative damage to protect your cells.

Since skipping those veggies and plant foods may have a double-whammy effect on health, first focus on increasing those rather than eliminating less healthy ones. What you're likely to find is that adding more anti-inflammatory foods makes the other two areas—eliminating inflammatory foods and restoring gut health—fall more in line without much effort.

a modified mediterranean diet approach

We've known that populations near the Mediterranean Sea are some of the healthiest, but the extent is pretty overwhelming (see Mediterranean Stats on page 23). Is it the olive oil or the red wine? Actually, it appears to largely be due to the overall anti-inflammatory effect of the foods emphasized in the Mediterranean diet.

Meals That Heal eating recommendations are patterned after the Mediterranean diet but also incorporate recent research findings from the DASH diet, the ketogenic diet, and the MIND diet, as well as plant-based diet effects and how glycemic impact affects various conditions. In fact, you won't find this exact "prescription" anywhere else. The next few pages share the general eating guidelines, and then Chapter 10 focuses on the most important aspects of the diet for various health conditions and provides menu plans.

eating recommendations

These general eating guidelines will help jump-start your new diet. In addition to the foods to avoid below, limit food and drink with added sugars (<6 teaspoons or 25 grams daily, and ideally <3 teaspoons or 12 grams.

	VEGETABLES	FRUITS	HIGH-FIBER, LOW-CARBS	PROTEIN
AMOUNT	5 to 9 servings daily	2 to 4 servings daily	2 to 6 servings daily*	4 to 8 ounces daily*
FOODS TO INCLUDE	Try to incorporate 1 to 2 servings at every meal. Focus on variety and color.	Focus on variety and color.	Choose high-fiber, low-GI whole grains, starchy vegetables, and peas and beans. See page 26 for specific foods. *Intake varies on activity level and health focus. See Chapter 10 for specific meal plans.	Incorporate a variety of protein sources, and look for opportunities to substitute plant-based proteins. See page 28 for specific guidelines. *Intake varies on needs and health focus. See Chapter 10 for specific meal plans.

keep within moderation

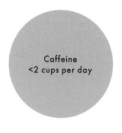

Caffeine <2 cups per day

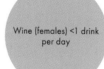

Wine (females) <1 drink per day

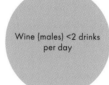

Wine (males) <2 drinks per day

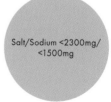

Salt/Sodium <2300mg/ <1500mg

HEALTHY OILS AND FATS

Daily

Incorporate healthy, less-processed oils and fats in most meals, emphasizing omega-3 fatty acids.

See page 30 for specific recommendations.

DAIRY

1 to 3 servings daily

Milk, unsweetened yogurt, kefir, cheese, unsweetened plant-based milks and yogurts

MEDITERRANEAN STATS

The data to support the health benefits of the Mediterranean diet are pretty strong and hard to dispute. Here are some of the strongest associations:

- Significant risk reduction for cardiovascular disease (particularly for those at high risk)
- Significant risk reduction for type 2 diabetes
- Improvement in metabolic syndrome components (blood lipids like HDL and LDL, blood glucose, etc.)
- Possible risk reduction for autoimmune diseases and/or easing of symptoms
- Possible improvements in memory and cognition, reduced risk of decline in brain functioning, as well as degenerative brain diseases like Alzheimer's

avoid or greatly limit

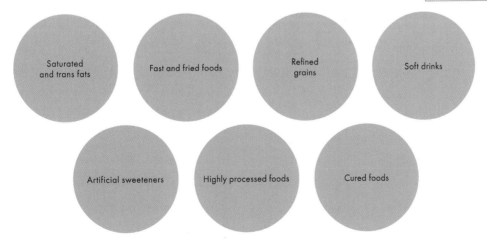

Saturated and trans fats

Fast and fried foods

Refined grains

Soft drinks

Artificial sweeteners

Highly processed foods

Cured foods

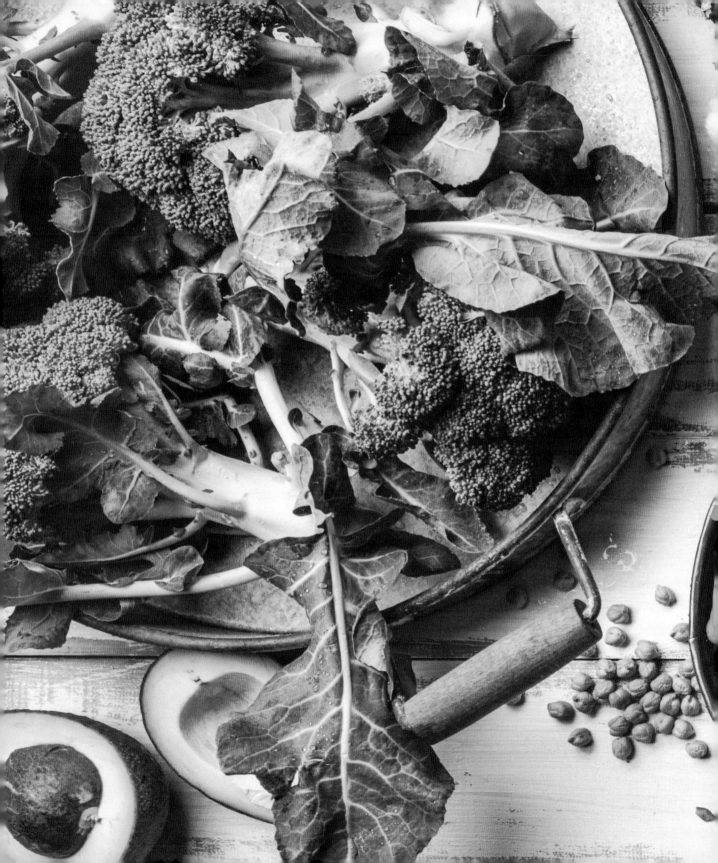

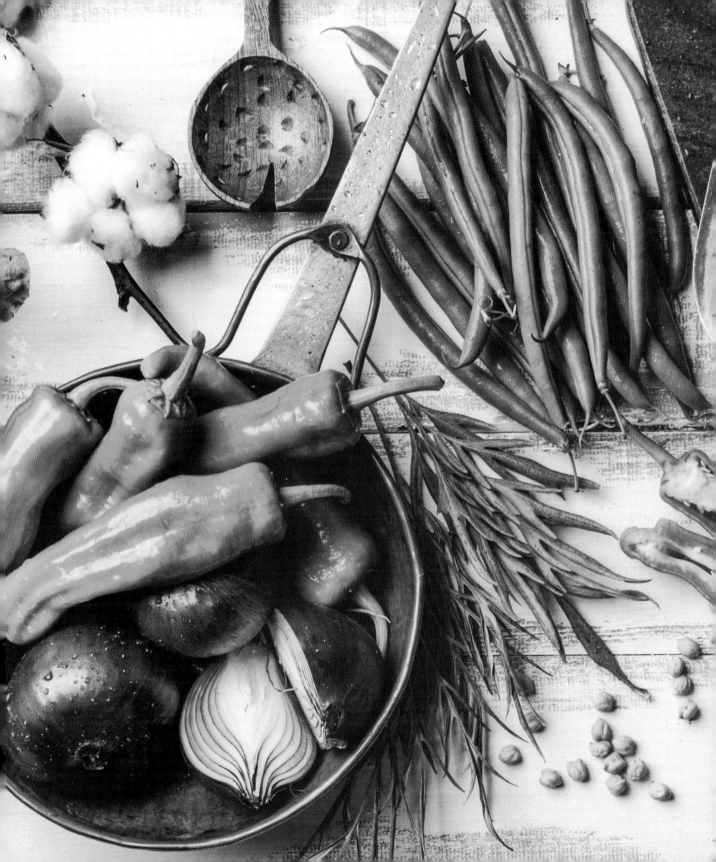

shift your macronutrient mind-set

A key component to increasing your intake of anti-inflammatory foods is shifting your outlook when it comes to carbs, protein, and fats and their proportion on a dinner plate. All three macronutrients are needed daily for energy and health, but you may not be consuming them in ideal amounts—and a higher proportion of these nutrients is coming from less healthy foods with inflammatory components.

best carb choices

The "Best Choices" listed below are all high-fiber, carbohydrate-rich foods with lower glycemic loads (the impact of glycemic index based on amount eaten). These carbohydrate foods are some of the most nutrient-dense sources, and they provide a slow, steady stream of glucose into the bloodstream when eaten, preventing peaks and dips in blood sugar levels. Try to opt for "Best Choices" for 80 percent or more of your carbohydrate needs.

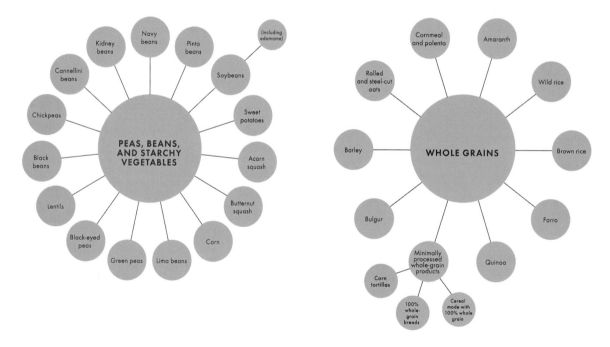

PEAS, BEANS, AND STARCHY VEGETABLES: Kidney beans, Navy beans, Pinto beans, Cannellini beans, Soybeans (including edamame), Chickpeas, Sweet potatoes, Black beans, Acorn squash, Lentils, Butternut squash, Black-eyed peas, Corn, Green peas, Lima beans

WHOLE GRAINS: Cornmeal and polenta, Amaranth, Rolled and steel-cut oats, Wild rice, Barley, Brown rice, Bulgur, Farro, Minimally processed whole-grain products, Corn tortillas, 100% whole-grain breads, Cereal made with 100% whole grain, Quinoa

carbs to watch and moderate

PASTAS
(UNLESS LEGUME-BASED OR 100% WHOLE GRAIN)

BREADS THAT AREN'T LABELED "100% WHOLE GRAIN"

INSTANT OR QUICK OATS

WHITE POTATOES

RED POTATOES

carbs to avoid or greatly minimize

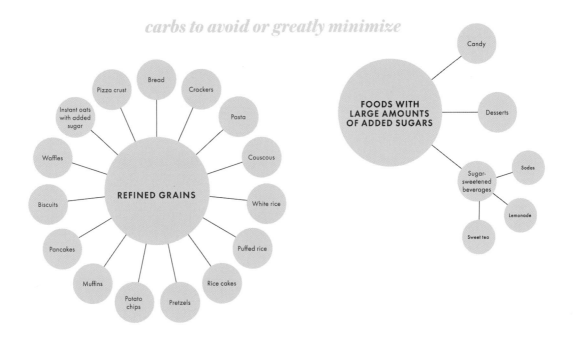

REFINED GRAINS

Pizza crust · Bread · Crackers · Pasta · Couscous · White rice · Puffed rice · Rice cakes · Pretzels · Potato chips · Muffins · Pancakes · Biscuits · Waffles · Instant oats with added sugar

FOODS WITH LARGE AMOUNTS OF ADDED SUGARS

Candy · Desserts · Sodas · Lemonade · Sweet tea · Sugar-sweetened beverages

best protein choices and frequencies

Protein in the typical American diet often comes from meat and poultry sources. In fact, many carnivores (myself included) considered plant-based proteins to be strictly a way for vegetarians to get adequate protein, not as a possible protein option at meals. However, research suggests that not getting protein from a larger variety of sources—particularly plants and fish—and overconsuming meat and poultry are key contributors to chronic inflammation. Based on current health recommendations and research, here are the best protein choices and the frequency with which they should be eaten.

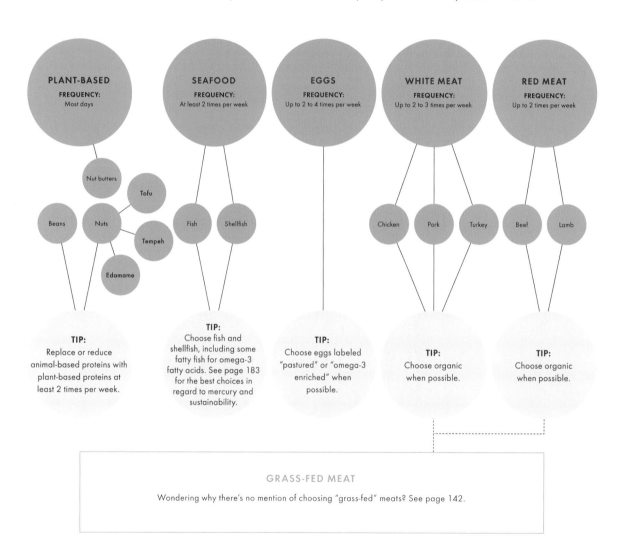

PLANT-BASED
FREQUENCY:
Most days

Nut butters
Tofu
Beans
Nuts
Tempeh
Edamame

TIP:
Replace or reduce animal-based proteins with plant-based proteins at least 2 times per week.

SEAFOOD
FREQUENCY:
At least 2 times per week

Fish
Shellfish

TIP:
Choose fish and shellfish, including some fatty fish for omega-3 fatty acids. See page 183 for the best choices in regard to mercury and sustainability.

EGGS
FREQUENCY:
Up to 2 to 4 times per week

TIP:
Choose eggs labeled "pastured" or "omega-3 enriched" when possible.

WHITE MEAT
FREQUENCY:
Up to 2 to 3 times per week

Chicken
Pork
Turkey

TIP:
Choose organic when possible.

RED MEAT
FREQUENCY:
Up to 2 times per week

Beef
Lamb

TIP:
Choose organic when possible.

GRASS-FED MEAT

Wondering why there's no mention of choosing "grass-fed" meats? See page 142.

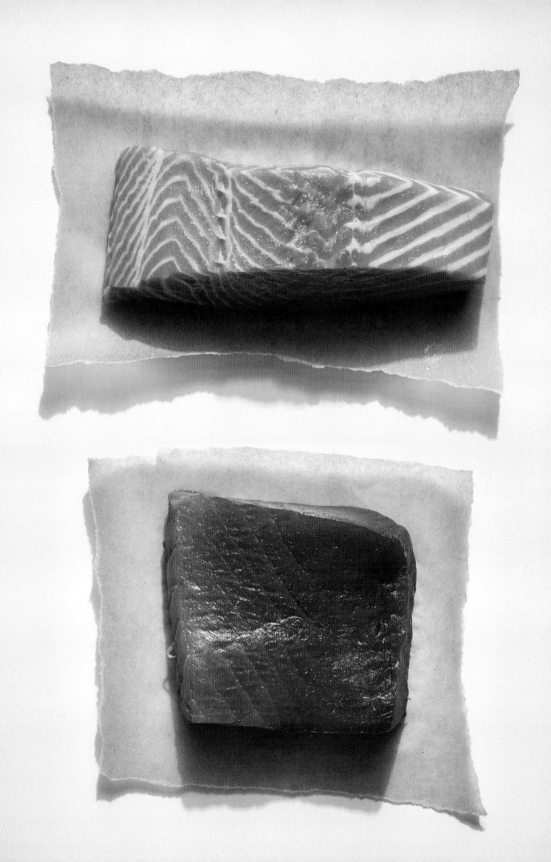

best fat and oil sources

Let go of the "fat-free" and "low-fat" brainwashing because new research suggests there's little benefit to those low-fat eating approaches. The new approach suggests that focusing on the quality of fat is most important, followed by moderating amounts to avoid excessive intake. Fat sources can either have beneficial and anti-inflammatory effects on health (such as unsaturated ones with high levels of omega-3s) or harmful, inflammatory effects (such as trans fats, saturated fats, excessive omega-6 fats, and a lack of omega-3 fats). There's still ongoing research to fully understand the relationship between health and saturated fat intake, as well as balance between omega-3 and omega-6 fatty acid intakes.

FAT RECOMMENDATIONS	WHY?	GOOD FATS AND OILS TO MEET RECOMMENDATIONS
Get omega-3 sources weekly	Adequate intake of omega-3 fatty acids are essential for preventing and reducing inflammation. Most individuals' intake is below recommendations.	Fatty fish (salmon, sardines, black sea bass, mackerel, freshwater trout) Sea vegetables Flaxseed, flax oil, walnuts, walnut oil, chia seeds Pastured or other omega-3-rich eggs
Choose oils higher in omega-3s or with other anti-inflammatory benefits when possible.	These unsaturated fat sources vary in their omega-6-to-3 ratio, but are still good sources to use regularly. Some, like extra-virgin olive oil, even out additional health benefits from antioxidants and phytochemicals.	Extra-virgin olive oil, canola oil, avocado oil, peanut oil, corn oil Olives Avocado Nuts (almonds, pecans, cashews, peanuts) Most mayonnaise types Most oil-based salad dressings
Choose less refined fats and oils	These are gathered by crushing or grinding the nut, seed, or grain. This avoids chemical solvents from being used in the processing and retains more of the oils, antioxidants, and phytochemicals.	Oils that include "extra-virgin" or "expeller-pressed"

FATS TO MINIMIZE AND AVOID		
Minimize and moderate intake of saturated fats	Some recent studies have questioned just how bad this notoriously "bad" fat is, and the truth is we aren't sure. For now, focus on the healthier fats and keep intake moderate or minimized.	Animal fat on meat and poultry Butter, lard, bacon Tropical oils such as coconut oil and palm oil
Avoid all trans fats	Trans fats are unsaturated oils that have been chemically altered—the result of which is a processed fat that is directly linked to increasing inflammation and risks for diabetes, heart disease, and other chronic diseases.	Fast food and fried foods Any type of "hydrogenated" or "partially hydrogenated"—look for in processed food products like margarines, snack foods, and packaged desserts Shortening

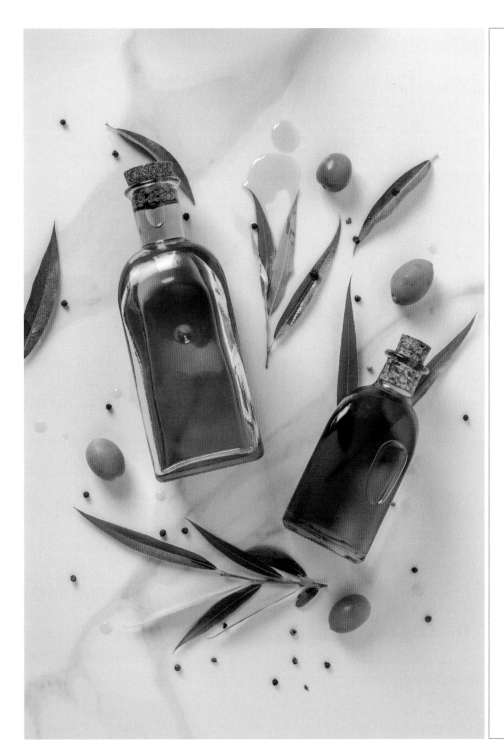

EVOO VS. REFINED OLIVE OIL

Extra-virgin olive oil is one of the primary oils used in recipes throughout this book, and this is for several reasons. First, EVOO undergoes little to no chemical or heat refining, which allows it to retain more antioxidants like vitamin E—which means the body has more ammunition in fighting oxidative stress and protecting cells from damage caused by free radicals.

Second, EVOO's lack of refining preserves more of the compound oleocanthal found in olives, which research suggests has a natural inflammation-suppressing effect.

Finally, olive oil is predominantly a monounsaturated fat and contains more omega-6 fatty acids, something that may seem contradictory to my recommendation to choose more omega-3 fatty acid sources (see opposite), but this is when you have to factor in an oil's or fat's chemical stability. Olive oil's high predominance of omega-6 fatty acids means it is much more stable and less likely to break down and re-create harmful chemicals in the body when heated, compared to those with a higher predominance of omega-3 fats. This stability factor combined with its inflammation-fighting compounds make EVOO my first choice for fresh or minimally cooked dishes.

I may opt for something different when I am cooking at higher heats or for longer periods of time. In these situations, it's best to use an oil with a higher smoke point, essentially an oil that can be heated to higher temps before breaking down. EVOO has a smoke point around 325°F, but refined olive oils are closer to 400°F or 425°F, often making them a better choice than EVOO. Other oils like avocado, sunflower seed, peanut, and corn all have smoke points above 400°F, so these can be good cooking options, too.

omega 6-to-3 ratio

The ratio of fats and oils that you consume containing omega-6 fatty acids versus omega-3 is a consideration when it comes to quality and health effects. Both are found in unsaturated fats, but omega-6 fatty acids are way overconsumed and in a much higher proportion to omega-3s.

This is thanks to the heavy use of vegetable oils like corn, soybean, and sunflower in most processed foods and other common grocery items. Some research suggests that overconsumption of omega-6 fatty acids increases inflammation within the body, but others argue that this is a side effect of underconsuming omega-3 fatty acids, which are vital for health and have an anti-inflammatory effect on the body. Regardless of the true answer, most of us need to increase our intake of omega-3s, so look for ways to use them in place of fats and oils containing predominantly omega-6 fatty acids.

key lifestyle components

Our sleep, stress, and activity are lifestyle components that, along with diet, can make one more prone to or exacerbate chronic inflammation.

REGULAR ACTIVITY: Individuals who get regular activity have lower levels of inflammatory blood markers; being sedentary is a risk factor for inflammation.

STRESS: It ranges from physical to emotional to psychological, and research suggests that ongoing stress reduces the body's ability to regulate the immune system, which doesn't help a body that's already irritated and inflamed. It's worth the time—and your health—to find ways to reduce and regulate stress, such as exercise, meditation, journaling, yoga, and staying in regular contact with friends and family (unless they are the stressor!).

SLEEP: Both too little and too much sleep are associated with increased inflammation in the body. Aim for 7 to 8 hours of continuous sleep to restore the body and to reduce inflammation. Catch up on sleep when you've been sleep-deprived, and set an alarm for those days off if you're apt to sleep the morning away.

rethinking the dinner plate

So are you wondering how to pull all the guidelines together to get a healthy (and good-tasting!) anti-inflammatory meal? Most people don't have trouble learning how to fit in some of their favorite foods—or cut out some of the inflammatory foods—but do have to practice shifting their mind-set a little when it comes to what an anti-inflammatory full meal looks like. Here are a few visuals to think about when planning or plating meals.

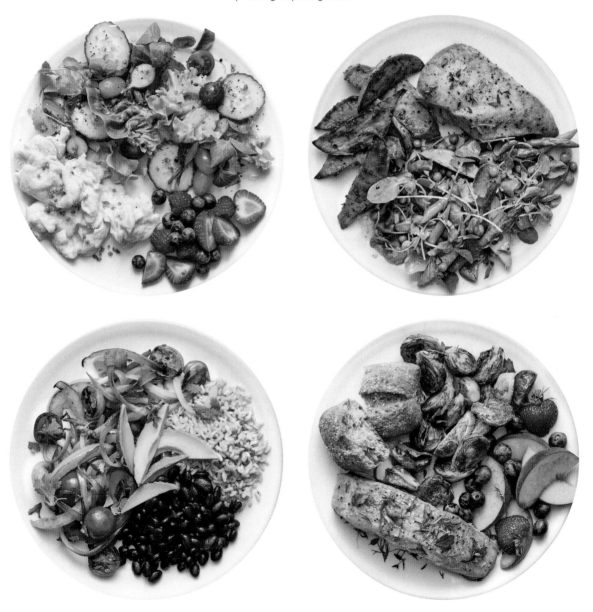

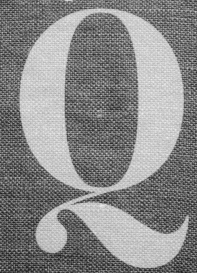

F

Got questions?

A

We've got answers.

Q

anti-inflammatory FAQs

These are the most common questions I get asked by people beginning an anti-inflammatory eating protocol. They're also some of the same ones that I had when I began researching inflammation and diet, but couldn't seem to find consistent answers to. This challenged me to delve deeper into the research so I could share straightforward, research-based answers with others. Though researchers still have a lot to discover in some areas, these recommendations are based on what the latest research findings suggest.

do I have to make everything from scratch?

Not at all, and I don't expect you to, because I sure don't! In fact, there's nothing that I love more than finding a new packaged food product to shave time and work off dinner prep. However, to do this and follow an anti-inflammatory lifestyle, it is **key** that you start looking closer at labels to choose more minimally processed products. In Chapter 2, you'll find my Store-Bought Product Buying Guide (page 72), which walks you through what to look for on packaging. Scattered throughout this book, you'll also find guidelines to help you select prepared cereals, breakfast foods, side dishes, salad dressings, snacks, and desserts—as well as a few of my family's favorite brands and products.

I've heard that dairy is inflammatory, so do I need to eliminate all dairy foods?

Contrary to popular belief, dairy products appear to have an anti-inflammatory effect in most people. In fact, yogurt is recommended to reduce inflammation by supporting gut health. Since saturated fat can contribute to inflammation, moderate intake is best, as well as choosing lower-fat versions. However, those with a dairy allergy or sensitivity should avoid dairy, since it will trigger their bodies' inflammatory responses when consumed, negating dairy's anti-inflammatory effects.

To accommodate a wide range of needs, most *Meals That Heal* recipes are either dairy-free or provide a dairy-free ingredient substitute. If you think that you may have a sensitivity to dairy, eliminate dairy from your diet during the Detox & Restore phase. Then slowly reintroduce it, watching for any symptoms.

what's the story on gluten?

It's trendy to be gluten-free, but most health professionals advise that only those with a wheat allergy or celiac disease (an autoimmune disease in which gluten causes damage to the small intestine) really need to avoid it. The idea that there may be some individuals who also suffer from a gluten sensitivity, a much milder intolerance for which there's no real way to screen or diagnose, has also been dismissed for years.

However, there's growing evidence that gluten sensitivity may be a real thing, and although damage doesn't occur to the intestines as in celiac disease, a sensitivity may trigger subtle inflammatory symptoms. Some may have a true sensitivity while others may be sensitive due to the body being irritated and inflamed already—a situation where food components that normally wouldn't trigger irritation (like gluten) cause further irritation due to the existing inflammation.

Based on the latest research, as well as recommendations from a host of medical organizations and universities, my approach to gluten when it comes to meal plans and eating guidelines in *Meals That Heal* is this:

- Avoid or greatly limit gluten during the Detox and Restore phase (or for your first several weeks of anti-inflammatory eating). This is temporary and gives the body time to calm down as irritants are removed and gut microbes are restored.
- Once potential irritants have been removed for at least two weeks, then you may want to try adding back a whole grain that contains gluten (such as whole wheat bread or farro). If you do add gluten back to your diet, do it slowly and monitor for any subtle side effects, such as bloating, gas, headaches,

and joint pain, and don't add back two potential irritants at the same time (such as dairy and gluten). The exception to this is if you choose a meal plan for a medical condition that may benefit continued avoidance of gluten such as an autoimmune condition.

- All *Meals That Heal* recipes are gluten-free to accommodate all diet needs.
- Gluten-free eating can be healthy or unhealthy depending on your approach. A healthier approach is to focus on swapping processed, gluten-containing foods and refined grains for vegetables, beans, starchy vegetables, fruits, and gluten-free whole grains like quinoa and coarse-ground cornmeal. This leads to a more nutrient-dense, less inflammatory diet because of the overall improved diet quality—not necessarily due to gluten avoidance. Simply swapping gluten-containing foods for processed foods labeled "gluten-free" does not improve diet quality or decrease inflammation.

should I avoid nightshades?

Nightshade vegetables, such as tomatoes, eggplant, peppers, and potatoes, are often blamed for arthritis inflammation due to a compound they contain called solanine. However, there's no conclusive research that nightshades trigger inflammation. These veggies are packed full of anti-inflammatory nutrients, so don't avoid nightshades—unless eating a specific one triggers pain or inflammation symptoms. If it does, the issue likely isn't the nightshade family, but rather a sensitivity to one specific food, which can be eliminated.

can I have a glass of wine?

Since any food or food component can irritate the body further when it's inflamed, it's ideal to eliminate or greatly reduce alcohol intake during the Detox and Restore phase. This gives the body time to calm down. After this phase, you can add an occasional drink, if desired, since alcohol—wine, beer, or liquor—when consumed in moderation can be a part of anti-inflammatory eating and living. "Alcohol and Inflammation" on page 275 explains both the anti-inflammatory and inflammatory potential that alcoholic drinks can have.

is some added sugar okay?

Well, I hope so, because I'm definitely not giving up dessert for the rest of my life! But at the same time, I can't ignore that Americans' consumption of excess added sugars is contributing to inflammation and the development of most all chronic diseases. And what's scary is that most individuals are unaware of just how much added sugar they consume on a daily basis. Because of this, I strongly encourage you to begin by eliminating all added sugars—something that will start to clean up your diet and also illustrate just how prevalent they are in our food supply. Use my Store-Bought Product Buying Guide (page 72) to walk you through what to look for on the packaging and exactly how added sugars may be disguised on labels.

Once individuals are more aware of added sugar prevalence, then I am all about incorporating some added sugars in moderation. Since it's easy for "moderation" to quickly cross the line into excess, I've found that many (myself included) need specific parameters of what moderate intake should be. A good goal is to aim to keep added sugar intake to less than 3 teaspoons or 12 grams on most days. When this is your norm the majority of days, then it's not a big deal to occasionally indulge. See "How to Eat Sugar" on page 256 for how to do this and how to make the most of those times!

are artificial sweeteners good substitutes for sugar?

All must be deemed relatively safe by the Food and Drug Administration to be on the market, but my concern surrounding artificial sweeteners is that the prominent ones that you see on restaurant tables and in food products are sweet-tasting chemical compounds (like aspartame and saccharine) made in a lab. And while deemed safe now, we haven't had time to collect long-term data to really know the effects that consuming these chemicals for fifty or sixty years will have on the body.

From an anti-inflammatory standpoint, the body may consider these foreign bodies or irritants—particularly if there's already some low-level inflammation. Additionally, while they may not be contributing calories or added sugar, research suggests that some artificial sweeteners negatively impact the body's glucose and insulin management, which could also encourage existing inflammation.

My approach is to limit artificial sweeteners in general. When I do need to use one, I opt for a low-calorie, plant-based sweetener (such as stevia).

A sweetener from a plant, rather than a chemistry lab, seems like a safer and healthier option. Also, research surrounding stevia is positive, even suggesting it may improve glycemic response following a meal.

my friend follows an anti-inflammatory plan that involves fasting. should I be fasting?

Intermittent fasting (IF) is a popular eating trend that centers around alternating between short periods of fasting (consuming little to no food for some portion of the day) and periods of regular food intake. A common approach to IF is eating only during an 8-hour window during the day, meaning you fast the remaining 16 hours. Not only does IF appear to decrease inflammation in some individuals, but research also suggests that it may reduce cardiovascular risk, improve insulin sensitivity, and maintain or improve metabolic rate. However, IF is definitely not for everyone, and much more research is needed. So if the thought of fasting seems dreadful, don't sweat it. Focus on the other dietary aspects with substantial research backing. But if you're not a breakfast eater or tend to go long periods without eating, you're on-trend and don't necessarily need to change anything in terms of your eating frequency.

top 8 anti-inflammatory foods

None of these has magical healing powers—or even the ability to reduce inflammation by themselves. But these are the top foods that I've found repeatedly pop up in research when it comes to offering anti-inflammatory effects to the body.

	LEAFY GREENS	OLIVE OIL	BERRIES	CRUCIFEROUS VEGETABLES
FOODS TO INCLUDE	Lettuces (like romaine, red leaf, green leaf, radicchio, arugula), cruciferous greens (like kale, mustard, turnip), spinach, Swiss chard, watercress, and dandelion greens	**BEST:** extra-virgin olive oil **NEXT BEST:** virgin olive oil, cold-pressed, or olive oil from a first pressing **SKIP:** ones labeled "light" or "pure"	Blueberries, strawberries, raspberries, blackberries, boysenberries, and cranberries	Broccoli, Brussels sprouts, cauliflower, cabbage, collard greens, kale, mustard greens, watercress, kohlrabi, bok choy, rutabaga, turnips, arugula, radish, and watercress
	At least 6 cups per week	Daily as part of fat intake	At least 2 cups per week	At least 5 servings per week
REASONS	The research behind the health benefits of eating leafy greens is some of the strongest with suggested risk reduction of heart disease, type 2 diabetes, some cancers, and brain deterioration. In fact, the risk may decrease with each additional serving consumed. Leafy greens are also packed with folate and phytochemicals with additional antioxidant and anti-inflammatory effects.	This pantry staple delivers the inflammation-suppressing compound oleocanthal, plus a small amount of omega-3s. Health benefits that research associates with olive oil include reduced risk of heart attack, stroke, cancer development, joint deterioration, and neurological diseases.	All berries are loaded with anthocyanins and antioxidants, which sweep up harmful free radicals that promote inflammation. This directly reduces the risk of heart disease, brain deterioration, and cancer. They're also packed with fiber that reduces cholesterol values and slows the digestive process to keep blood sugar in check.	What separates this crunchy family from other vegetables are sulfur-containing compounds called glucosinolates. Indoles and isothiocyanates are two types of powerful glucosinolates that appear to lower inflammatory markers in the body, lower cancer risk, and possibly initiate the death of cancer cells. On top of that, most cruciferous veggies are packed with antioxidants like vitamin C and beta-carotene, and other anti-inflammatory phytochemicals.

FATTY FISH	GREEN TEA	GUT-HEALTH PROMOTERS	NUTS AND SEEDS
Salmon, anchovies, butterfish, sea bass, mackerel, and sardines	Green, white, oolong, and black teas	Cultured and fermented foods, such as yogurt, kimchi, kombucha, miso, and sauerkraut, as well as prebiotics (see page 18)	Almonds, Brazil nuts, cashews, chia seeds, flaxseed, hazelnuts, macadamia nuts, pecans, pine nuts, pistachios, sunflower seeds, walnuts
8 to 12 ounces per week	At least 1 cup per day	Daily or at least several times per week	Include 1 ounce, 5 or more days per week
The omega-3 fats DHA and EPA in salmon and other oily fish play key roles in suppressing inflammation and boosting production of anti-inflammatory compounds. DHA and EPA appear to have a particularly strong link to heart and neurological disease prevention, and fattier fish are one of the few dietary sources.	Research suggests that regular intake of this antioxidant-rich beverage may suppress both the development and growth of cancer cells, promote the growth of good bacteria, and block or slow the plaque formation associated with Alzheimer's development. This is all thanks to compounds called catechins that appear to be one of the most effective antioxidants in preventing free radical damage. Very few negatives are associated with green tea intake, just watch caffeine intake.	The exact role that "good" microbes play is still unclear, but current research suggests that the relationship between gut health and disease prevention is substantial. Consuming foods with "good" bacteria regularly and consuming a variety of strains are the best ways to encourage a healthy gut—not to mention that these foods are usually nutrient-rich sources of antioxidants, too. Another plus of live cultures in yogurt: The live bacteria produces lactic acid that inhibits the growth of bad bacteria in the gut.	Not only is regular intake associated with healthier body weight, but nuts are packed with omega-3s, antioxidants like vitamin E, protein, and slow-digesting carbohydrates, which support better blood sugar regulation and improve insulin sensitivity. Walnuts and almonds are considered some of the best, but all nuts are good to incorporate as part of daily fat intake.

STEP #1

Assess

STEP #2

Detox and Restore

STEP #3

Target or Reassess

STEP #4

Eat and Feel Good!

getting started/how to use this book

Not sure where to begin? Let me help you get started! These four simple steps will walk you through the process of slowly healing your body and creating a personalized plan specific to your health concerns. Then use the guidelines in this chapter, as well as the information and meal plans in Chapter 10, to make anti-inflammatory eating quick, easy, and delicious!

step #1: assess

The first step is to identify what the biggest "issues" are in your current diet. To do this, think through your food intake over the past week or track your normal eating for a few days. Then, see how many of the following you eat in 3 to 5 days.

_____ Refined grains
_____ Highly processed foods and ready-to-eat foods
_____ Fast food and fried foods
_____ Added sugars (think coffee drinks, soft drinks, cereals, grain products, condiments, etc.)
_____ How many days did you have more than two caffeinated drinks?
_____ Men: How many days did you have more than two alcoholic drinks? Women: How many days did you have more than one alcoholic drink?
_____ Cured or processed meats (bacon, sausage, lunch meats, hot dogs, etc.)
_____ Other
_____ Other

_____ Total vegetables
_____ Beans, legumes, and peas
_____ Leafy greens
_____ Fruit (other than dried or in syrup) _____ How many of those were berries?
_____ How many meals do you eat a plant-based protein in place of an animal protein?
_____ Fish _____ How many of those were fatty fish?
_____ Nuts
_____ Other

semi-homemade is okay

Cooking dinner from scratch every night is often seen as the ultimate pinnacle of healthy eating. However, this isn't a realistic expectation for many of us today, and it shouldn't be the standard we hold ourselves to or that causes ongoing guilt—even though I felt it for years. I know as a dietitian that it's the quality of the food that I serve my family that matters—not whether every single item was peeled, steamed, emulsified, or spiralized by my own hands.

The key for me is finding the healthy balance between convenience and health, and to do this I rely on some minimally processed foods and food products (think canned beans, frozen sweet potato wedges, and corn tortillas). Combining these items with prepped staples or quick-cooking foods allows me to have a healthy meal made from high-quality foods usually in 20 minutes or less. While it may not be completely "from scratch," the end result is the same—or maybe better—and much healthier than the alternative.

step #2: detox and restore

Your next step to healing your body is to focus for two weeks on consuming foods that supports the body's natural detoxification process.

what this means

- Eating foods with nutrients that support the liver and the body's natural detoxification processes
  - o Whole or minimally processed foods (see page 72 for what this means)
  - o Lots of vegetables, fruit, herbs, and spices
  - o Increasing the proportion of healthier fats, carbs, and proteins
- Ridding the diet of toxins and irritants
  - o Unnecessary additives like colorings, artificial sweeteners, chemicals, and pesticides when possible
  - o Irritants like gluten, added sugars, alcohol, excessive caffeine, etc. (Don't worry—many of these are temporary!)
- Restoring, balancing, and nourishing gut bacteria
  - o Probiotic foods—those rich in "good" bacteria strains
  - o Prebiotic foods

what detox and restore doesn't mean

- Eliminating food group(s) unless you have specific allergies or sensitivities
- Consuming only liquids, juices, or odd food combinations
- Severely restricting calories
- Cutting out flavor, taste, salt, or fat

defining your own plan

Do you have several issues to address, and don't know where to start? No worries, because your best bet is to start small! Here's how to define a personalized Detox and Restore plan:

- Choose two or three of your top "issues" or priorities that you identified in your assessment (priorities may include any of the inflammatory food items or habits on page 16, such as reducing fast food, reducing soda intake, eliminating artificial sweeteners, etc.).
- These top two or three priorities then define what you are detoxing (eliminating or greatly reducing) during the initial two weeks, while you're also increasing gut-health-promoting foods (page 39).
- At the end of the initial two weeks, add another top priority to eliminate or add to your existing detox plan (this may include additional inflammatory food items or habits from page 16). Don't forget that detox isn't just about elimination. You should start to incorporate more anti-inflammatory foods and habits as "priorities" in your plan, too.
- Stick with it! Remember that your body benefits from all changes, even small ones! And small ones can add up quickly to have a powerful impact.

The goal is to calm the body and restore key nutrients and bacteria, but this will mean something different to each individual. Choose to follow the Detox and Restore meal plans on pages 287–89 or define your own plan using the guidelines above.

step #3: target or reassess

Congrats! You've made it two weeks eating a cleaner, more anti-inflammatory diet. You next step to healing your body is to choose an action plan to focus even more anti-inflammatory healing on ailments or disease prevention. Or repeat step 2 to restrict additional toxins.

if you followed the detox and restore plan as written, then you are ready to:

- Start healing your body by targeting specific diseases and health conditions using Chapter 10's meals plans and guidelines (page 283).
- Continue to Detox and Restore (page 287) for an additional one to two weeks.

if you defined your own plan, then you are ready to:

- Continue detoxing and restoring by adding an additional one or two focus areas to eliminate or incorporate for another two weeks. Continue this process until you have addressed most of the concerns from the assessment.
- Start healing your body by targeting specific diseases and health conditions using Chapter 10's meals plans and guidelines (page 283).

step #4: eat and feel good!

Enjoy the food, the improvement in energy, the easing of symptoms, and, most important, the process! Sure, the healthy guidelines are the basis for healing your body, but these two components are essential for continuing long-term.

- Progress, not perfection: If you're like me, then you're probably tempted to try overhauling your diet in one day, but this isn't the goal—nor is it recommended. Research suggests that incorporating gradual, small changes is more manageable and something you're more likely to continue. Don't take an all-or-nothing approach. Instead, focus on progress, and then on maintaining and growing that progress.

- 80/20 living: Your short-term goal is to gradually "clean up" your diet. Your long-term goal is to make anti-inflammatory eating your natural eating "norm" at least 80 percent of the time. But let's be completely honest: All of us are going to eat added sugars again, be in a situation where we have less-than-healthy options, or maybe want a big, juicy steak. And this is okay 20 percent of the time, if you're eating your best the other 80 percent.

the healing kitchen

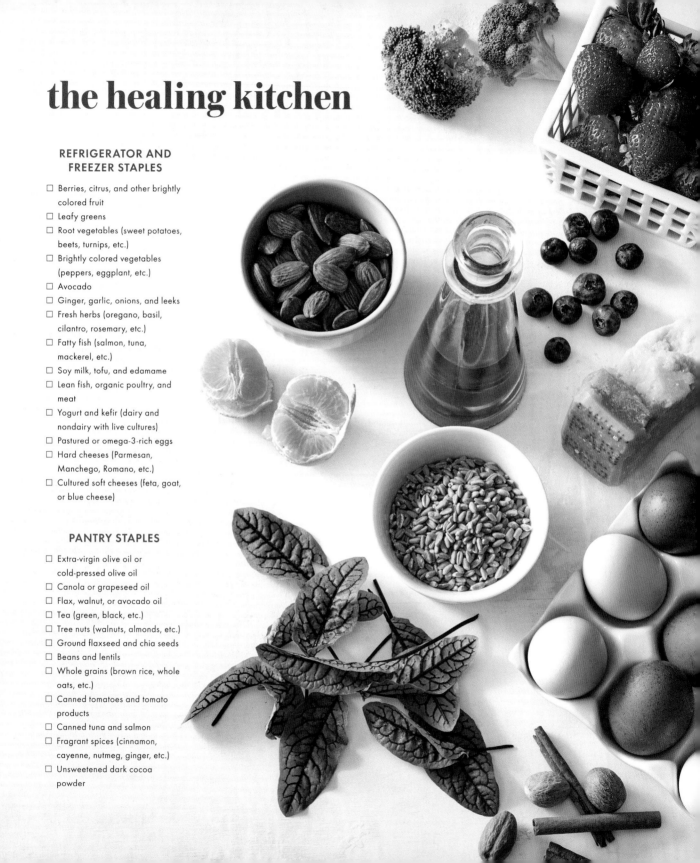

REFRIGERATOR AND FREEZER STAPLES

☐ Berries, citrus, and other brightly colored fruit

☐ Leafy greens

☐ Root vegetables (sweet potatoes, beets, turnips, etc.)

☐ Brightly colored vegetables (peppers, eggplant, etc.)

☐ Avocado

☐ Ginger, garlic, onions, and leeks

☐ Fresh herbs (oregano, basil, cilantro, rosemary, etc.)

☐ Fatty fish (salmon, tuna, mackerel, etc.)

☐ Soy milk, tofu, and edamame

☐ Lean fish, organic poultry, and meat

☐ Yogurt and kefir (dairy and nondairy with live cultures)

☐ Pastured or omega-3-rich eggs

☐ Hard cheeses (Parmesan, Manchego, Romano, etc.)

☐ Cultured soft cheeses (feta, goat, or blue cheese)

PANTRY STAPLES

☐ Extra-virgin olive oil or cold-pressed olive oil

☐ Canola or grapeseed oil

☐ Flax, walnut, or avocado oil

☐ Tea (green, black, etc.)

☐ Tree nuts (walnuts, almonds, etc.)

☐ Ground flaxseed and chia seeds

☐ Beans and lentils

☐ Whole grains (brown rice, whole oats, etc.)

☐ Canned tomatoes and tomato products

☐ Canned tuna and salmon

☐ Fragrant spices (cinnamon, cayenne, nutmeg, ginger, etc.)

☐ Unsweetened dark cocoa powder

guide to anti-inflammatory eating away from home

Not that any of us probably need scientific evidence to confirm this, but research suggests that eating food prepared in your own home is almost always healthier than eating out. In fact, meals prepared outside of the home—whether that's fast food, quick-service, or fancier table service—are typically higher in saturated fat, calories, and sodium. Combine that with the fact that you've got little input on the quality or preparation of the ingredients used, and this equates to meals that range from "not so healthy" to "very unhealthy and inflammatory."

Yet here's the reality: We are all going to eat at a restaurant, order takeout, and probably even run through a drive-through window again, and that's okay. The secret is being aware so it's not a daily or frequent habit, as well as giving a little thought to your options before you go eat out.

Restaurants vary by region and, as you'll soon learn, individually or locally owned restaurants are often a better choice—two things that make giving specific menu-item recommendations difficult. But here are some general guidelines to use to steer you toward healthier, less inflammatory choices when eating out.

- **GO LOCAL:** Restaurants with multiple (or hundreds of) locations often rely heavily on prepared products and standardized methods to ensure product consistency, and they have little ability to make changes based on freshness, quality, or seasonality. Chefs and cooks at locally owned restaurants with a single location, or even a few locations, usually have much more freedom to creatively incorporate locally grown and in-season produce, organic ingredients, and homemade items. Though eating local doesn't always guarantee a healthier meal, it's my first choice when it comes to healthfulness, as well as freshness and taste.

- **LOOK FOR SPECIAL DIETS:** Choosing items that meet special diet requirements—even though you may not

have a dairy allergy or gluten sensitivity—can sometimes mean dishes that are healthier and less inflammatory. These dishes are often prepared with a little more attention to quality and ingredients. They may also contain more fresh or homemade sauces or seasonings to steer clear of those dietary components that are often in prepared products.

- **ORDER SIMPLE:** Basic preparation techniques like baking, roasting, grilling, and sautéing are often healthier in terms of saturated fat and sodium. But keeping your order simple (for example, grilled fish with steamed vegetables or a baked sweet potato) also helps you focus on a balanced plate (see page 33). It's even more important when eating out to make sure that at least half of your meal is made up of fresh or cooked produce.

- **THINK FISH:** All fish, but particularly those rich in omega-3s (see page 39), are vital for health and reducing inflammation. Yet fish isn't something that people tend to prepare at home as often as meat and poultry. Use eating out as an opportunity to get one of your weekly servings of fish to boost health and to minimize the body's inflammatory response.

- **EXPLORE GLOBALLY:** Whether it's Greek, Thai, Japanese, Indian, South American, or Italian, each cuisine centers around its own assortment of spices, herbs, and fresh ingredients. Sure, preparation plays a big role, but many times it's easier to find vegetable-forward dishes with less emphasis on animal proteins at ethnic restaurants. Cuisines like Indian also pack an anti-inflammatory punch thanks to turmeric and curry blends, and some Asian cuisines incorporate probiotic-rich kimchi and seaweed greens.

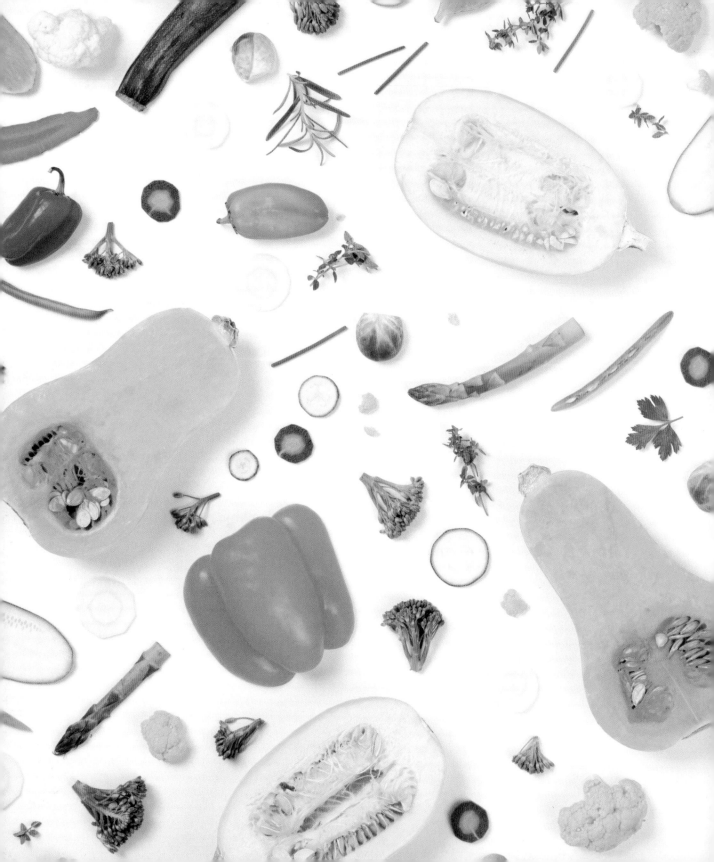

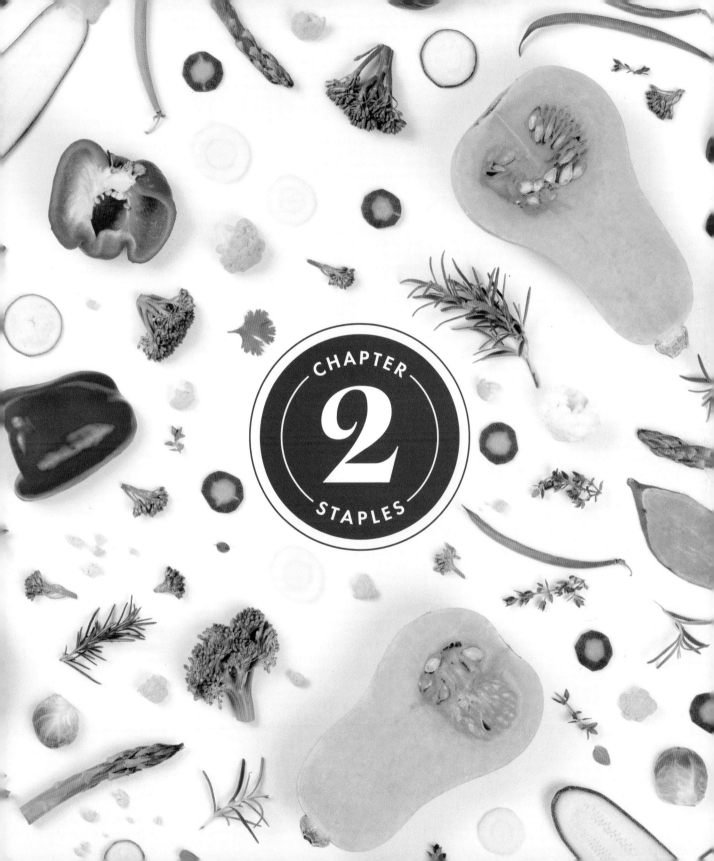

CHAPTER

2

STAPLES

Anti-inflammatory eating sounds great in theory:

It slows the aging process, reduces or prevents future illness and diagnoses, and soothes current symptoms.

But how do you sustain this type of eating long-term (or at least beyond Monday)?

Today, most of us live high-speed lifestyles; the need for convenience is essentially how the American diet got where it is today.

SIMPLE
staples

With my background in nutrition, I've fed my family pretty healthfully (most days, at least). However, I still felt like our diet was chronically low in veggies and other key anti-inflammatory nutrients, and higher than I liked to admit in refined carbs, added sugars, and processed food items. But this was also my reality:

- I had little to no time to plan meals each week;
- I had little time in the evenings—and on some days, little desire or energy—to cook dinner from scratch;
- I wasn't willing to devote my Sunday afternoons to hours of cooking;
- I hadn't had great—or appetizing, at least—success with freezer or slow-cooker meals.

So I became determined to figure out how to provide nutritious meals that make us healthy now as well as long-term, **but** without spending hours planning, prepping, and cooking. It took a few years, lots of trials and failures, and a few last-minute runs through our local Chick-fil-A drive-through, but I finally figured out a system. I rely on Simple Staples.

Simple Staples are key foods that I buy every week and key ingredients that I prep. They are not fully cooked meals, but rather components I keep at the ready to use in lots of different meals during the week. They take minimal prep time, and they allow me to cook only two or three nights a week—something my friends are probably surprised to learn! Simple Staples are my solution for quick lunches and family dinners in a matter of minutes, and some weeks they are the only way I am able to get healthy meals in lunch boxes and on the table.

how do simple staples work?

STOCK UP: On the weekend or at the start of the week, make a grocery trip to stock up on fresh and frozen vegetables and fruits, lean proteins, and dairy-case items, as well as pantry items like whole grains, beans, minimally processed canned goods, healthy oils and condiments, spices, and other shelf-stable foods that are part of weekly meals.

PREP: Find just 30 minutes to 1 hour to spend prepping at least two vegetables or veggie dishes and one protein food—and maybe a seasoning or dressing if there's time.

PULL TOGETHER AND ENJOY: Using the key items you purchased and prepped, you have all you need to create a different healthy meal every day without sacrificing taste or time. This book will show you exactly how to do this!

what are your simple staples?

There's no exact prescription for Simple Staples other than that they should be nutrient-dense foods. In fact, Simple Staples should be tailored to your needs and preferences, and the concept can be used for any type of special diet. The key is to focus on prepping or making those healthy foods that you tend to skimp on when busy.

Answer these questions to determine where your focus should be when stocking and prepping. I've given my answers below as an example.

WHAT <u>ANTI-INFLAMMATORY</u> FOODS DO YOU NEED TO EAT MORE REGULARLY? WHAT <u>ANTI-INFLAMMATORY</u> FOODS DOES YOUR DIET USUALLY CONTAIN *LESS* OF WHEN YOU'RE BUSY AND NOT AS PREPARED?
Pick your top priority followed by one or two others. This is where you want to start your Simple Staples prep work. These are the main foods that you want to focus on making super accessible and ready-to-go for the coming week, and emphasize those foods in your answer to the second question.

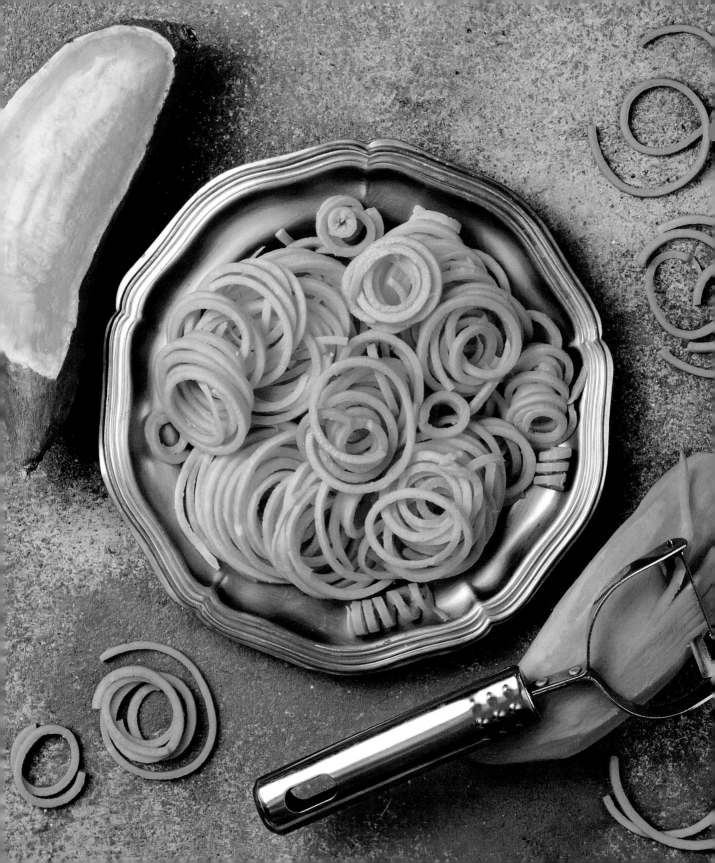

MY ANSWER: Getting the recommended servings of produce (or at least close to it) is what I consider the most important, followed by healthy protein and omega-3 fat sources. And when I'm busy or less prepared, vegetables fall by the wayside—without a doubt! This is followed by seafood or plant-based protein sources.

WHAT THIS MEANS: I need to have vegetables ready to reheat or toss into dishes so they are an easier food choice to grab and use in a meal. My grocery "essentials" to buy each week are leafy greens (two or three containers), two or three other vegetables (one of which can be used as a "base" for bowls, like spaghetti squash, cauliflower rice, or veggie noodles), two or three lean proteins (at least one of which is plant-based or seafood), and omega-3-rich snacks or condiments (nuts, oils, avocado, etc.). I also try to roast a batch of vegetables, make a veggie-carb substitute (see page 52), and have a healthy oil-based dressing on hand.

WHAT <u>INFLAMMATORY</u> FOODS DOES YOUR DIET CONTAIN *MORE* OF WHEN YOU'RE BUSY AND LESS PREPARED?

These are usually foods to avoid buying because they are what we tend to use as a "crutch" when we're tired or busy. Having these on hand will detract from other foods that are now just as quick and healthier.

MY ANSWER: Refined grains, as well as whole grains that are easy to overconsume like pasta, sauces, and sides that are more processed. My protein sources also tend to be limited to meat and poultry.

WHAT THIS MEANS: I avoid buying refined snack foods and grains like pasta and bread products. Having these items on hand makes it too easy to ignore healthier items. To incorporate carbs, I focus on keeping on hand whole grains like brown rice and quinoa, corn tortillas, canned beans, and starchy vegetables like sweet potatoes.

SIMPLE STAPLES = SIMPLE MEALS

Here's an example of how a little prep gives me lots of quick meal options.

SIMPLE STAPLES PREPPED: spaghetti squash, cooked chicken breast, quinoa

SIMPLE STAPLES IN PANTRY: canned beans, canned tuna, chickpea pasta

SIMPLE STAPLES PURCHASED: corn tortillas, salad greens, cherry tomatoes, avocado, store-bought dressing, cheese, and a few extra fresh or frozen fruits or vegetables

MEALS THAT I CAN MAKE IN 20 MINUTES OR LESS:

(1) Warm Spinach Breakfast Bowl (page 93)

(6) Chopped Greek Salad Bowls with Chicken (page 114)

(2) Sweet or Savory Quinoa Breakfast Bowl (page 96)

(7) Spinach-Quinoa Bowls with Chicken and Berries (page 121)

(3) Avocado-Chicken Salad (page 105)

(8) Lemony Black Bean–Quinoa Salad (page 191)

(4) Tuna, White Bean, and Arugula Salad (page 109)

(9) Huevos Rancheros Tostadas (page 195)

(5) Black Bean and Spinach Quesadillas (page 110)

(10) Quick Roasted Tomato Pasta (page 200)

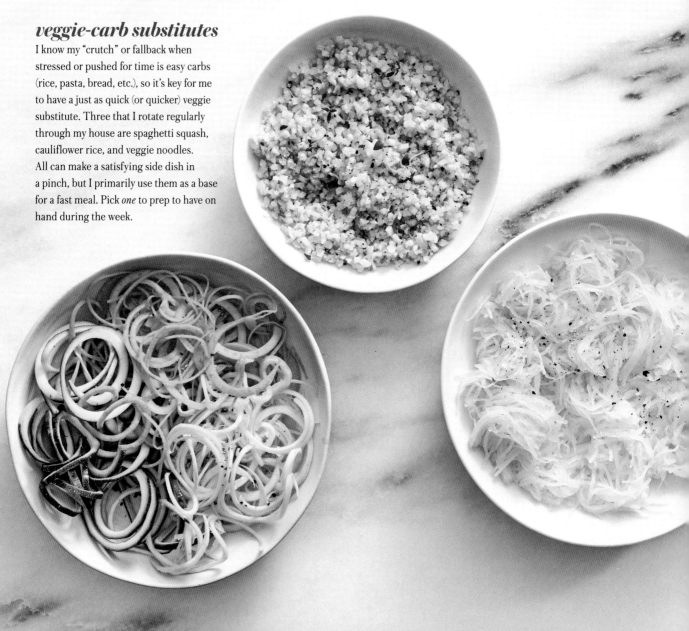

veggie staples

Even when I have the best healthy eating intentions at the start of the week, I have learned that my veggie intake falls by the wayside unless I have a variety of easily accessible, quick options. I try to have at least one of each of these staples ready to go at the start of my week: a veggie-carb substitute, a seasoned cooked vegetable, and leafy greens. Let me walk you through the prep and give you some ideas on how to use them.

veggie-carb substitutes

I know my "crutch" or fallback when stressed or pushed for time is easy carbs (rice, pasta, bread, etc.), so it's key for me to have a just as quick (or quicker) veggie substitute. Three that I rotate regularly through my house are spaghetti squash, cauliflower rice, and veggie noodles. All can make a satisfying side dish in a pinch, but I primarily use them as a base for a fast meal. Pick *one* to prep to have on hand during the week.

spaghetti squash

The long strands from this large yellow squash are not only a gluten-free substitute for rice and pasta, but also a way to pack in more veggies. Prep at the beginning of the week to yield 4 to 6 cups of strands; then reheat and toss with protein, veggies, herbs, cheese, or sauce for super-fast entrées and sides. The options this low-calorie, low-carb veggie offers are endless.

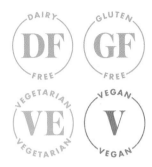

1 Preheat the oven to 350°F. Cut the squash in half lengthwise. Scrape out and discard the seeds and membranes. Place the halves, cut sides down, in a large baking dish; add water to a depth of ¼ inch.

2 Bake for 45 to 50 minutes or until tender. Remove the squash from the oven. Turn the cut sides up; cool for 10 minutes. Scrape the flesh of the squash with a fork into spaghetti-like strands. Discard the skins.

3 Heat a large skillet over medium heat. Add the oil to the pan; swirl to coat. Add the squash strands and cook for 2 minutes or until warm throughout. Season lightly with salt and pepper. Serve or store in an airtight container in the refrigerator.

(SERVING SIZE: 1 CUP): CALORIES 62; FAT 3G (SAT 0G, UNSAT 2G); PROTEIN 1G; CARB 10G; FIBER 2G; SUGARS 4G (ADDED SUGARS 0G); SODIUM 108MG; CALC 3% DV; POTASSIUM 4% DV

IN THE MICROWAVE: Pierce the squash using a knife, making 6 to 8 cuts (about ½ inch deep). Place the whole squash in the microwave on its side and cook on HIGH for 4 minutes. Rotate the squash and cook on high for an additional 4 to 6 minutes, or until the outside of the squash gives slightly when touched. Carefully cut the squash in half lengthwise, placing the halves cut sides up, and cool for 10 minutes. Scrape out and discard the seeds and membranes. Then, scrape the flesh of the squash with a fork into spaghetti-like strands. Discard the skins.

IN THE MULTICOOKER: Follow the directions for preparing the squash in the microwave, but place the whole pierced squash and 1 cup water in the multicooker. Close and lock the lid on the multicooker, and pressure-cook for 15 minutes. Once done, release the steam and open the multicooker as directed by the manufacturer. Carefully cut the squash in half lengthwise, placing the halves cut sides up, and cool for 10 minutes. Scrape out and discard the seeds and membranes. Then, scrape the flesh of the squash with a fork into spaghetti-like strands. Discard the skins

1 (3-pound) spaghetti squash
1 to 2 tablespoons extra-virgin olive oil
Salt and black pepper

---

5 QUICK SPAGHETTI SQUASH BOWLS

Reheat 1 to 2 cups of the lightly seasoned spaghetti squash and then top with other staples, produce, and pantry items you have on hand—anything you might top pasta with. You've got a complete meal in less than 5 minutes!

TACO: Add seasoned taco meat or meatless crumbles + tomatoes + olive oil vinaigrette + avocado

PESTO SHRIMP: Add cooked shrimp + fresh tomatoes + wilted spinach + pesto

CAPRESE "PASTA": Add tomatoes + fresh mozzarella cheese + fresh basil + balsamic vinaigrette

BLACK BEAN ENCHILADA: Add black beans + corn + enchilada sauce + cheddar cheese + shredded lettuce

BUILD YOUR OWN: Add ½ cup lean protein + 1 cup cooked or raw veggies + up to 3 tablespoons dressing, sauce, cheese, or other flavor extra

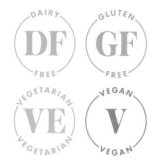

cauliflower rice

Another fave to use as a carb substitute is cauliflower rice. It's almost as versatile as spaghetti squash and, due to its popularity, is now available in a variety of forms. Season as "rice" or mash to create a mashed potato substitute.

1 to 2 tablespoons extra-virgin olive oil
4 cups riced cauliflower
Salt and black pepper

Heat a large skillet over medium-high heat. Add the oil to the pan; swirl to coat. Add the cauliflower and cook, stirring frequently, for 5 to 7 minutes or until the cauliflower is cooked to the desired texture. Season lightly with salt and pepper. Serve or store in an airtight container in the refrigerator.

(SERVING SIZE: 1 CUP): CALORIES 51; FAT 4G (SAT 1G, UNSAT 3G); PROTEIN 2G; CARB 4G; FIBER 2G; SUGARS 2G (ADDED SUGARS 0G); SODIUM 146MG; CALC 2% DV; POTASSIUM 5% DV

IN THE MICROWAVE: You can also steam frozen or fresh riced cauliflower in the microwave following the package directions. Season lightly and sauté in a skillet for 1 to 2 minutes as directed above.

where do you get riced cauliflower?

BUY FRESH: Look for 12-ounce bags of cauliflower rice in the produce section near the precut vegetables.

BUY FROZEN: Look for 12-ounce bags of frozen cauliflower rice; thaw and let stand on paper towels for 10 minutes before cooking to remove any excess moisture.

MAKE YOUR OWN: Cut 1 cauliflower head, leaves removed, into florets. Place in the food processor and pulse for 10 to 15 seconds or until the cauliflower has been coarsely chopped into small pieces about the size of rice. Remove any larger pieces that don't get chopped properly. Empty the grated cauliflower from the bowl, and return any larger pieces to the food processor. Pulse for a few seconds or until the remaining cauliflower is properly chopped.

4 cups cauliflower "rice" = 1 (12-ounce) fresh or frozen bag or from 1 cauliflower head

---

5 QUICK MEALS WITH CAULIFLOWER RICE

Steam, sauté, or reheat 1 to 1½ cups of the lightly seasoned cauliflower rice. Then add ingredients that you might ordinarily combine with rice or another grain. You've got a complete meal in less than 10 minutes!

GREEK: Add baby spinach + chickpeas + cucumber + feta + tzatziki sauce or olive oil vinaigrette

SPRING SALMON: Add steamed sugar snap peas + steamed asparagus + cooked salmon + pesto

SOUTHWESTERN: Add taco seasoned ground turkey + tomato + corn + Avocado-Cilantro Dip and Dressing (page 70) or guacamole

GINGER PORK: Add cooked pork loin + scallions + roasted broccoli or green beans + ginger or soy vinaigrette

BUILD YOUR OWN: Add ½ cup lean protein + 1 cup cooked or raw veggies + up to 3 tablespoons dressing, sauce, cheese, or other flavor extra

zucchini noodles

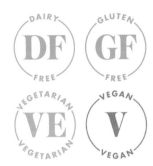

Zucchini has a mild flavor that pairs well with other ingredients—not to mention that you can just wash and spiralize it with the peel. Other veggies like sweet potatoes, butternut squash, and beets can be spiralized to make "noodles" too, but typically need peeling and a slightly longer cooking time.

Heat a large skillet over medium-high heat. Add the oil to the pan; swirl to coat. Add the zucchini and cook, stirring frequently, for 2 minutes or until the noodles are just tender. Season lightly with salt and pepper. Serve or store in an airtight container in the refrigerator.

(SERVING SIZE: 1 CUP) CALORIES 64; FAT 5G (SAT 1G, UNSAT 4G); PROTEIN 2G; CARB 4G; FIBER 1G; SUGARS 3G (ADDED SUGARS 0G); SODIUM 172MG; CALC 2% DV; POTASSIUM 8% DV

1 tablespoon olive oil
3 cups zucchini noodles or spirals
Salt and black pepper

where do you get veggie noodles?

BUY FRESH SPIRALS: Most grocery stores now offer several types of spiralized vegetables in the precut produce section.

MAKE YOUR OWN: Make veggie noodles by using a spiralizer or a vegetable peeler. Wash and dry the produce. If using a spiralizer, follow the manufacturer's directions. If using a julienne peeler, make ribbons by peeling the zucchini lengthwise into strips, stopping at the inside part containing the seeds; discard the seeds.

3 cups "noodles" = 1 (10.7-ounce) package or 1 pound vegetables (before being trimmed and cut)

---

5 QUICK "NOODLE" BOWLS

Reheat 1 to 2 cups of the lightly seasoned zucchini, sweet potato, or other veggie noodles. Use the veggie noodles like you would spaghetti squash—pretty much anywhere you might use pasta! "Quick Spaghetti Squash Bowls" recipes (page 53) work well for most veggie noodles, as do these combinations!

SALMON TERIYAKI: Add cooked salmon + edamame + carrots + scallions + teriyaki sauce

LEMONY SHRIMP: Add sautéed shrimp + black beans + baby spinach + tomato + citrus or lemon vinaigrette

CHICKEN BLT: Add cooked chicken breast + tomato + wilted baby spinach + uncured bacon crumbles

TOFU CURRY: Add sautéed tofu + red bell pepper + sugar snap peas + curry sauce

BUILD YOUR OWN: Add ½ cup lean protein + 1 cup cooked or raw veggies + up to 3 tablespoons dressing, sauce, cheese, or other flavor extra

seasoned vegetables

I like to cook a batch of a single veggie—or a mix of veggies—at the start of the week to keep in my fridge so that they are so convenient, it is almost impossible not to use them. Steam, sauté, roast—many methods work—but my favorite and "staple" method is roasting.

roasted vegetables

Most vegetables are better roasted, a cooking technique that is almost as simple as steaming. Not only does the high temp caramelize the vegetable's natural sugars, but roasting slightly crisps the veggie's outside. Roasted vegetables don't take long to prepare and are good straight from the oven, as well as reheated later in the week. Here's how: Cover your sheet pan with foil for super-easy cleanup, then preheat the oven to 425°F. Slice, cut, or trim the vegetables, making sure they are all about the same size for even roasting (see opposite for even more roasting tips). Then toss with a little olive oil, salt, pepper, and garlic powder and roast (see the chart below for vegetable-specific times)! Stir once about two-thirds of the way through the cooking time.

how to use leftovers

Need ideas on how to use the veggies you've created? Here are a few ways I like to use them.

- Add to a salad
- Stir into grits or a savory breakfast bowl
- Use in scrambled eggs, an omelet, or a frittata
- Top a pizza
- Toss with a hot grain or pasta and sauce for a quick meal
- Stuff a sweet potato or baked potato

VEGETABLE	TIME
Asparagus	10 to 12 minutes
Broccoli	15 to 20 minutes
Brussels sprouts	15 to 20 minutes
Carrots, baby	25 to 30 minutes
Carrots, whole	30 to 35 minutes
Cauliflower	18 to 22 minutes
Green beans	12 to 15 minutes
Peppers	12 to 15 minutes
Small red potatoes	30 to 35 minutes
Squash and zucchini	10 to 12 minutes
Sweet potatoes	30 to 35 minutes

TRICKS FOR PERFECTLY ROASTED VEGETABLES

① Cut the vegetables to a uniform size.

② Choose ones that have similar cooking times if combining vegetables.

③ Don't be afraid of oil and salt—just measure.

④ Get the oven hot!

⑤ Give the veggies some space—air circulation around the vegetables is key for browning.

⑥ Don't be afraid of a little browning.

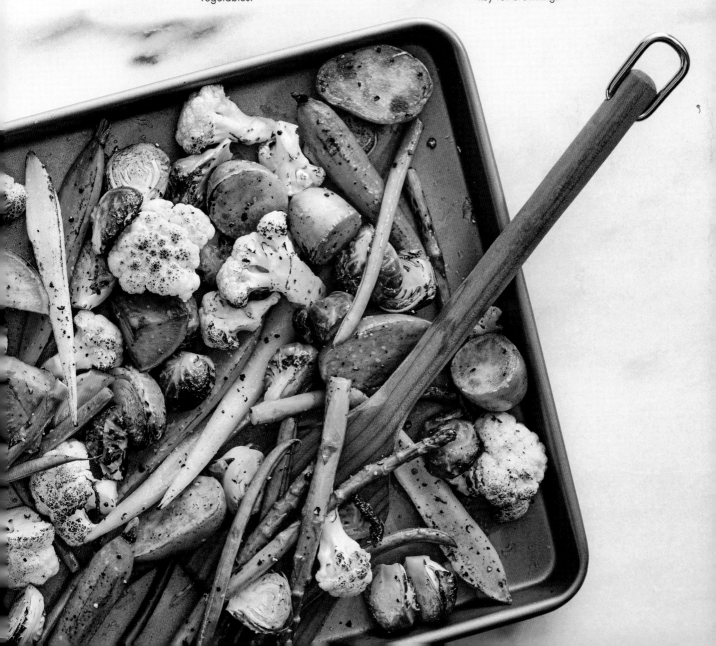

protein staples

Cooking a lean protein or two to keep on hand each week ensures you're never more than 5 minutes away from a healthy meal.

	CHICKEN BREASTS	CHICKEN THIGHS	FLANK STEAK OR SKIRT STEAK	PORK TENDERLOIN OR LOIN
COOKING METHODS	BAKE in the oven, GRILL, SEAR in a skillet, POACH in liquid	BAKE in the oven, GRILL, SEAR in a skillet	BROIL in the oven, GRILL, SEAR in a skillet	BAKE in the oven, GRILL
APPROXIMATE COOKING TIME	**BONELESS:** 18 to 35 minutes or 8 to 12 minutes per side* **BONE-IN:** 40 to 50 minutes or 11 to 17 minutes per side	**BONELESS:** 20 to 30 minutes or 5 to 8 minutes per side **BONE-IN:** 35 to 45 minutes or 7 to 11 minutes per side	6 to 12 minutes per side	20 to 28 minutes

*Cutlets and thinner breasts will be at the lower end of each time range; thicker breasts will be toward the upper end.

SALMON, TUNA STEAK, OTHER FISH

BAKE or BROIL in the oven, GRILL, SEAR in a skillet, POACH in liquid

10 minutes per inch (at thickest part), turning halfway through cooking

SHRIMP

BAKE or BROIL in the oven, GRILL, SEAR in a skillet, POACH in liquid

2 to 5 minutes

TOFU

BAKE in the oven or SAUTÉ

8 to 30 minutes, depending on cut size and method

ALMOST-INSTANT PROTEINS

And for those weeks when prep just doesn't happen, these proteins can help you quickly pull together a meal.

- Canned beans
- Frozen peeled shrimp
- Canned tuna and salmon
- Rotisserie chicken or baked salmon from your local grocery store
- Frozen edamame
- Eggs
- InstantPot shredded chicken or pork (follow the general guidelines on page 133 for chicken and page 153 for pork loin)

SIMPLE
grain staples

Whole grains are a key part of a healthy diet, and most cook in less than 30 minutes. This is doable some nights, but for those nights it's not, I like to get a head start by cooking a batch of one or two grains each week to store in the refrigerator. See page 63 for explanation of the cooking methods. I also provide some 10-Minutes-or-Less options on page 63 too.

	CORNMEAL (POLENTA)	OATS, OLD-FASHIONED	OATS, STEEL-CUT	QUINOA
AMOUNTS	4 cups liquid for 1 cup dry grain yields approximately 3 cups	1½ to 2 cups liquid for 1 cup dry grain yields approximately 2 cups	3½ to 4 cups liquid for 1 cup dry grain yields approximately 4 cups	1¼ cups liquid for 1 cup dry grain yields approximately 3 cups
COOK TIME AND METHOD	5 minutes with traditional method	5 minutes with pasta method	10 to 20 minutes with traditional method	12 minutes with traditional method

WHOLE GRAINS 101

Choosing a whole grain means opting for a grain whose entire kernel—the germ, endosperm, and bran—is intact or all three are kept within the grain mixture if ground or crushed. Refined grains are created when the germ and bran (the parts that contain fiber, protein, vitamins, and minerals) are stripped away, leaving only the starchy endosperm. The research to support eating whole grains as part of your regular diet and in place of refined grains is substantial and suggests the following health effects:

- Reduces risk of heart disease
- Reduces risk of type 2 diabetes
- Reduces risks of some cancers
- Improves gut and digestive health
- Reduces overall inflammation in the body

BULGUR	AMARANTH	MILLET	FREEKEH
2 cups liquid for 1 cup dry grain yields approximately 3 cups	2½ cups liquid for 1 cup dry grain yields approximately 3 cups	2 cups liquid for 1 cup dry grain yields approximately 3½ cups	2¼ cups liquid for 1 cup dry grain yields approximately 3½ cups
12 minutes with traditional method	20 minutes with traditional method	20 minutes with traditional method	20 to 25 minutes with traditional method

grain staples
(continued)

	FARRO	BROWN RICE	WILD RICE	HULLED BARLEY
AMOUNTS	6 cups liquid for 1 cup dry grain yields approximately 3 cups	8 cups liquid for 1 cup dry grain yields approximately 3½ cups	6 cups liquid for 1 cup dry grain yields approximately 3½ cups	8 cups liquid for 1 cup dry grain yields approximately 3½ cups
COOK TIME AND METHOD	25 to 60 minutes with pasta method	30 to 45 minutes with pasta method	45 to 50 minutes with pasta method	45 to 60 minutes with pasta method

WHEAT BERRIES	SPELT
8 cups liquid for 1 cup dry grain yields approximately 3 cups	8 cups liquid for 1 cup dry grain yields approximately 3 cups

50 to 60 minutes with pasta method	60 to 75 minutes with pasta method

TRADITIONAL METHOD

Bring the grain and liquid to a boil; cover, reduce the heat, and cook. For cornmeal and oats, bring the liquid to a boil, then add the grain. Cover, reduce the heat, and simmer. All (or most) of the liquid will be absorbed by the end of cooking.

PASTA METHOD

Bring the liquid to a boil in a large pot; add the grain. Reduce the heat and simmer. Drain the grain at the end of cooking.

OTHER OPTIONS

Cooking grains in a multicooker or pressure cooker can cut the cooking time by half or more. Refer to your specific cooker's manual since cook time can differ and additional liquid may be needed.

REFRIGERATOR STORAGE

5 to 7 days; add 1 to 2 tablespoons water before reheating if the grain seems dry.

FREEZER STORAGE

Up to 2 months; freeze in small batches that you can easily pull out to use as needed.

10-MINUTES-OR-LESS OPTIONS

- Instant boil-in-bag brown rice
- Ready-to-heat brown or wild rice
- Ready-to-heat quinoa, farro, or amaranth
- Ready-to-heat pilafs made with brown or wild rice, quinoa, farro, or amaranth
- Ready-to-heat lentil and grain pilafs
- Frozen brown rice and quinoa pilafs

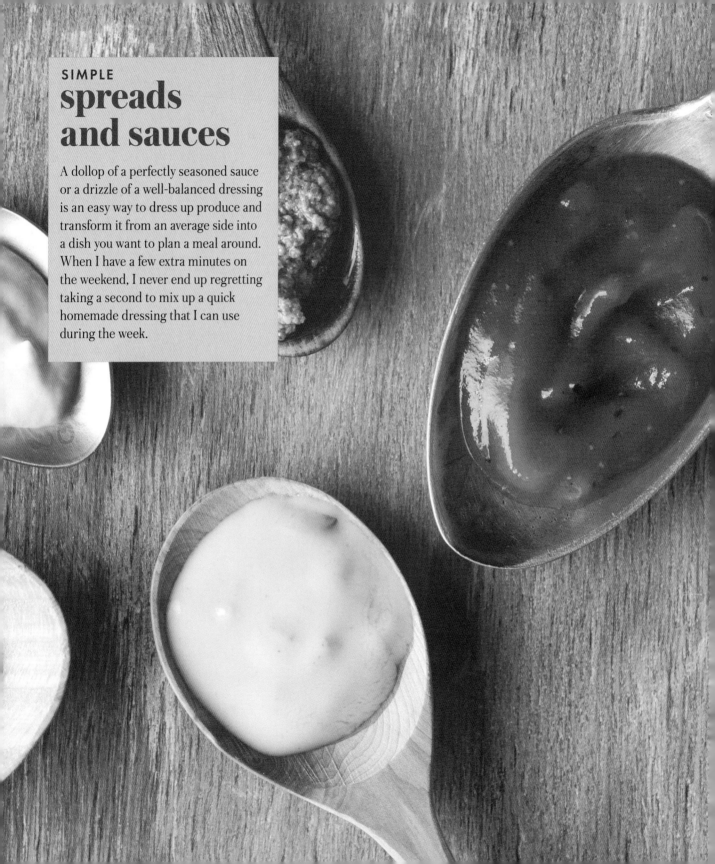

SIMPLE
spreads and sauces

A dollop of a perfectly seasoned sauce or a drizzle of a well-balanced dressing is an easy way to dress up produce and transform it from an average side into a dish you want to plan a meal around. When I have a few extra minutes on the weekend, I never end up regretting taking a second to mix up a quick homemade dressing that I can use during the week.

almond butter

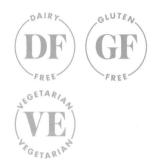

Roasting nuts is an easy way to add more flavor to homemade nut butters. For this recipe, purchase unsalted roasted almonds or roast raw almonds on a baking sheet at 350°F for 10 to 12 minutes.

1 Place the roasted almonds, honey, oil, water, and salt in a food processor and process until creamy, 4 to 8 minutes, scraping down the sides occasionally.

2 Store in a jar with a tight lid or in an airtight container in the refrigerator for up to 1 month.

(SERVING SIZE: 2 TABLESPOONS): CALORIES 218; FAT 19G (SAT 2G, UNSAT 16G); PROTEIN 7G; CARB 8G; FIBER 4G; SUGARS 3G (ADDED SUGARS 1G); SODIUM 121MG; CALC 9% DV; POTASSIUM 5% DV

4 cups roasted almonds

1 tablespoon honey or pure maple syrup

1 tablespoon coconut oil

1 to 2 teaspoons water

1 teaspoon kosher salt

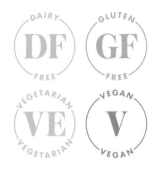

all-purpose taco seasoning

The blend of spices in taco seasoning may have been designed for tacos and fajitas, but it's also a quick way to add a touch of Southwestern flavor to black beans, skillet dinners, chicken, steak, seafood, and dressings. A batch of this recipe lasts me 3 to 4 months, costs pennies compared to organic options, and avoids excess sodium and fillers that can be found in others.

¼ cup chili powder

2 tablespoons ground cumin

1 tablespoon kosher salt

1 tablespoon paprika

1 tablespoon garlic powder

1 tablespoon cornstarch

2 teaspoons dried oregano

½ teaspoon cayenne pepper

1 Stir together all the ingredients in a small bowl.

2 Store in a jar or airtight container at room temperature for up to 3 months.

(SERVING SIZE: 1 TEASPOON): CALORIES 7; FAT 0G; PROTEIN 0G; CARB 1G; FIBER 1G; SUGARS 0G (ADDED SUGARS 0G); SODIUM 210MG; CALC 1% DV; POTASSIUM 1% DV

simple green pesto

If you love basil, but want to tone down its grassy flavor just a little, try blanching it (see below). Simply submerging it in boiling water for 5 seconds smooths out the raw herb's intense flavor, making it a little more kid-friendly. Try substituting sunflower seeds if the price of pine nuts is more than you care to spend.

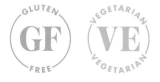

1 Place the basil, pine nuts, oil, salt, and garlic in a food processor; process until smooth.

2 Add the cheese; process until blended.

3 Store in a jar or airtight container in the refrigerator for up to 2 weeks.

(SERVING SIZE: 1 TABLESPOON): CALORIES 86; FAT 8G (SAT 1G, UNSAT 6G); PROTEIN 3G; CARB 1G; FIBER 0G; SUGARS 0G (ADDED SUGARS 0G); SODIUM 113MG; CALC 9% DV; POTASSIUM 2% DV

DAIRY-FREE AND VEGAN OPTION: Omit the cheese, and add an additional 2 tablespoons toasted pine nuts and 2 tablespoons nutritional yeast.

how to blanch basil

Bring a large Dutch oven filled two-thirds full with water to a boil. Fill a large bowl with ice water. Place the basil leaves in a metal strainer. Place the strainer in the pan, using tongs to quickly submerge all the basil leaves; cook for 5 seconds or just until the leaves turn bright green. Carefully remove the strainer with the leaves from the pan; drain. Immediately plunge the strainer with the leaves in the ice water. Let stand for 10 seconds. Remove the basil; drain well. Spread the basil leaves on a clean, dry dish towel; gently blot them dry with another towel.

6 cups fresh basil leaves

2 tablespoons pine nuts, toasted

5 tablespoons extra-virgin olive oil

¼ teaspoon kosher salt

2 garlic cloves

2 ounces finely grated Parmigiano-Reggiano cheese (about ½ cup)

condiment buying guide

The key to buying condiments at the grocery store is locating those that give you punches of flavor without adding excess sodium, added sugars, or unhealthy fats. Guidelines for selection are as unique as each condiment's flavor and purpose, but here are general tips to use when looking at the label.

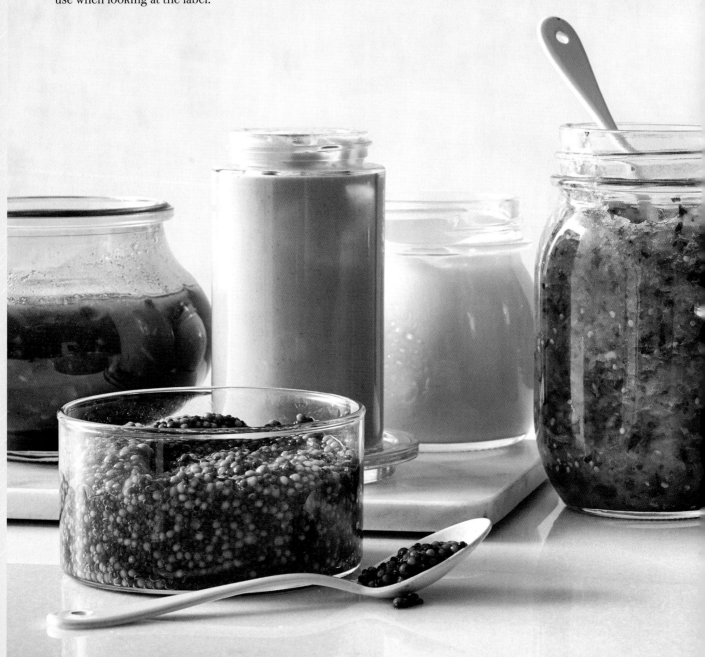

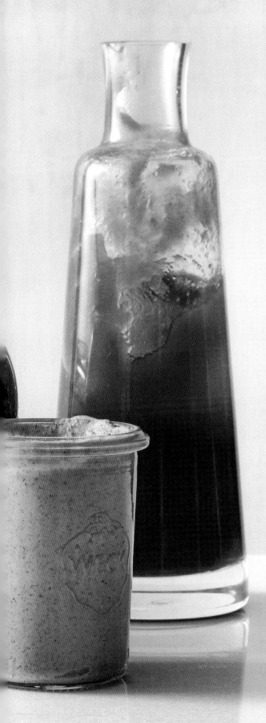

KETCHUP

SODIUM: ≤160mg sodium per tablespoon

SUGARS: ≤5 grams sugars per tablespoon

ADDED SUGAR TIP: Tomatoes contribute approximately 2 to 3 grams natural sugars per tablespoon. Any additional sugars are from added sugars.

TRY THESE BRANDS: Sir Kensington's Classic Ketchup, Annie's Organic Ketchup, Simply Balanced Organic Ketchup, Simply Heinz Ketchup, Primal Kitchen Organic and Unsweetened Kethcup

MUSTARD

SODIUM: ≤65mg sodium per teaspoon

TRY THESE BRANDS: Simply Balanced Yellow Mustard, Westbrae Natural Mustard, Annie's Horseradish & Yellow Mustards, Heinz Spicy Brown Mustard, 365 Organic German & Honey Mustards, Mustard Girl Stoneground Deli Mustard, Organicville Stoneground Mustard

MAYONNAISE

INGREDIENT QUALITY is the most important, not necessarily total fat grams.

TRY THESE BRANDS: Sir Kensington's Organic Mayonnaise, Hellmann's Avocado Oil Mayonnaise Dressing, Spectrum Mayonnaise with Extra-Virgin Olive Oil, Chosen Foods Avocado Oil Mayonnaise, Primal Kitchen Chipotle Lime Mayonnaise, Duke's Light Mayonnaise with Olive Oil

SALSA

SODIUM: ≤120mg sodium per 2 tablespoons

SUGARS: No added sugars in ingredient list

TRY THESE BRANDS: The variety of salsas is immense, but these are brands that have options that meet the guidelines: Newman's Own salsas, Muir Glen salsas, fresh refrigerated salsas (not brand specific), Green Mountain Gringo salsas

---

GENERAL CONDIMENT GUIDELINES

MINIMAL AND RECOGNIZABLE INGREDIENTS—typically the shorter the list, the better.

AVOID HYDROGENATED AND PARTIALLY HYDROGENATED OILS

AVOID ADDED SUGARS IF POSSIBLE; if not, added sugars should be located toward the end or in the second half of the ingredient list.

SIMPLE
salad dressings

Homemade dressing comes together in minutes and is far healthier, cheaper, and fresher than most bottled dressings with added sugars, chemicals, and fillers. Prep ahead and store in a covered jar or container in the refrigerator. But, if you don't have time, I've included a buying guide to help you find a smart store-bought variety.

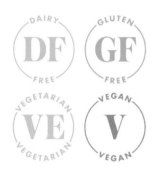

HANDS-ON: 5 MIN. // TOTAL: 5 MIN. // MAKES 1 CUP

avocado-cilantro dip and dressing

You know that sauce that you find yourself putting on everything? Well, this is mine! Salads, tacos, sandwich spread, dip for veggies, dressing for slaw—my list could go on. Bright green, creamy, and not "light" feeling at all, this thick, dip-like dressing has avocado to thank for its rich flavor and creamy texture. To make a thinner, more pourable dressing, add 1 tablespoon water at a time until you reach the desired consistency. Keep this in your fridge and use it for anything.

1 ripe avocado, peeled

½ cup fresh cilantro leaves

6 tablespoons milk, unsweetened nondairy milk, or water

1 garlic clove, minced

3 tablespoons olive oil

1½ tablespoons fresh lime juice

1½ teaspoons red wine vinegar

1 teaspoon honey

¼ teaspoon kosher salt

⅛ teaspoon black pepper

1 Place all the ingredients in a food processor or blender; process until smooth, about 30 seconds, stopping as needed to scrape down the sides.

2 Store in a jar or airtight container in the refrigerator for up to 1 week.

(SERVING SIZE: 1 TABLESPOON): CALORIES 40; FAT 4G (SAT 1G, UNSAT 3G); PROTEIN 0G; CARB 1G; FIBER 1G; SUGARS 0G (ADDED SUGARS 0G); SODIUM 35MG; CALC 1% DV; POTASSIUM 1% DV

buttermilk-chive dressing

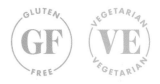

Ranch is the only dressing that I can get my picky-eater, Griffin, to touch, but I've had a hard time finding a bottled version that meets both my taste and health expectations. So I started playing around with a few ingredients in the kitchen. The result is this creamy, ranch-like dressing that kind of goes with everything. I'm also happy because it's free from fillers and that preservative aftertaste, and my picky tasting panel gave it three thumbs up!

1 Combine all the ingredients in a 1-quart glass jar with a tight-fitting lid.

2 Cover and shake vigorously to blend. Chill for 20 minutes before using or store in the refrigerator for up to 1 week.

3 Shake well before serving.

(SERVING SIZE: 1 TABLESPOON): CALORIES 36; FAT 4G (SAT 1G, UNSAT 3G); PROTEIN 0G; CARB 1G; FIBER 0G; SUGARS 1G (ADDED SUGARS 0G); SODIUM 79MG; CALC 1% DV; POTASSIUM 0% DV

½ cup buttermilk

¼ cup avocado oil mayonnaise or olive oil mayonnaise

2 teaspoons fresh lemon juice

1½ tablespoons finely chopped fresh chives

¼ teaspoon kosher salt

¼ teaspoon garlic powder

Black pepper

store-bought product buying guide

Thank goodness anti-inflammatory eating doesn't have to mean making all foods from scratch, because the concept of "semi-homemade" is one I rely on daily. Choosing products that are minimally processed is key. So how do you find those foods?

We often jump straight to the Nutrition Facts panel, which provides good nutrient info, but you get a better picture of a food's quality (and ultimately health effect) by looking at the ingredients list. It takes a little bit of investigative work and decoding, but here are the facts I look for in the ingredients list and what they mean.

level of processing

- Look for products that keep ingredients minimal. Typically, the shorter the ingredients list, the less processed the product.
- Choose those that you would expect the primary ingredients to be first in the list.
- Read through the ingredients. Do you recognize them as a food, spice, or seasoning? Does it make sense for the ingredient to be included? If so, this is a sign of less or minimal processing.
- Are ingredient names long, complex, or reminiscent of science class? Are there many ingredients that you've never heard of and/or don't know why are included? These are signs of a more processed food.

So I became determined to figure out how to provide nutritious meals that make us healthy now as well as long-term, **but** without spending hours planning, prepping, and cooking. It took a few years, lots of trials and failures, and a few last-minute runs through our local Chick-fil-A drive-through, but I finally figured out a system. I rely on Simple Staples.

amount of added sugars

Identifying sugars on labels can be confusing, so here's a trick that I use sometimes. When I can't determine the prevalence of added sugar in a food product, I find another brand of the same product that I know has no added sugars. Then, I compare the total grams of sugar between the two products. If the number is the same or very close, you can assume there are no added sugars in the product in question. Below are some more straightforward facts to look for.

- Ingredients are listed in descending order by weight, meaning the ingredient listed first is used in the highest quantity and the ingredient listed last is used in the least. The closer the added sugars or sweeteners fall toward the end of the ingredients list, the less added sugar is in the product.
- On the Nutrition Facts panel, the total sugar grams are a total of the natural sugars and the added sugars in a serving. This tells you very little about added sugars, especially if the food contains both added and natural, like yogurts. Until new labeling guidelines go into effect, the best way to assess added sugars is to identify added sugars in the ingredients list and look where they fall in the order of ingredients.
- Natural sugars refer to those that are naturally found in a food, but when those natural sugars (like honey) are used in other products, they are considered added sugars.

INGREDIENT NAMES OF ADDED SUGARS

Brown sugar, confectioners' sugar, invert sugar, raw sugar, sugar, white granulated sugar, cane sugar, cane crystals, beet sugar

Honey, maple syrup, molasses, nectars (such as agave or peach), corn syrup, corn syrup solids, high-fructose corn syrup (HFCS), malt syrup, rice syrup, evaporated cane juice, caramel

Dextrose, fructose, maltose, sucrose, lactose, glucose, xylose, or ends in "-ose"

---

whole-grain proportion

- Only products labeled "100% whole grain" are made completely of whole grains.
- Many products use a mix of whole and refined grains, so try to determine if the product is predominantly made of whole or refined grains. What you want to see is that whole-grain flours (whole wheat flour, whole oat flour, brown rice flour, etc.) are listed before refined flours (unbleached flour, wheat flour, etc.) in the ingredients list.
- Many products use a mix of whole and refined grains, so try to determine if the product is predominantly made of whole or refined grains. What you want to see is that whole-grain flours (whole wheat flour, whole oat flour, brown rice flour, etc.) are listed before refined flours (unbleached flour, wheat flour, etc.) in the ingredients list.
- Know which labeling terms actually mean something about the food quality and which are marketing fluff.

trans fats

Avoid any fat or oil with the words "hydrogenated" or "partially hydrogenated."

Label terms that always signify a whole grain: The words "whole" or "stone-ground whole" in front of a grain (whole wheat, whole oats, stone-ground whole wheat, etc.).

Others: oats, oatmeal, brown rice, wheat berries Labels you probably can't trust to be all or predominantly whole grains: Stone-ground, multigrain, wheat, flour, durum flour, semolina flour, organic wheat flour

Label terms that never indicate whole grains: Enriched flour, self-rising flour, cake flour, bran, germ, de-germinated

---

Throughout this book, you'll find item-specific buying guides and brand recommendations. Here's a list for quick reference:

- Condiment Buying Guide (page 68)
- Salad Dressing Buying Guide (page 76)
- Breakfast Food Buying Guide (page 98)
- Side Dish Buying Guide (page 242)
- Snack Buying Guide (page 280)

mason jar vinaigrettes

Basic but flavorful oil-and-vinegar-based dressings are easy to whip up in 5 minutes or less, but there are some secrets to creating a balanced homemade one.

- **A GENERAL OIL-TO-ACID RATIO** for dressings is 2:1 or, as in the recipes opposite, 6 tablespoons oil to 3 tablespoons acid. This will vary slightly based on other ingredients and doesn't always apply to creamy dressings.
- **BALANCE STRONGER ACIDS** (think lemon juice, white vinegar, balsamic vinegar) with a little natural or added sweetness like honey, maple syrup, or orange juice. Don't worry—this added sugar will be extremely minimal per serving.

- **DON'T BE AFRAID OF USING SALT** in your dressing; a little is essential to bringing out the rich flavors in the oils and usually results in needing less dressing overall.
- **MEASURE!** Dressings are delicate balances and aren't as forgiving as other recipes. When I try to eyeball amounts, I usually end up scrapping the emulsion and starting over.
- **FLAVORS TYPICALLY GET BETTER AFTER** sitting. I like to combine the ingredients, top with the lid, shake, and then refrigerate for several hours or up to a day before using.

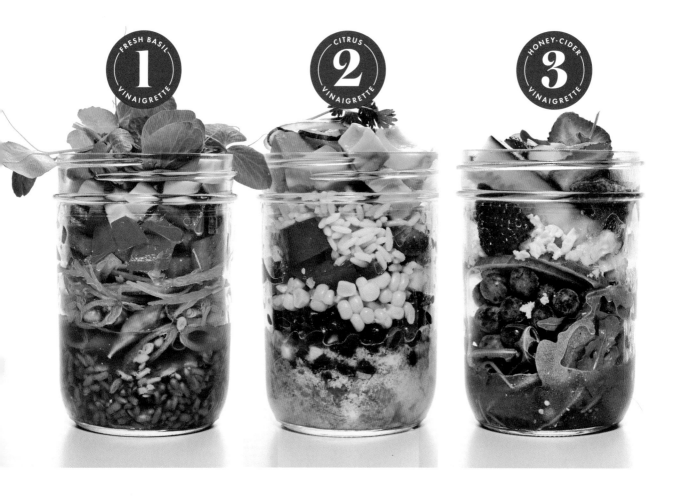

FRESH BASIL **1** VINAIGRETTE

CITRUS **2** VINAIGRETTE

HONEY-CIDER **3** VINAIGRETTE

① FRESH BASIL VINAIGRETTE

ACID: 3 tablespoons white wine vinegar

OIL: 6 tablespoons extra-virgin olive oil or walnut oil

FLAVOR BOOSTERS: 2 teaspoons honey, 2 tablespoons chopped fresh herb such as basil, salt and black pepper

② CITRUS VINAIGRETTE

ACID: 3 tablespoons fresh lemon juice

OIL: 6 tablespoons extra-virgin olive oil or avocado oil

FLAVOR BOOSTERS: 3 tablespoons fresh orange juice, 1 tablespoon Dijon mustard, salt and black pepper

③ HONEY-CIDER VINAIGRETTE

ACIDS: 2 tablespoons apple cider vinegar, 1 tablespoon white wine vinegar

OIL: 6 tablespoons grapeseed, avocado, or mild olive oil

FLAVOR BOOSTERS: 1 tablespoon coarse-grain mustard, 1 tablespoon honey, salt and black pepper

④ ASIAN VINAIGRETTE

ACID: 2 tablespoons rice vinegar, 1 tablespoon fresh lime juice

OIL: ¼ cup olive oil or avocado oil, 2 tablespoons sesame oil

FLAVOR BOOSTERS: 1 tablespoon low-sodium soy sauce, 2 teaspoons honey, 1 tablespoon finely grated fresh ginger

⑤ MAPLE-BALSAMIC VINAIGRETTE

ACIDS: 2 tablespoons balsamic vinegar, 1 tablespoon apple cider vinegar

OIL: 6 tablespoons extra-virgin olive oil or walnut oil

FLAVOR BOOSTERS: 1½ tablespoons pure maple syrup, 1½ teaspoons Dijon mustard, salt and black pepper

⑥ RED WINE VINAIGRETTE

ACID: 3 tablespoons red wine vinegar

OIL: 6 tablespoons extra-virgin olive oil

FLAVOR BOOSTERS: 1 tablespoon Dijon mustard, salt and black pepper

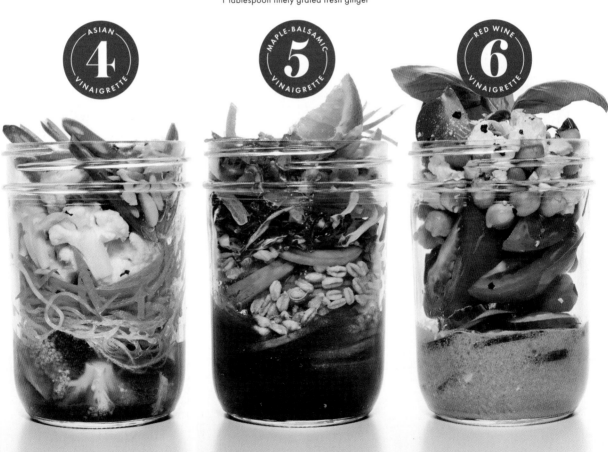

salad dressing buying guide

Even though I always have the highest healthy-eating aspirations Monday morning, I've learned that being prepared also means being realistic—meaning there are days where a homemade dressing just isn't in the cards. To keep this from being a roadblock to healthy eating, I keep an assortment of store-bought dressings in my fridge to drizzle on salads and veggies, or use as a last-minute marinade, when needed.

TOTAL FAT

A dressing is supposed to be fat-based, so don't compare fat grams among brands. And skip fat-free varieties. If you want to focus on fat, then check out the type(s) used in the ingredient list.

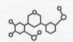

ADDED SUGARS

A touch of sweetness is sometimes needed to balance flavors, but make sure the dressing has <3 grams total sugars per serving.

SODIUM

<250mg per serving (ideally <200mg per serving)

INGREDIENT LIST

Look for those that contain the same or very similar ingredients to what might be in a homemade recipe. These will typically be your less processed.

TYPES OF FATS AND OILS

Avoid hydrogenated or partially hydrogenated oils. Find a dressing using flaxseed oil, olive oil, avocado oil, or walnut or other nut oils since they have more omega-3 to omega-6 fatty acids.

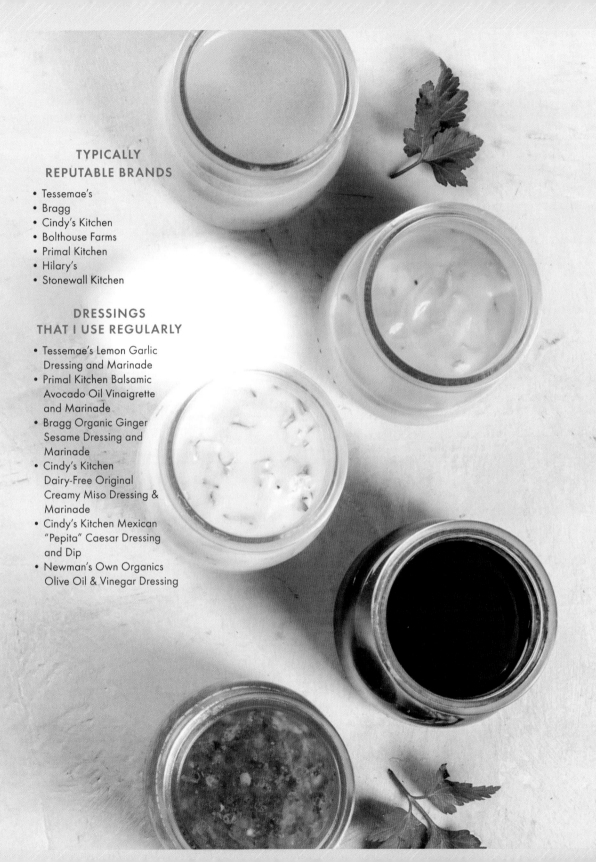

TYPICALLY
REPUTABLE BRANDS

- Tessemae's
- Bragg
- Cindy's Kitchen
- Bolthouse Farms
- Primal Kitchen
- Hilary's
- Stonewall Kitchen

DRESSINGS
THAT I USE REGULARLY

- Tessemae's Lemon Garlic Dressing and Marinade
- Primal Kitchen Balsamic Avocado Oil Vinaigrette and Marinade
- Bragg Organic Ginger Sesame Dressing and Marinade
- Cindy's Kitchen Dairy-Free Original Creamy Miso Dressing & Marinade
- Cindy's Kitchen Mexican "Pepita" Caesar Dressing and Dip
- Newman's Own Organics Olive Oil & Vinegar Dressing

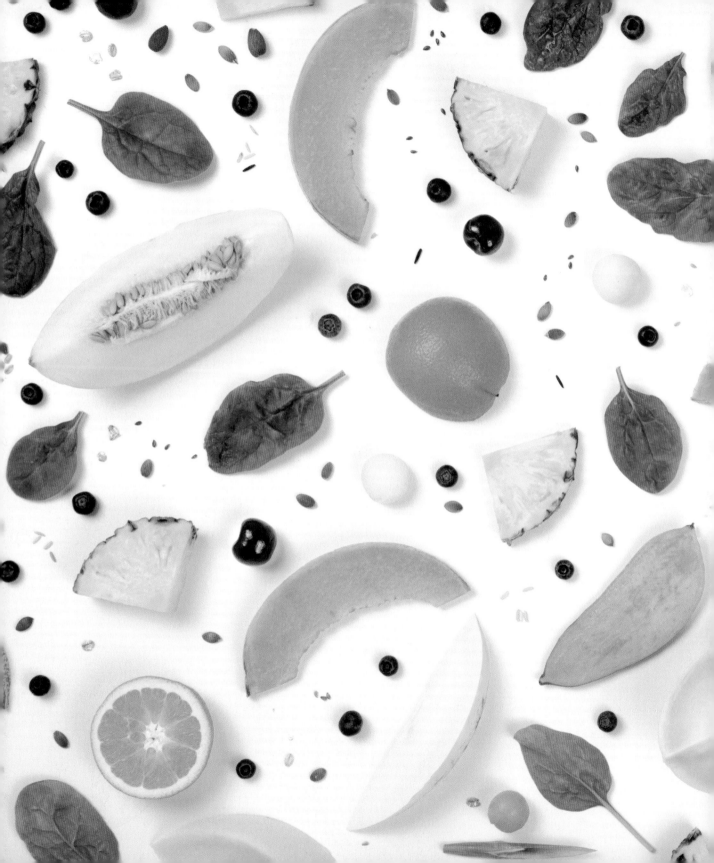

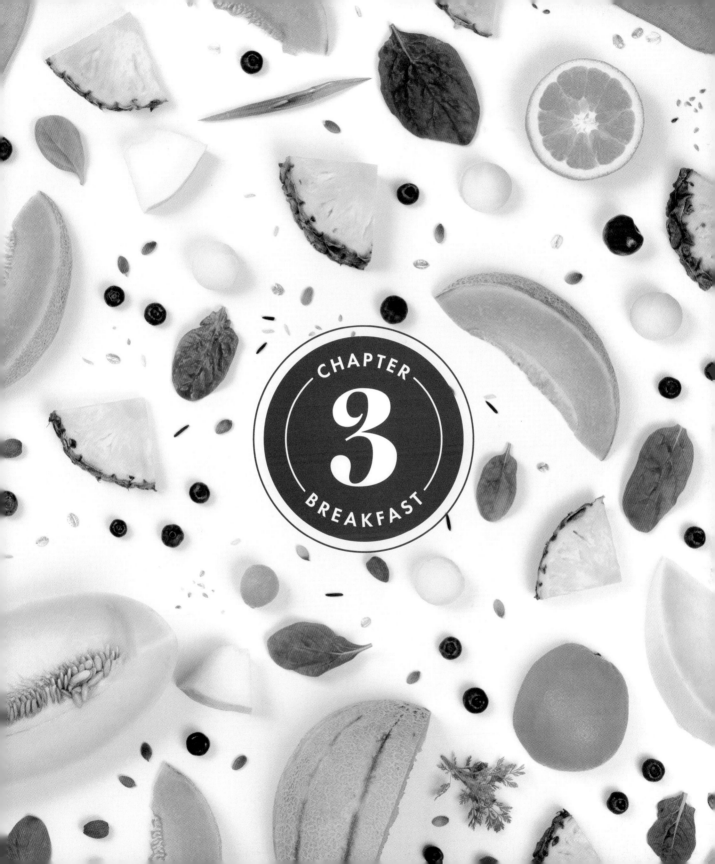

CHAPTER

3

BREAKFAST

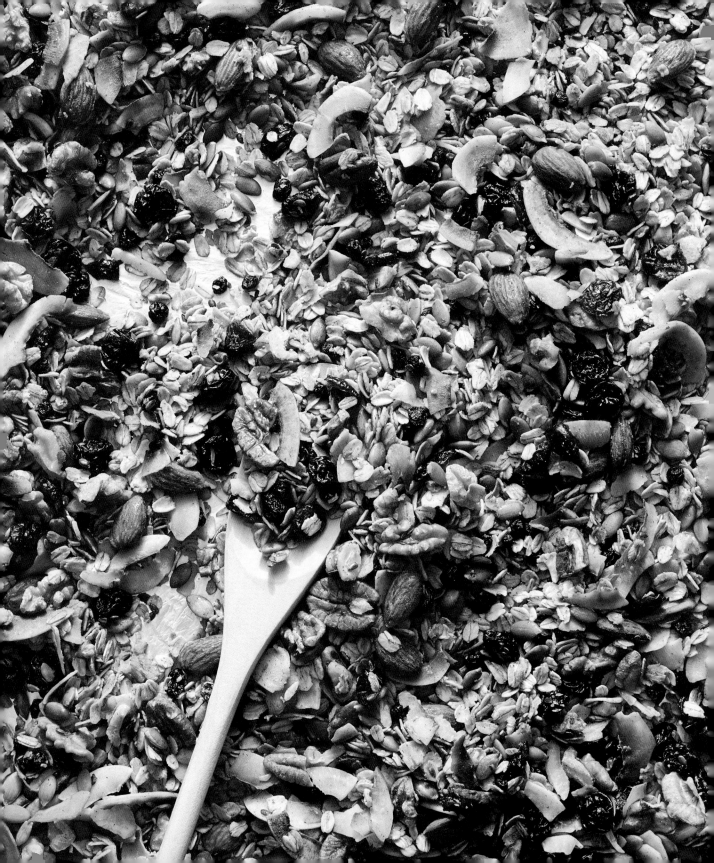

easy make-ahead granola

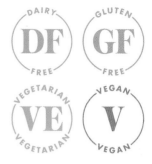

This basic granola recipe uses just a touch of sweetness (½ teaspoon of added sugar per serving) and is loaded with the good stuff: nuts, coconut flakes, and dried fruit. Serve with yogurt, sprinkle over a smoothie bowl, or just grab a handful to snack on. Watch the oven time closely—you want the mixture to get toasty and fragrant and the nuts to begin to release their oils. But be careful to not leave it in too long, or the oats and nuts darken and can develop a slightly bitter taste.

1 Preheat the oven to 350°F. Line a large rimmed baking sheet with aluminum foil and lightly coat the foil with cooking spray.

2 Combine the oats, nuts, coconut, and pumpkin seed kernels in a large bowl. Place the maple syrup in a small microwavable bowl. Microwave on HIGH until warm, about 15 seconds. Add the oil, salt, and cinnamon to the syrup; whisk to combine. Pour the syrup mixture over the oat mixture, stirring well to coat. Spread the oat mixture in a single layer on the prepared baking sheet. Sprinkle with the flaxseed.

3 Bake until golden, about 18 minutes, stirring after 12 minutes. Let cool completely, about 30 minutes. Add the dried fruit, if desired; toss to combine. Store in an airtight container at room temperature for up to 1 week.

(SERVING SIZE: ¼ CUP): CALORIES 134; FAT 8G (SAT 2G, UNSAT 6G); PROTEIN 3G; CARB 13G; FIBER 3G; SUGARS 3G (ADDED SUGARS 2G); SODIUM 62MG; CALC 2% DV; POTASSIUM 2% DV

GRAIN-FREE OPTION: Omit the oats, and increase the nuts to 4 cups, the coconut to 1½ cups, and the pumpkin seed kernels to ⅔ cup. Proceed with the recipe as directed.

flaxseed

Both flaxseed and flax oil are rich in omega-3 fats. Research tells us that getting an adequate amount of these fats in your diet can significantly reduce the risk of heart disease, decrease the risk of dementia and brain diseases, and ease some autoimmune conditions and arthritis. The actual flaxseed—compared to just flax oil—also contains bioactive compounds known as lignans, which may further reduce the risk of heart disease and bone and joint issues, as well as possibly reduce the risk of hormone-related cancers such as breast and ovarian. Whole seeds can pass through the GI tract not fully digested, so it's thought that choosing ground flaxseed is best to get all the seed's benefits. You can also grind whole seeds yourself. Sprinkle flaxseed in yogurt, trail mixes, hot cereals, and the batter for baked goods.

Cooking spray

3 cups uncooked old-fashioned rolled oats

1½ cups chopped unsalted raw nuts (such as almonds, pecans, walnuts, or a mixture)

⅔ cup unsweetened flaked coconut

⅓ cup raw unsalted pumpkin seed kernels (pepitas)

¼ cup pure maple syrup

2 tablespoons canola or coconut oil

¾ teaspoon kosher salt

½ teaspoon ground cinnamon

3 tablespoons ground flaxseed

1 cup dried fruit (such as raisins, cherries, blueberries, or cranberries; optional)

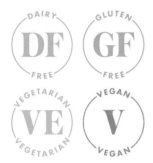

DAIRY FREE **DF** / GLUTEN FREE **GF**

VEGETARIAN **VE** / VEGAN **V**

- 1 cup frozen wild blueberries or mixed berries
- ½ cup fresh baby spinach leaves
- 2 tablespoons fresh orange juice
- 2 tablespoons water
- 1 (5.3-ounce) container plain 2% Greek yogurt or plain soy yogurt
- 1 medium ripe banana, sliced

HANDS-ON: 5 MIN. // TOTAL: 5 MIN. // SERVES 1

berry green smoothie

Incorporating a protein source in your smoothie will help keep you fueled all morning. To prepare a dairy-free version, make sure to choose a soy yogurt, which has comparable protein to Greek yogurt, or a plant-based yogurt like almond or flax with at least 5g of protein per serving.

Place the berries, spinach, orange juice, water, yogurt, and banana in a blender; blend until smooth. Serve immediately.

(SERVING SIZE: ABOUT 1¾ CUPS): CALORIES 297; FAT 4G (SAT 2G, UNSAT 2G); PROTEIN 18G; CARB 54G; FIBER 8G; SUGARS 33G (ADDED SUGARS 0G); SODIUM 75MG; CALC 23% DV; POTASSIUM 20% DV

wild blueberries

Blueberries have long been touted as a "superfood" but there's a specific type known as wild blueberries that may provide even more health benefits. Research suggests that wild blueberries (as compared to ordinary or conventional ones) not only contain higher levels, but greater diversity, of phytochemicals—something that makes their antioxidant activity rank at the top when compared to other berries and produce.

While consumption of all blueberries is associated with reducing risk of heart disease, cancer, and memory loss, eating wild blueberries may deliver even more in return due to their concentrated nutrients and compounds. Research suggests that wild blueberries may lower blood pressure, improve insulin sensitivity, improve brain activity in children and teens related to memory and concentration, and promote good bacteria to improve gut health.

How do you know if your blueberries are wild? Most are frozen immediately after harvest to preserve nutrients, so they are typically found near other frozen berries and fruit. Simply look for "wild" on packaging, and then use just as you would other frozen fruits for smoothies, or thaw to stir into batter for muffins, pancakes, and breads or to toss in oatmeal or yogurt.

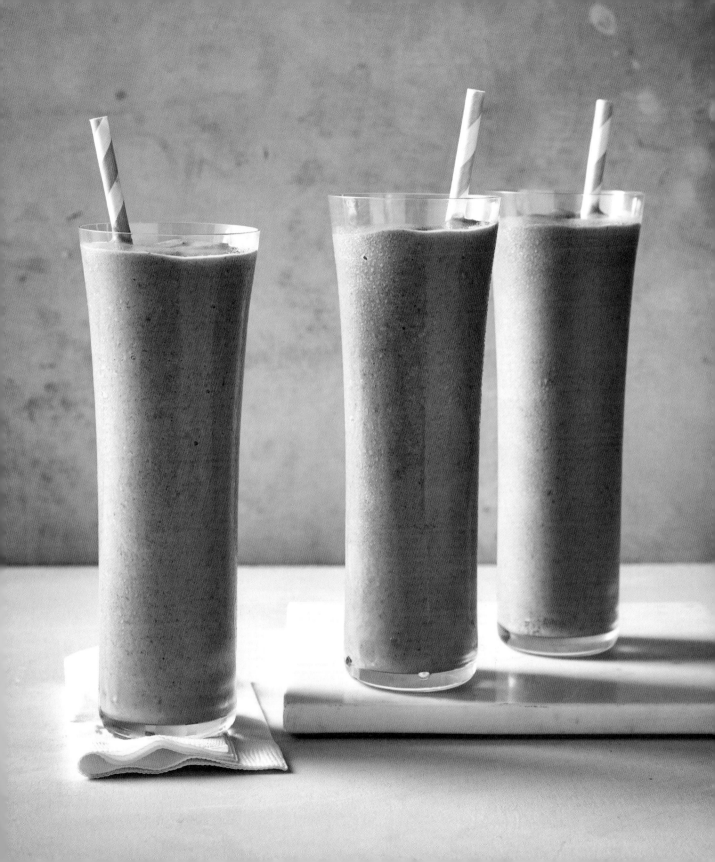

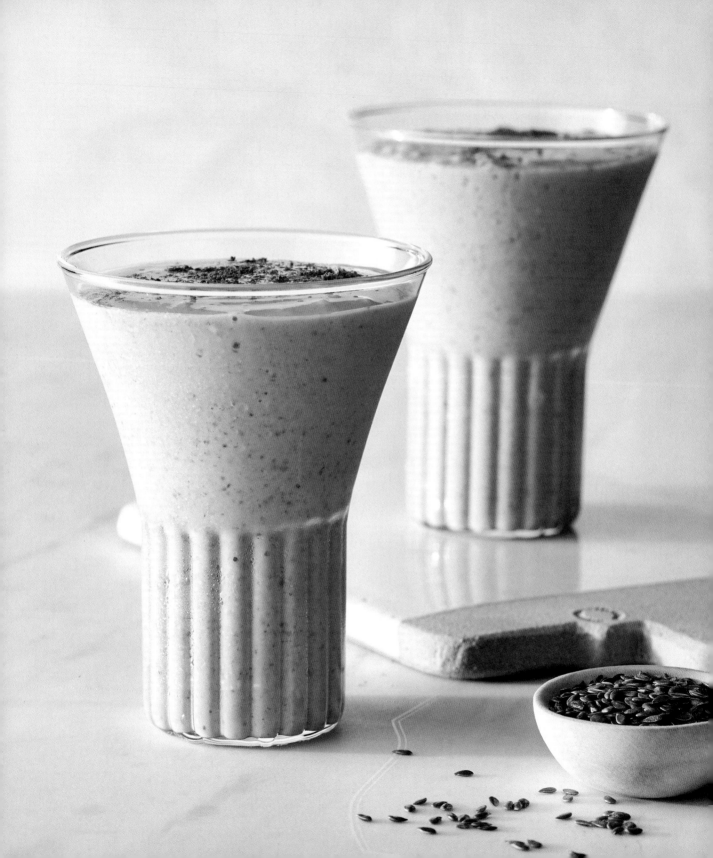

cherry power smoothie

Choosing a ripe banana adds just the right amount of sweetness; opting for frozen cherries makes the smoothie thick and icy. My kids love this for breakfast or a snack, and I love it sprinkled with a touch of dark chocolate shavings for a more decadent treat.

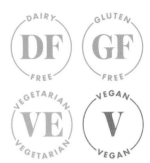

Place the banana, cherries, yogurt, milk, lemon juice, flaxseed, and honey in a blender; blend until smooth, about 30 seconds. Serve immediately.

(SERVING SIZE: 1 CUP): CALORIES 207; FAT 3G (SAT 1G, UNSAT 1G); PROTEIN 6G; CARB 41G; FIBER 4G; SUGARS 32G (ADDED SUGARS 6G); SODIUM 63MG; CALC 17% DV; POTASSIUM 13% DV

1 small ripe banana

1½ cups frozen pitted dark sweet cherries

½ cup plain 2% Greek yogurt or drained soft tofu

⅓ cup 2% milk or unsweetened nondairy milk

1 tablespoon fresh lemon juice

2 teaspoons ground flaxseed

2 teaspoons honey, or ½ teaspoon liquid stevia

cherries

Both sweet and tart varieties lower inflammatory blood proteins, and cherries may even offer pain relief comparable to ibuprofen. When cherries aren't in season, try tart cherry juice in smoothies and salad dressings.

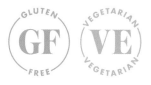

yogurt-granola breakfast bark

What's better than a super-quick, healthy breakfast that kids enjoy? One that the kids can serve themselves! Tangy and cold, with just the right amount of sweetness, it's like a yogurt ice pop but in handheld form and provides a healthy dose of probiotics, antioxidants, and fiber. These melt quickly, so keep them stored in the freezer, pull out only what you need, and eat fast.

1 (7-ounce) container plain 2% Greek yogurt

2 tablespoons honey or pure maple syrup, or ½ to 1 teaspoon liquid stevia

1 tablespoon fresh lemon juice (optional)

½ cup fresh or frozen wild blueberries

⅔ cup whole-grain, gluten-free granola (such as Kind Maple Quinoa Clusters with Chia Seeds) or Easy Make-Ahead Granola (page 81)

1 Combine the yogurt, honey, lemon juice (if using), and blueberries in a small bowl. Stir well to combine, mashing the blueberries against the side of the bowl.

2 Line a rimmed baking sheet or shallow storage container with aluminum foil. Pour the yogurt mixture onto the prepared baking sheet or into the container, spreading the mixture to ¼-inch thickness. Sprinkle evenly with the granola, breaking apart any large clusters. Freeze for at least 1 hour before serving. Store in the refrigerator until ready to serve. Just before serving, break into pieces. Return leftover pieces to the freezer. To serve, remove the pieces from freezer, and eat immediately.

NOTE: You can use 1 cup of yogurt in place of a 7-ounce container.

(SERVING SIZE: ¼ OF BARK): CALORIES 129; FAT 2G (SAT 1G, UNSAT 1G); PROTEIN 6G; CARB 21G; FIBER 0G; SUGARS 13G (ADDED SUGARS 7G); SODIUM 38MG; CALC 7% DV; POTASSIUM 1% DV

fat, dairy, and health

We've been told for years to choose fat-free or lower-fat dairy products in order to reduce saturated fat intake, which in turn will decrease cardiovascular risk and inflammation from those fats. However, research suggests that the level of fat in dairy doesn't make much difference on health. In fact, most studies that have compared full-fat to lower-fat dairy intake show no real difference in cardiovascular risk. A few even suggested that higher-fat dairy intake may even be beneficial. Additionally, the overwhelming research consensus is that dairy has an anti-inflammatory effect in the body. Only those with a dairy allergy or intolerance should skip dairy to avoid inflammation.

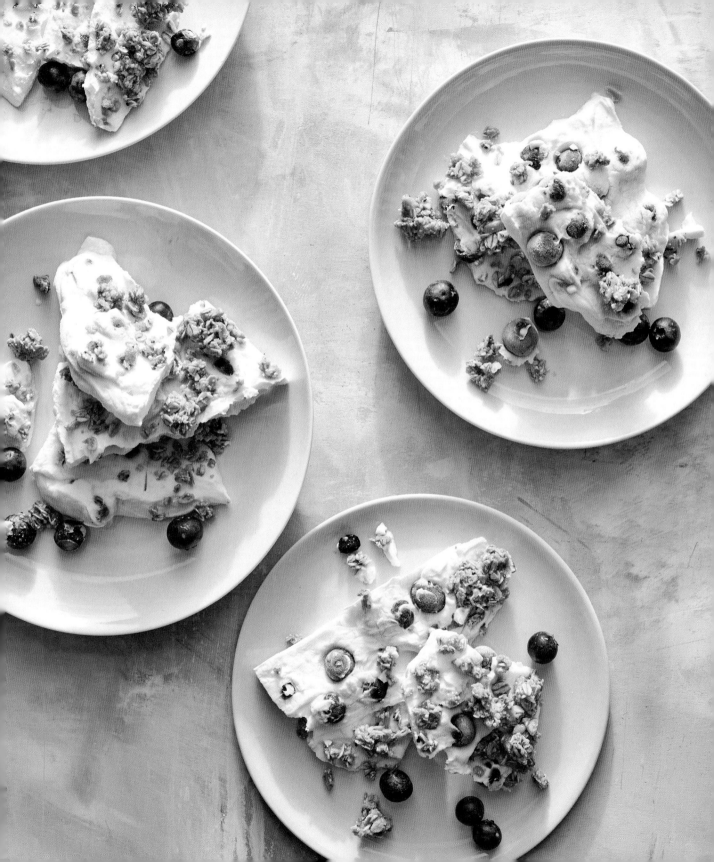

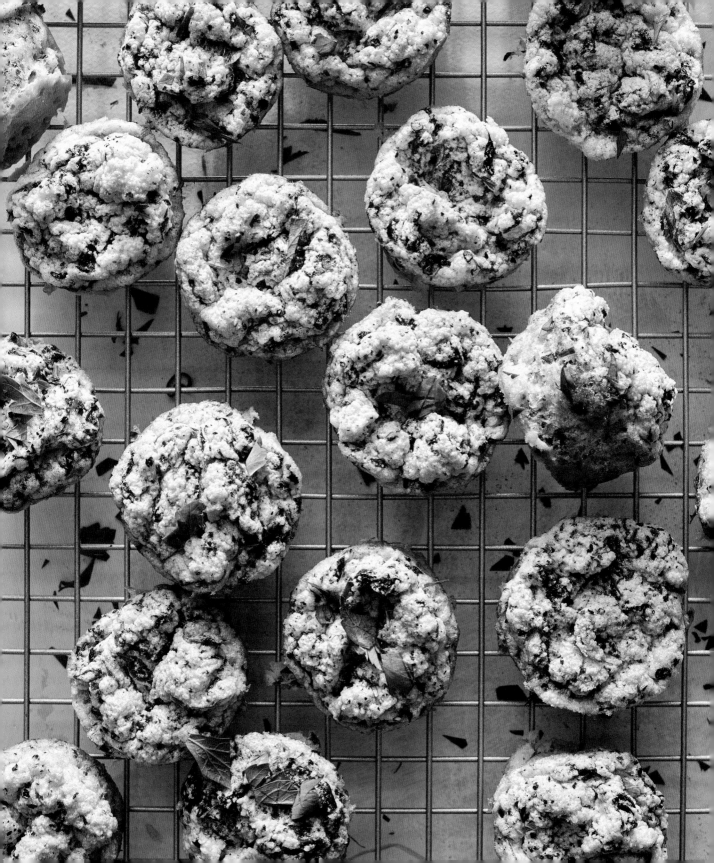

super green frittata bites

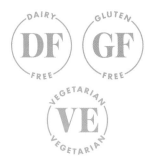

Light, airy, and slightly custardy, these are like mini soufflés for breakfast! And don't worry—whipping the egg whites is all that's required to get a soufflé-like effect. If you don't mind a little dairy, then definitely check out the "cheesy" option with feta or Parmesan cheese below.

1 Preheat the oven to 350°F. Lightly coat a 24-cup mini-muffin pan with cooking spray. Place the broccoli in a small microwavable bowl. Cover with plastic wrap and microwave on high until just tender, about 2 minutes. Let cool completely, about 15 minutes.

2 Combine the egg yolks, spinach, scallions, parsley, salt, pepper, and broccoli in a large bowl and whisk to combine.

3 Place the egg whites in a medium bowl. Beat with an electric mixer on high speed until stiff, about 2 minutes. Fold one-third of the egg whites into the yolk mixture; repeat twice with the remaining egg whites. Spoon the egg mixture into the prepared muffin pan, filling each cup completely.

4 Bake until the centers are set, about 8 minutes. Let cool in the pan for 2 minutes. Remove the bites from the pan and transfer to a wire rack. Serve warm, or let cool completely, about 20 minutes, and store in an airtight container in the refrigerator for up to 5 days.

(SERVING SIZE: 4 FRITTATA BITES): CALORIES 112; FAT 7G (SAT 2G, UNSAT 4G); PROTEIN 9G; CARB 2G; FIBER 1G; SUGARS 1G (ADDED SUGARS 0G); SODIUM 270MG; CALC 7% DV; POTASSIUM 4% DV

CHEESY SUPER GREEN FRITTATA BITES: Stir ¼ cup crumbled feta cheese or grated Parmesan cheese into the egg mixture after folding in the egg whites in step 3. Proceed with the recipe as directed.

kitchen hack

Fold the whipped egg whites immediately into the yolk mixture (don't let the egg whites stand too long before adding) to get the soufflé effect.

Ingredients

Cooking spray
1 cup finely chopped broccoli florets
2 tablespoons water
8 large eggs, separated
½ cup frozen chopped spinach, thawed and squeezed dry
¼ cup chopped scallions
¼ cup chopped fresh parsley
½ teaspoon kosher salt
½ teaspoon black pepper

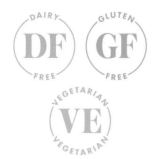

sweet potato home fries with eggs

Skip step 1 by making extra roasted sweet potato wedges for dinner to heat up in the skillet for breakfast the next morning. Another option is to cook frozen roasted sweet potato like Earthbound Farms Organic Roasted Sweet Potato Slices with Sea Salt and Olive Oil.

1 large sweet potato

1 teaspoon olive oil

¼ teaspoon salt

⅛ teaspoon garlic powder

Cooking spray

2 large egg whites

3 large eggs

Black pepper (optional)

Fresh thyme (optional)

1 Prick the potato in several spots with a fork; microwave on high for 5 minutes. Let cool for 5 minutes, then chop into ½-inch cubes.

2 Heat the oil in a medium skillet over medium-high. Add the sweet potato cubes and sprinkle with ⅛ teaspoon of the salt and the garlic powder; cook for 6 minutes or until crisp and brown on the outside. Remove from the pan; keep warm.

3 Coat the same skillet with cooking spray. Whisk together the egg whites, eggs, and remaining ⅛ teaspoon salt in a medium bowl. Add to the pan; cook over medium for 3 minutes or until soft-scrambled. Serve with the potatoes; top with pepper and thyme, if desired.

(SERVING SIZE: 1 CUP POTATOES AND ABOUT ⅔ CUP EGG MIXTURE): CALORIES 240; FAT 11G (SAT 3G, UNSAT 8G); PROTEIN 15G; CARB 22G; FIBER 3G; SUGARS 5G (ADDED SUGARS 0G); SODIUM 518MG; CALC 6% DV; POTASSIUM 10% DV

are eggs okay?

Once seen as a cholesterol-raising heart attack causer, the egg is back and considered part of a healthy diet. In fact, the American Heart Association says it's okay for most people to eat one egg daily. Its combination of fat and protein—one egg has about 7 grams of protein and 5 grams of fat—make it a healthy food that also keeps you full until lunch. Some research suggests that eating eggs for breakfast can help you eat less later in the day, too.

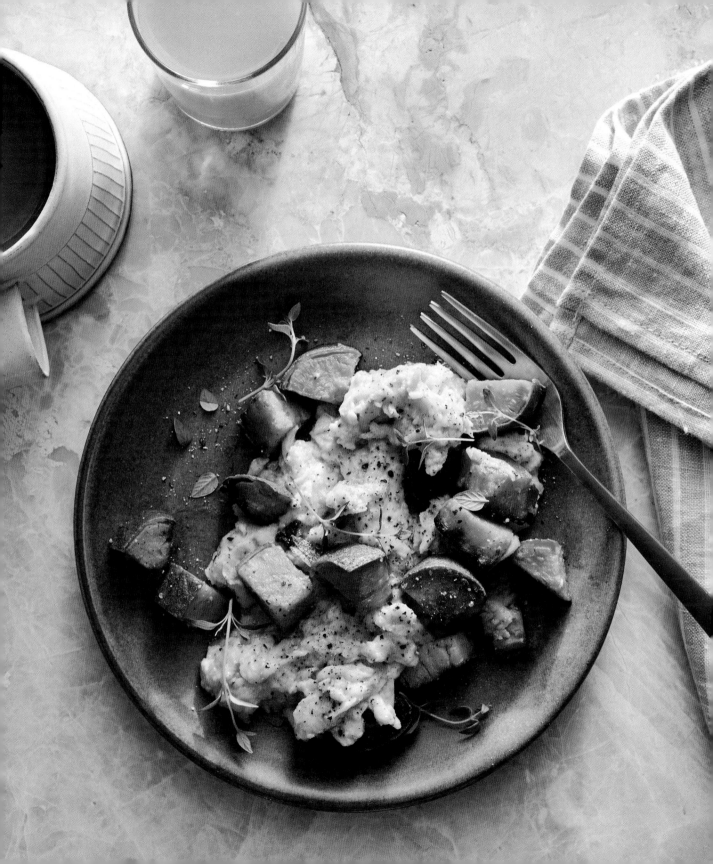

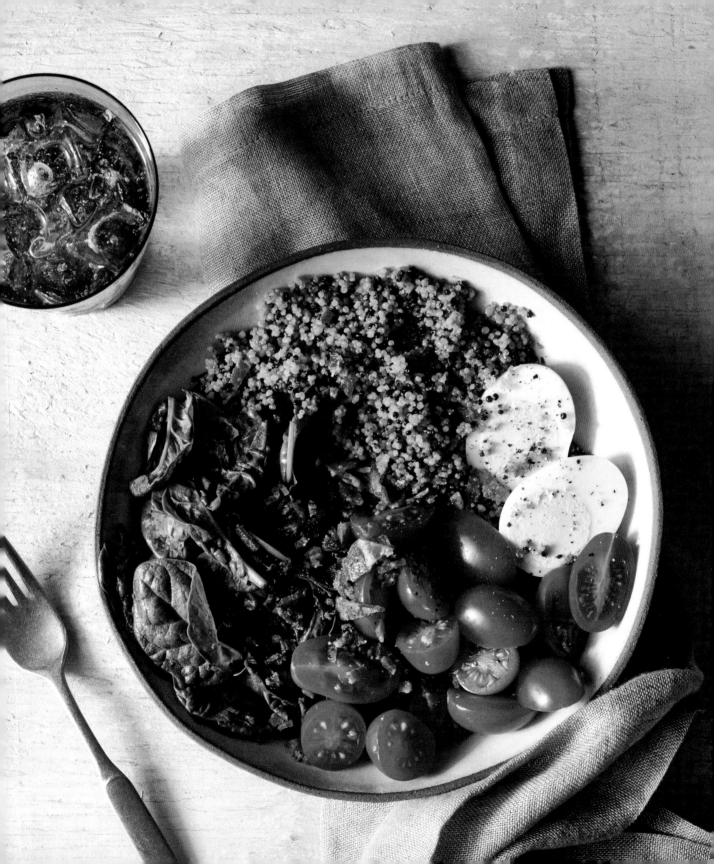

warm spinach breakfast bowl

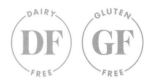

Greens for breakfast? Wilted baby spinach with a tangy vinegar-bacon dressing makes the perfect savory base for a satisfying breakfast bowl with quinoa and eggs. Use quinoa or other leftover cooked whole grains, and add a poached egg with a runny yolk to "dress" the quinoa.

1 Cook the bacon in a skillet over medium, turning occasionally, until crisp, 4 to 5 minutes; transfer the bacon to a paper towel–lined plate to drain, reserving the drippings in the skillet. Reduce the heat to low and add the vinegar and ⅛ teaspoon of the salt to the reserved drippings; whisk to combine.

2 Add the spinach to the skillet, tossing to coat. Cook, tossing occasionally, until the spinach wilts, about 1 minute. Divide the spinach evenly between two bowls; add ⅔ cup of the quinoa, ¼ cup of the tomatoes, and a cooked egg to each bowl. Crumble the bacon. Top the bowls evenly with the bacon crumbles and sprinkle evenly with the pepper and remaining ⅛ teaspoon salt.

(SERVING SIZE: 1 BOWL): CALORIES 296; FAT 10G (SAT 3G, UNSAT 5G); PROTEIN 18G; CARB 32G; FIBER 7G; SUGARS 2G (ADDED SUGARS 0G); SODIUM 544MG; CALC 16% DV; POTASSIUM 8% DV

- 2 uncured bacon slices
- 2 tablespoons red wine vinegar or sherry vinegar
- ¼ teaspoon kosher salt
- 4 cups chopped fresh baby spinach
- 1⅓ cups cooked quinoa
- ½ cup halved grape tomatoes
- 2 large eggs, hard-cooked and halved, fried, or poached
- ⅛ teaspoon black pepper

is breakfast essential?

We've been trained to believe skipping breakfast is unhealthy and can slow metabolism, but recent research suggests breakfast may not be as important as once believed. This research, largely driven by interest in the health effects associated with intermittent fasting (see page 37), states that eating (or not eating) breakfast appears to have little effect on metabolism or daily energy balance. However, while there appears to be little impact on metabolism, eating breakfast has been associated with having a healthier diet in general and better long-term success losing and maintaining weight. People who typically eat breakfast also have better insulin sensitivity and lower fasting cholesterol compared to skippers.

So what does this mean? Right now, there's no clear-cut answer on what's healthier—eating breakfast or not. Your best bet is to determine what works for you in terms of energy, hunger, and schedule.

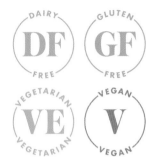

strawberry overnight oats with crunch

I love tricks to streamline time in the kitchen, and making these ahead in individual serving containers has breakfast ready in only a minute. It also allows everyone to customize their own oatmeal—something that seems to make mornings go a lot smoother! I like to add a touch of sweetness, a little fresh fruit, and a bit of crunch. Top it off with a dash of sea salt, ground cinnamon or nutmeg, or unsweetened cocoa powder.

1 cup 2% milk or plain unsweetened almond or soy milk

½ cup uncooked steel-cut oats

2 teaspoons pure maple syrup

1 cup sliced fresh strawberries

¼ cup Easy Make-Ahead Granola (page 81) or store-bought whole-grain granola (crunch)

1 Combine the milk and oats in an airtight container; seal. Refrigerate for 8 hours or up to overnight.

2 Add the maple syrup to the oat mixture. Divide the oat mixture evenly between two bowls; top evenly with the strawberries and granola.

(SERVING SIZE: ABOUT ⅔ CUP OATS MIXTURE, ½ CUP STRAWBERRIES, AND 2 TABLESPOONS GRANOLA): CALORIES 336; FAT 9G (SAT 3G, UNSAT 4G); PROTEIN 11G; CARB 54G; FIBER 7G; SUGARS 16G (ADDED SUGARS 5G); SODIUM 90MG; CALC 19% DV; POTASSIUM 11% DV

favorite flavor combinations

- **APPLE CRUMBLE OATMEAL:** 2 teaspoons brown sugar + ¼ cup granola + ¼ cup toasted walnuts + 1 cup diced Granny Smith apple
- **BANANA-ALMOND OATMEAL:** 2 teaspoons honey + 3 tablespoons almond butter + 1 sliced banana or 1 cup blueberries
- **CITRUS-BERRY OATMEAL:** 2 teaspoons pure maple syrup + ⅓ cup granola + 1 tablespoon toasted unsweetened coconut + ½ cup orange wedges + ½ cup fresh or thawed frozen wild blueberries

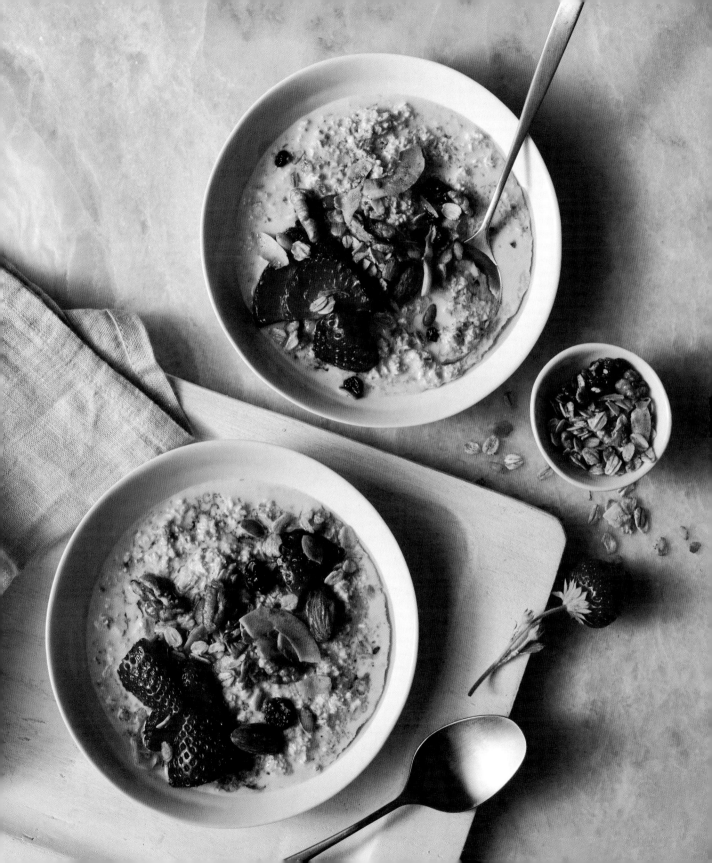

HOW TO
make a breakfast bowl

There's little time on weekday mornings to follow a recipe. I've got to have quick options to grab-and-go or assemble quickly, which is exactly why I fell in love with breakfast bowls. There's no precise recipe, so there's no way to mess them up. This also means each one is unique, and the options for breakfast bowls—sweet and savory—are endless when you think outside the norms of just a bowl of cereal or oats. Here's my formula for creating a healthy and filling breakfast bowl:

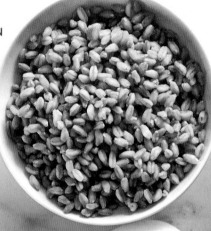

START WITH A WHOLE-GRAIN OR VEGGIE BASE

BASE IDEAS: Oats, quinoa, brown rice, barley, farro, grits; veggies like baby spinach, kale, salad blends, baked sweet potato

ADD PROTEIN

PROTEIN IDEAS: Eggs, nuts, nut butters, shredded cooked chicken breast, yogurt, beans, smoked salmon, tofu

③ ADD FRUITS OR VEGETABLES

FRUIT IDEAS: Berries, sliced strawberries, citrus sections, banana slices, chopped apple, pineapple chunks, kiwi slices, canned pumpkin, raisins, dried cranberries, other dried fruit

VEGETABLE IDEAS: Cherry tomatoes, fresh or wilted greens, leftover roasted vegetables, chopped cucumber, diced avocado, sliced radishes, black beans, chickpeas, corn kernels, scallions, slivered onions, sun-dried tomatoes

④ TOP IT OFF
(THINK A DASH OF SWEET OR SAVORY AND MAYBE A LITTLE CRUNCH)

SWEET: Honey, maple syrup, peanut butter or other nut butter, ground cinnamon, cocoa, Greek yogurt

SAVORY: Pesto, fresh salsa, mashed avocado, tzatziki sauce, Sriracha, feta cheese, cheddar cheese, kalamata olives, fresh herbs, Greek yogurt

CRUNCH IDEAS: Toasted almonds, toasted pecans, chopped pistachios, pumpkin seed kernels, toasted coconut, crumbled uncured bacon

breakfast bowl ideas

	BASE	PROTEIN	FRESH	EXTRAS
SWEET	Oatmeal	Kefir or milk	Strawberry slices	Dash of cinnamon, sprinkle of toasted walnuts
	Quinoa	Milk	Canned pumpkin	Dash of cinnamon, drizzle of maple syrup and sprinkle of toasted pecans
	Cooked sweet potato	Almond butter and yogurt	Fresh or thawed frozen wild blueberries	Toasted pecans and dash of cinnamon
	Brown rice	Peanut butter or almond butter and milk	Chopped apple	Dash of cinnamon, drizzle of maple syrup, and sprinkle of toasted walnuts
	Chia seeds	Yogurt	Chopped pineapple and kiwi slices	Toasted coconut and drizzle of maple syrup
	Granola	Yogurt	Strawberry slices	Drizzle of maple syrup and sprinkle of toasted walnuts
	Farro	Kefir or milk	Diced pear	Drizzle of honey and sprinkle of chopped pistachios
	Oats	Milk	Citrus sections or banana slices	Sprinkle of granola and drizzle of maple syrup
SAVORY	Oats	Milk or chicken broth or bone broth	Cherry tomatoes and scallions	Grated sharp cheddar cheese
	Quinoa	Salmon	Wilted greens and cherry tomatoes	Drizzle of Greek yogurt mixed with dill
	Brown rice	Yogurt (mixed with lime juice and cumin) and black beans	Fresh salsa and sliced radishes	Pumpkin seed kernels and diced avocado
	Greens	Chickpeas and/or egg	Cherry tomatoes and slivered onion	Tzatziki sauce and sprinkle of crumbled feta cheese
	Grits	Scrambled egg	Diced tomato and chives	Crumbled uncured bacon
	Barley	Chicken broth or bone broth and chickpeas	Wilted greens and sun-dried tomatoes	Sprinkle of kalamata olives and crumbled feta cheese
	Farro	Egg	Cherry tomatoes and wilted greens	Diced avocado
	Roasted sweet potato wedges	Egg and/or black beans	Wilted greens and diced tomato	Avocado-Cilantro Dip and Dressing (page 71) or mashed avocado and salsa

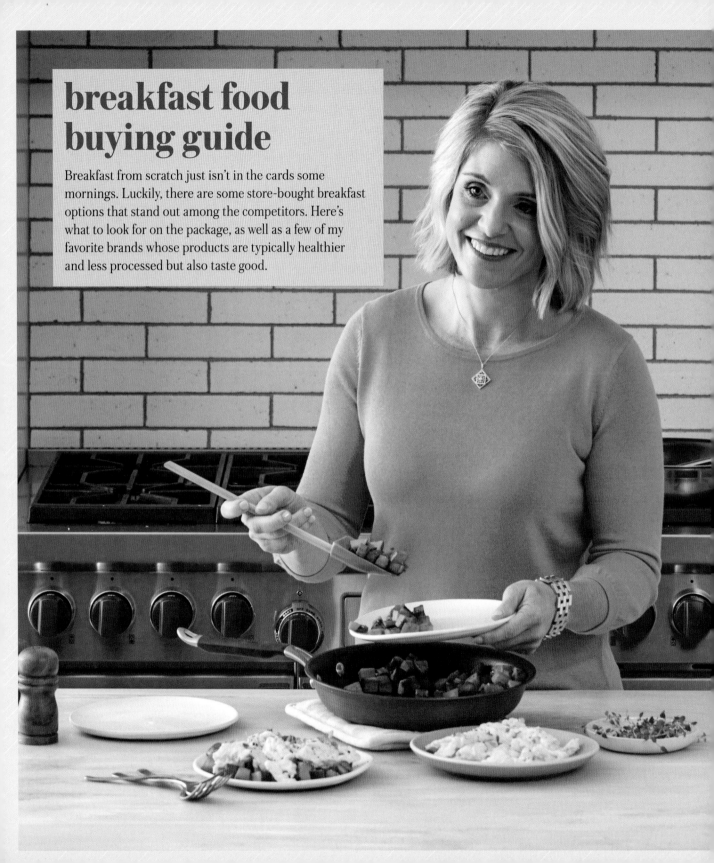

breakfast food buying guide

Breakfast from scratch just isn't in the cards some mornings. Luckily, there are some store-bought breakfast options that stand out among the competitors. Here's what to look for on the package, as well as a few of my favorite brands whose products are typically healthier and less processed but also taste good.

CEREALS AND GRANOLA

FIBER: ≥3 grams

PROTEIN: ≥5 grams

CALORIES: Check the calories in comparison to serving size. Does it seem reasonable?

WHOLE GRAINS: Are they predominantly overrefined? (See page 72 for how to determine.)

ADDED SUGARS: 8 grams for grain and/or nut varieties; 12 grams for grain and/or nut varieties with dried fruit

TRY THESE BRANDS: The variety of cereals are too immense to list, so these are brands that often have cereals that meet the guidelines: Nature's Path, Nature Valley, Purely Elizabeth, Cascadian Farms, Kashi, Bear Naked, Simply Balanced, Barbara's Puffins, Special K Protein, KIND, Udi's Gluten-Free

PANCAKES AND WAFFLES

SATURATED FAT: ≤3.5 grams

FIBER: ≥3 grams

PROTEIN: ≥3 grams

SODIUM: Ideally 200 to 300mg per serving, but definitely <500mg

ADDED SUGARS: Minimal (see page 72 for how to determine)

WHOLE GRAINS: Predominant (see page 72 for how to determine)

TRY THESE BRANDS: 365 Organic Multi-Grain Waffles, Earth's Best Organic Mini Blueberry Waffles, Nature's Path Gluten-Free Homestyle Waffles, Van's Multigrain 8 Whole Grains Waffles, Nature's Path Gluten-Free Wheat-Free Dark Chocolate Chip Waffles, 365 Organic Whole-Wheat Pancakes, De Wafelbakkers Whole-Grain Blueberry Pancakes, De Wafelbakkers A+ Cinnamon Sweet Potato Whole-Grain & Spelt Pancakes, Earth's Best Organic Mini Homestyle Pancakes

MUFFINS AND SANDWICHES

SATURATED FAT: ≤7 grams meals, <3.5 grams muffins and sides

FIBER: ≥3 grams

PROTEIN: ≥5 grams

SODIUM: <500mg meals, <300mg muffins and sides

ADDED SUGARS: Minimal (see page 72 for how to determine)

WHOLE GRAINS: Predominant (see page 72 for how to determine)

TRY THESE BRANDS: Amy's Tofu Scramble, Jimmy Dean's Turkey Sausage Bowl, Good Food Made Simple Fruit & Berries Oatmeal, Garden Lites Carrot Berry Muffins, Amy's Breakfast Burrito, Evol's Egg and Smoked Gouda Sandwich

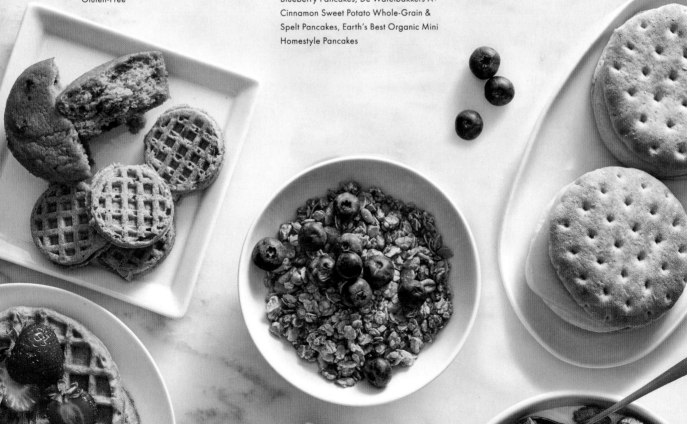

yogurt buying guide

We've got more options than ever when it comes to yogurt, but this can also make choosing which one to buy confusing. The key steps to selecting a healthy yogurt are below.

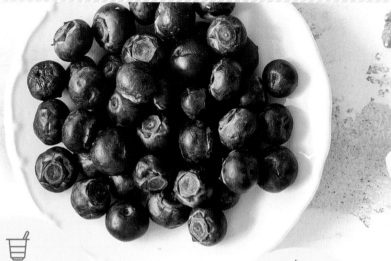

TYPE

Greek, regular, and nondairy yogurts: All three are healthy types and have different uses. Greek is thicker and higher in protein due to being strained more than regular yogurt. Nondairy is good for those with dairy or lactose allergies or sensitivities.

PACKAGING

"Live and active cultures": Make sure you see these words since bacteria need to be alive to benefit the body. Some yogurts may undergo pasteurization after the bacteria cultures are added, which kills them.

INGREDIENT LIST

A pretty short list: Yogurt is made of milk and bacterial cultures so they don't need to contain much else.

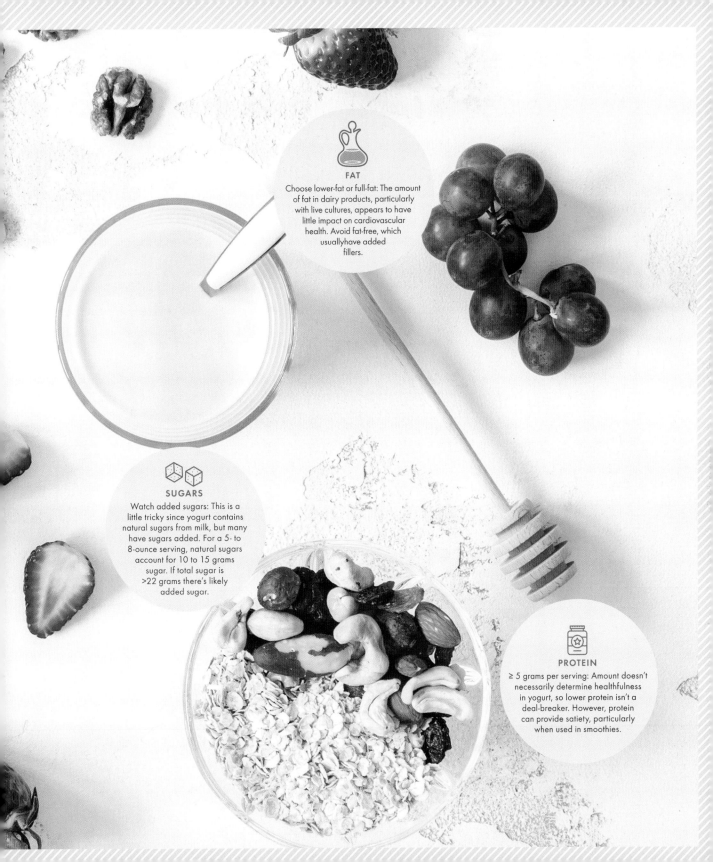

FAT

Choose lower-fat or full-fat: The amount of fat in dairy products, particularly with live cultures, appears to have little impact on cardiovascular health. Avoid fat-free, which usuallyhave added fillers.

SUGARS

Watch added sugars: This is a little tricky since yogurt contains natural sugars from milk, but many have sugars added. For a 5- to 8-ounce serving, natural sugars account for 10 to 15 grams sugar. If total sugar is >22 grams there's likely added sugar.

PROTEIN

≥ 5 grams per serving: Amount doesn't necessarily determine healthfulness in yogurt, so lower protein isn't a deal-breaker. However, protein can provide satiety, particularly when used in smoothies.

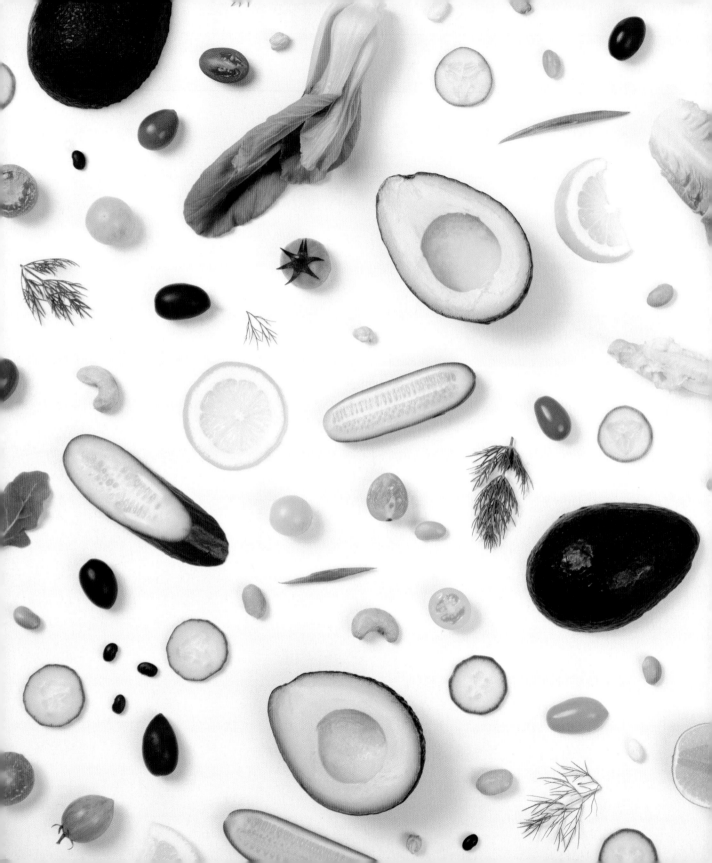

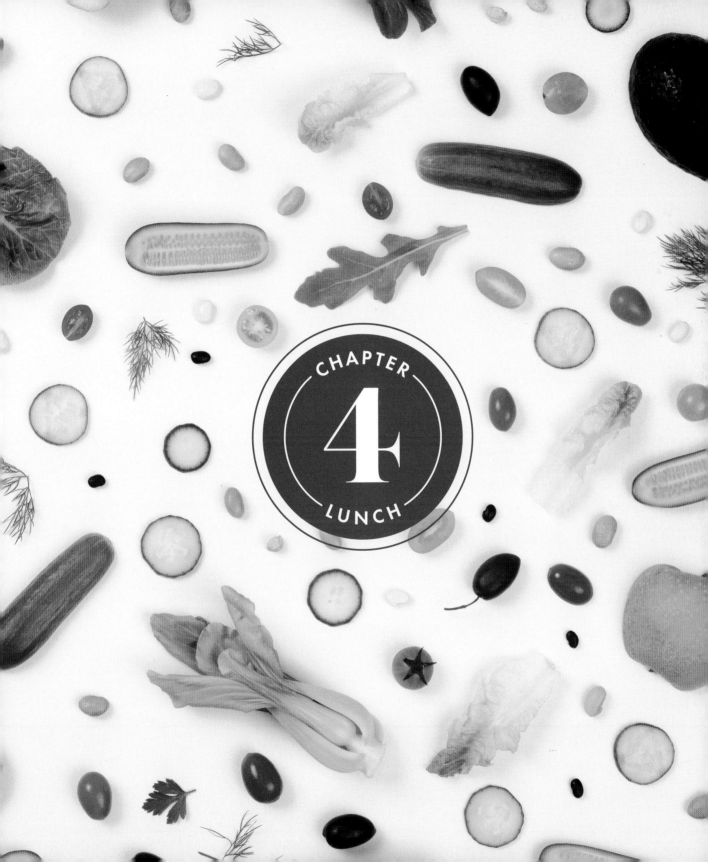

CHAPTER

4

LUNCH

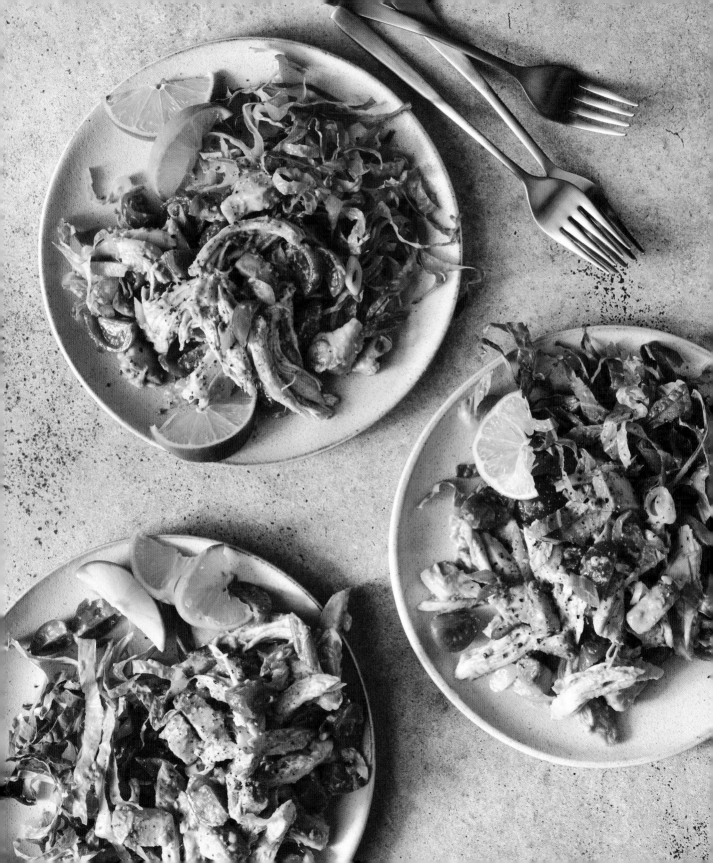

avocado-chicken salad

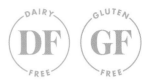

This clean chicken salad is quick and satisfying with a subtle Southwestern flavor thanks to cumin and lime—all reasons why it's often my go-to lunch at the start of the week. Mashed avocado is a nice sub for traditional mayo, and a rotisserie chicken from the market makes this salad a breeze to pull together. I like to save a little avocado to chop and fold in for texture, and then serve the salad over a bed of baby spinach or greens.

Place the chicken, tomatoes, and scallions in a large bowl. Coarsely chop three-fourths of the avocado and add the chopped avocado to the chicken mixture. Place the remaining one-fourth of the avocado in a small bowl; mash with the back of a fork. Add the lime juice, oil, salt, and cumin to the mashed avocado, whisking with the fork to combine. Pour over the chicken mixture, stirring gently to combine well. Cover and refrigerate until ready to serve, up to 2 hours.

(SERVING SIZE: ¾ CUP): CALORIES 227; FAT 13G (SAT 2G, UNSAT 9G); PROTEIN 23G; CARB 5G; FIBER 3G; SUGARS 1G (ADDED SUGARS 0G); SODIUM 298MG; CALC 3% DV; POTASSIUM 9% DV

- 2 cups shredded cooked chicken breast
- ⅔ cup cherry tomatoes, quartered
- ⅓ cup chopped scallions
- 1 ripe avocado
- 2 tablespoons fresh lime juice
- 1½ tablespoons extra-virgin olive oil
- ½ teaspoon kosher salt
- ½ teaspoon ground cumin

avocado

This creamy fruit soothes inflammation in the body thanks to monounsaturated fats and antioxidants. And avocado may even counteract eating some inflammatory foods: In one study, people who topped their hamburger with avocado had lower inflammatory markers than those who ate just the burger.

One avocado is more than you'll need at one meal, so the trick is learning how to keep the unused portion fresh until your next meal or the next day; avocados will begin to brown once cut. Try these options to preserve freshness.

- Keep the skin and seed intact and rub the exposed areas with lemon or lime juice; wrap in plastic wrap and refrigerate.
- Mash the whole avocado with lime juice and salt to make a quick guacamole. Cover with plastic wrap that you press down on the surface and refrigerate.

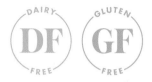

chicken salad with apple, cashews, and basil

The slightly tart crispness of a Granny Smith pairs perfectly with the creamy basil dressing, but feel free to substitute another apple, as well as nut, if desired. Use leftover or rotisserie chicken, or quickly poach chicken as directed below.

¼ cup olive or avocado oil mayonnaise

2 tablespoons chopped fresh basil

1 tablespoon water

¼ teaspoon kosher salt

⅛ teaspoon black pepper

2 cups chopped cooked chicken breast

⅔ cup diced Granny Smith apple

3 tablespoons chopped toasted cashews

Stir together the mayonnaise, basil, water, salt, and pepper in a large bowl. Add the chicken, apple, and cashews to the dressing; toss gently to combine. Cover and refrigerate until ready to serve.

(SERVING SIZE: ½ CUP): CALORIES 218; FAT 12G (SAT 2G, UNSAT 9G); PROTEIN 23G; CARB 5G; FIBER 1G; SUGARS 2G (ADDED SUGARS 0G); SODIUM 293MG; CALC 2% DV; POTASSIUM 5% DV

quick chicken tip

Poaching is an easy way to cook chicken to use in recipes like this one because it's quick, and the liquid keeps the chicken from drying out. To get 2 to 3 cups diced or shredded cooked chicken, purchase 1 to 1¼ pounds raw skinless, boneless breasts. Pat the chicken dry with paper towels and pound the breasts to an even thinness. Place the chicken in a large saucepan and add water or low-sodium broth to cover by ½ inch. Add salt and pepper, if desired, and bring to a gentle simmer. Cook for 8 to 10 minutes or until no trace of pink remains. Transfer to a bowl of ice water for 5 minutes. Drain, pat dry, and dice or shred the chicken.

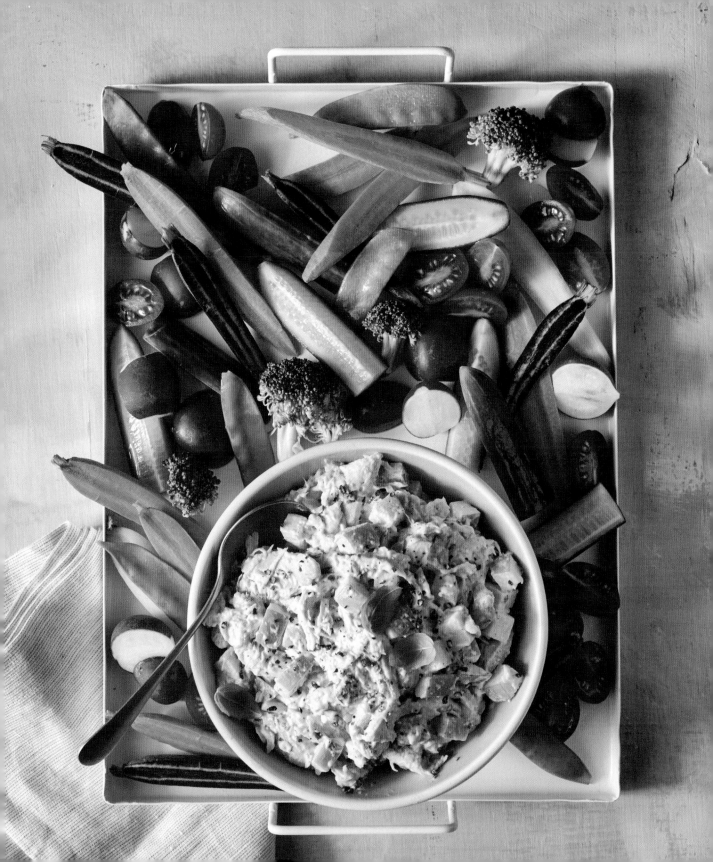

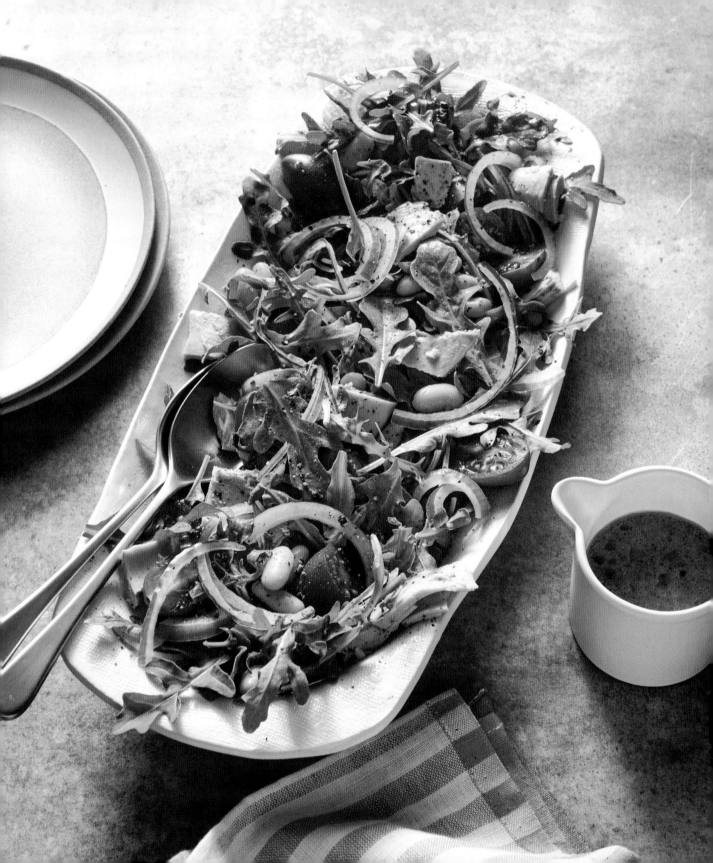

tuna, white bean, and arugula salad

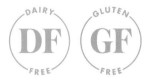

Lemon, olive oil, tomatoes, and arugula quickly transform tuna from a pouch into a lunch that's high in protein and fiber. If you're worried about mercury, the FDA lists canned light tuna as one of the "best choices"—fish whose nutritional benefits when consumed two or three times per week outweigh any potential risk (see page 183 for Best Fish Choices).

Whisk together the oil, lemon zest, lemon juice, mustard, salt, and pepper in a large bowl. Add the beans, tomatoes, onion, tuna, and arugula; toss well. Cover and refrigerate until ready to serve.

(SERVING SIZE: ½ OF SALAD): CALORIES 316; FAT 12G (SAT 2G, UNSAT 9G); PROTEIN 30G; CARB 21G; FIBER 6G; SUGARS 3G (ADDED SUGARS 0G); SODIUM 364MG; CALC 9% DV; POTASSIUM 14% DV

tuna terminology

Shelf-stable canned or pouch tuna varieties are a healthy lean protein that's portable and ideal to keep on hand for quick meals. Plus, tuna is packed with omega-3 fatty acids and vitamin D, key anti-inflammatory nutrients, as well as the antioxidant selenium. To maximize those nutrients' benefits and minimize risk, make sure you purchase "light" tuna rather than "white." Chunk "light" comes from small skipjack, which contain about 60 percent less mercury than albacore, the tuna that "white" comes from. Also, drain the water to reduce the sodium, and opt for less-salt or low-sodium varieties.

1½ tablespoons extra-virgin olive oil

½ teaspoon lemon zest

1 tablespoon fresh lemon juice

½ teaspoon Dijon mustard

¼ teaspoon kosher salt

⅛ teaspoon black pepper

1 cup canned no-salt-added cannellini beans, rinsed and drained

½ cup grape tomatoes, halved

¼ cup thinly sliced red onion

1 (6.4-ounce) pouch low-sodium chunk light tuna in water, drained and broken into chunks

2 cups firmly packed arugula

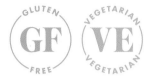

black bean and spinach quesadillas

Even when the cupboards look bare, there are a few staples that I usually have on hand: beans, greens, tortillas, and some type of cheese. On one of those days, I came up with these quick quesadillas, which have become a hit—even when the shelves are stocked. You can also cook these quesadillas under the broiler or in a toaster oven for 1 minute on each side or until the cheese is melted.

½ cup canned no-salt-added black beans, rinsed and drained

2 tablespoons refrigerated fresh salsa

4 (6-inch) corn tortillas

½ cup finely chopped fresh baby spinach

6 tablespoons shredded cheddar cheese

Cooking spray

1 Heat a large skillet over medium.

2 Combine the beans and salsa in a small bowl; mash with a fork. Layer 1 tortilla with half the bean mixture and half the spinach. Sprinkle with 3 tablespoons of the cheese; top with another tortilla. Repeat the procedure to make another quesadilla.

3 Lightly coat the tops of the quesadillas with cooking spray; place the coated side of 1 quesadilla in the skillet. Cook for 2 minutes. Lightly coat the top of the quesadilla with cooking spray; carefully turn it over with a spatula. Cook for 1 to 2 minutes or until lightly browned and the cheese is melted. Repeat the procedure.

(SERVING SIZE: 1 QUESADILLA): CALORIES 264; FAT 10G (SAT 4G, UNSAT 2G); PROTEIN 11G; CARB 33G; FIBER 6G; SUGARS 2G (ADDED SUGARS 0G); SODIUM 237MG; CALC 24% DV; POTASSIUM 5% DV

corn vs. flour

Most flour tortillas are made with some, if not all, refined grain flour, which has been linked to increases in blood sugar and inflammation. Switch to corn tortillas to pack in more nutrients for fewer calories and an increased satiety due to more stable blood glucose. Look for tortillas made with "whole corn" or "whole corn flour" for a healthier, whole-grain option. If you see "degerminated" or "degermed," keep shopping since this indicates part of the grain has been removed.

	TWO CORN TORTILLAS	TWO 6-INCH FLOUR TORTILLAS
CALORIES	110	185
SAT FAT	0g	2g
CARBS	22g	30g
FIBER	3g	2g
SODIUM	20mg	440mg

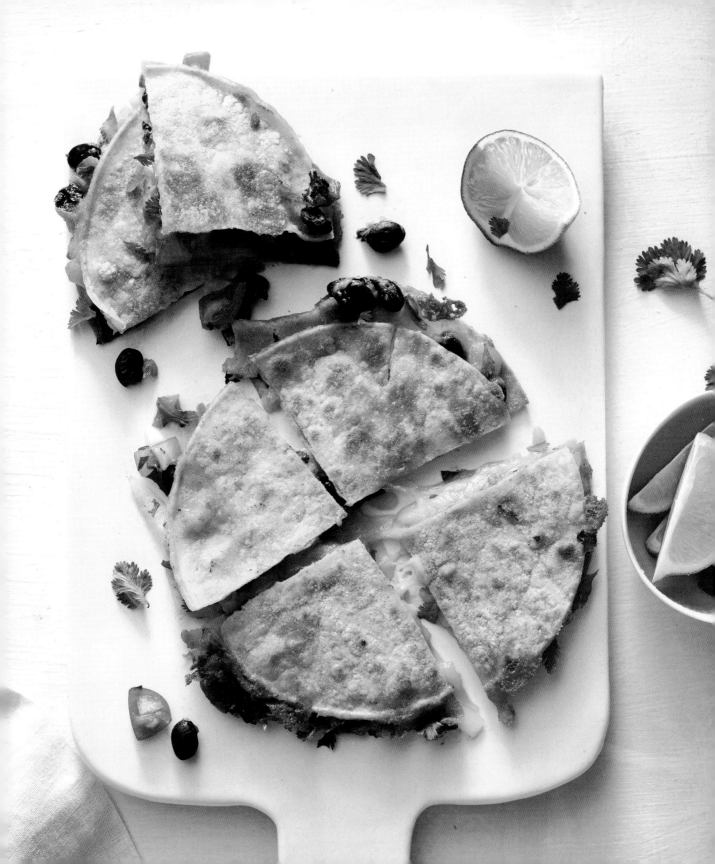

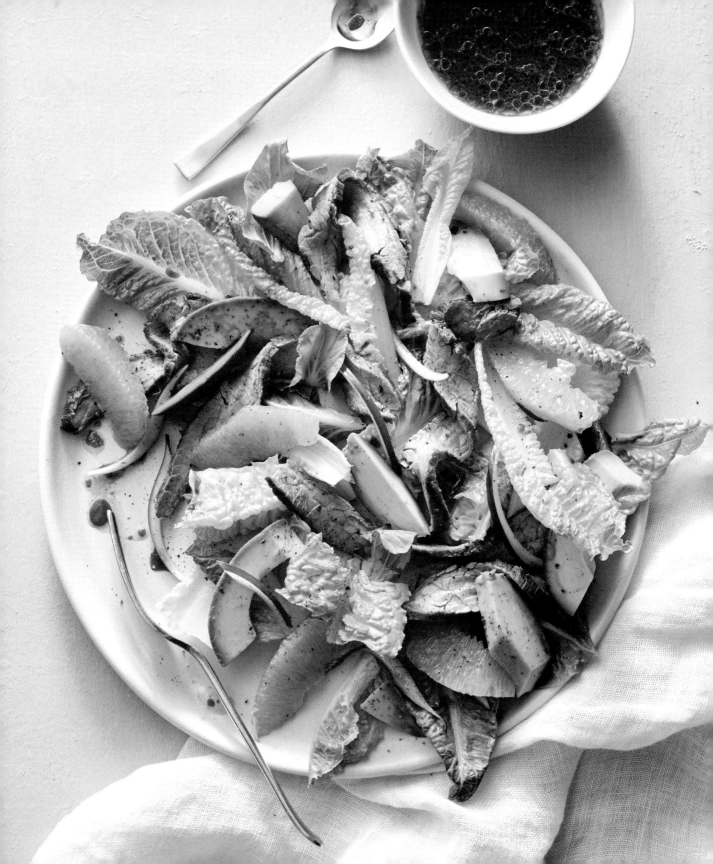

citrus-balsamic steak salad

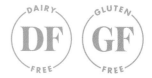

Got a great bottle of olive oil and balsamic vinaigrette? Skip the homemade dressing by adding 3 tablespoons of store-bought dressing to the orange juice instead. If you're afraid of having onion breath, soak the slices in cold water for a few minutes to remove some of the pungent bite, or swap out the onion for chopped cucumber.

1 Evenly divide the romaine, onion, and steak between two serving bowls or storage containers.

2 Peel and section the orange in a bowl; cut the sections in half. Arrange the orange pieces evenly over the salads, reserving the juice in the bowl. Add the oil, vinegar, mustard, and salt to the juices in the bowl; whisk to combine. Drizzle the dressing evenly over the salads. Top with the avocado just before serving; toss and serve immediately.

(SERVING SIZE: 1 SALAD): CALORIES 410; FAT 27G (SAT 5G, UNSAT 20G); PROTEIN 27G; CARB 17G; FIBER 7G; SUGARS 9G (ADDED SUGARS 0G); SODIUM 332MG; CALC 8% DV; POTASSIUM 19% DV

why are there no sandwiches?

Wondering where the sandwich and wrap recipes are and why I've included only "un-sandwich" lunch ideas? Don't get me wrong—there's nothing better some days than a PB&J or melted cheese on toasted focaccia. But I realized that sandwiches—even if they're made with whole-grain breads or wraps—are always an easy lunch fallback for me. I also noticed that when I relied on a sandwich, I tended to get in fewer vegetables. However, when my lunch is something other than a sandwich or wrap—a salad with protein or beans or a serving of last night's dinner, for example—my overall diet quality tends to improve, and I usually get more veggies and fiber and less sodium.

3 cups chopped romaine lettuce

⅓ cup very thinly sliced red onion

6 ounces cooked lean flank steak, warmed and cut into bite-size pieces

1 orange

2 tablespoons extra-virgin olive oil

1 tablespoon balsamic vinegar

½ teaspoon Dijon mustard

¼ teaspoon kosher salt

½ ripe avocado, chopped

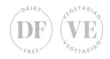

chopped greek salad bowls with chicken

I'm not sure why I didn't discover chopped salads earlier since they're so easy to make and a lot easier to eat. Chopping and assembling takes just a few minutes, and then you can toss with the dressing when you're ready to eat. Substitute 4 ounces of grilled fish, canned tuna, or other lean protein in place of the chicken, if desired.

6 cups chopped hearts of romaine lettuce

½ cup canned no-salt-added chickpeas, rinsed and drained

½ cup cherry or grape tomatoes, halved

½ cup chopped cucumber

2 tablespoons finely chopped red onion

4 pitted kalamata olives

4 ounces sliced grilled chicken breast

3 tablespoons crumbled feta cheese

3 tablespoons Citrus Vinaigrette (page 75) or store-bought olive oil vinaigrette or balsamic vinaigrette

Evenly divide the romaine between two serving bowls or storage containers. Arrange the chickpeas, tomatoes, cucumber, onion, olives, chicken, and feta on top in sections. Drizzle 1½ tablespoons of the dressing over each salad just before serving, and toss.

(SERVING SIZE: 1 SALAD): CALORIES 334; FAT 19G (SAT 4G, UNSAT 13G); PROTEIN 25G; CARB 18G; FIBER 6G; SUGARS 6G (ADDED SUGARS 0G); SODIUM 433MG; CALC 15% DV; POTASSIUM 15% DV

DAIRY-FREE OPTION: Omit the cheese. Increase the chickpeas to ⅔ cup. If desired, sprinkle with 1 tablespoon toasted pine nuts or other nut.

VEGETARIAN OPTION: Omit the chicken. Increase the chickpeas to ⅔ cup and add ⅔ cup cooked quinoa or brown rice to the chickpea mixture.

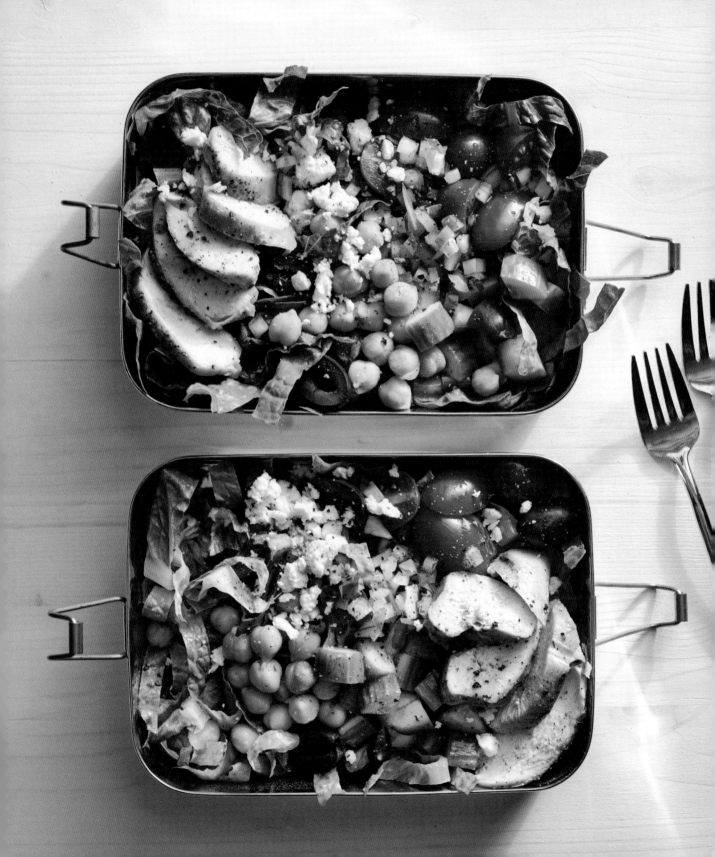

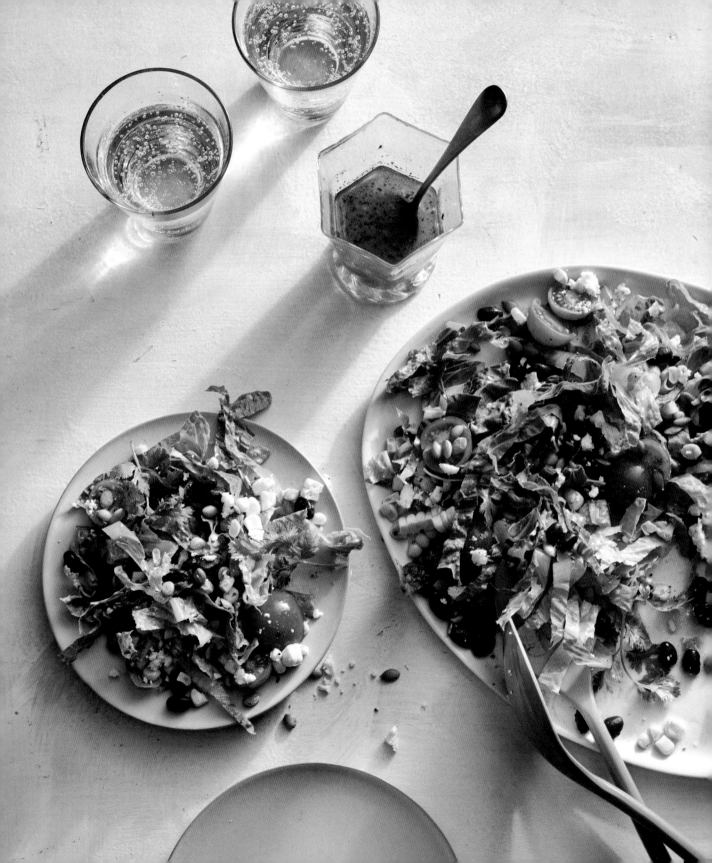

chopped southwestern salad

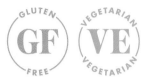

Quick to assemble and pack, this colorful salad is impossible to mess up. Crumble some tortilla chips over the top for added crunch, or add a little grilled chicken or shrimp to make it more substantial. You could even stuff this tossed salad mixture into a burrito to eat on the go.

1 Divide the lettuce, tomatoes, corn, beans, and cilantro evenly between two 1-quart airtight containers. Divide the cheese and pumpkin seed kernels evenly between the salads. Cover with the lids and chill until ready to serve.

2 Just before serving, whisk together the oil, lime juice, honey, salt, and cumin in a small bowl. Divide the dressing evenly between the salads and toss to coat; serve immediately.

(SERVING SIZE: 1 SALAD): CALORIES 320; FAT 18G (SAT 4G, UNSAT 12G); PROTEIN 13G; CARB 32G; FIBER 9G; SUGARS 10G (ADDED SUGARS 3G); SODIUM 375MG; CALC 18% DV; POTASSIUM 17% DV

DAIRY-FREE OPTION: Substitute ¼ cup cubed avocado for the queso fresco.

6 cups chopped romaine lettuce

½ cup cherry tomatoes, halved

½ cup fresh or thawed frozen corn kernels

⅔ cup canned no-salt-added black beans, rinsed and drained

2 tablespoons chopped fresh cilantro

1 ounce queso fresco (fresh Mexican cheese), crumbled (about ¼ cup)

2 tablespoons roasted unsalted pumpkin seed kernels (pepitas)

4 teaspoons extra-virgin olive oil

2 tablespoons fresh lime juice (from 1 lime)

1 teaspoon honey or maple syrup

¼ teaspoon kosher salt

¼ teaspoon ground cumin

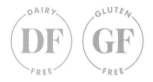

thai salmon–brown rice bowls

Heartier greens like bok choy and romaine are good choices to prep ahead because they stay crisp and tend not to wilt, unlike more delicate leaves. You can substitute an equivalent amount of any cooked whole grain in place of the rice, as well as an equivalent amount of lean protein for the fish. Got a peanut allergy in the house? Use an alternate nut butter like almond.

1⅓ cups cooked brown rice

¼ cup matchstick-cut carrot

⅓ cup steamed shelled edamame

½ cup shredded bok choy or romaine lettuce

6 ounces broiled salmon or drained canned salmon

1 tablespoon creamy peanut butter

1 tablespoon gluten-free lower-sodium soy sauce or tamari

2 teaspoons rice vinegar

2 teaspoons sesame oil

2 teaspoons fresh lime juice

1 Place the rice, carrot, edamame, and bok choy in a large bowl; toss to combine. Divide evenly between two bowls and top each evenly with the salmon.

2 Just before serving, whisk together the peanut butter, soy sauce, vinegar, oil, and lime juice in a small bowl. Drizzle the dressing over the bowls just before serving. Serve immediately.

(SERVING SIZE: 1 BOWL): CALORIES 435; FAT 18G (SAT 3G, UNSAT 14G); PROTEIN 30G; CARB 37G; FIBER 5G; SUGARS 1G (ADDED SUGARS 0G); SODIUM 381MG; CALC 6% DV; POTASSIUM 15% DV

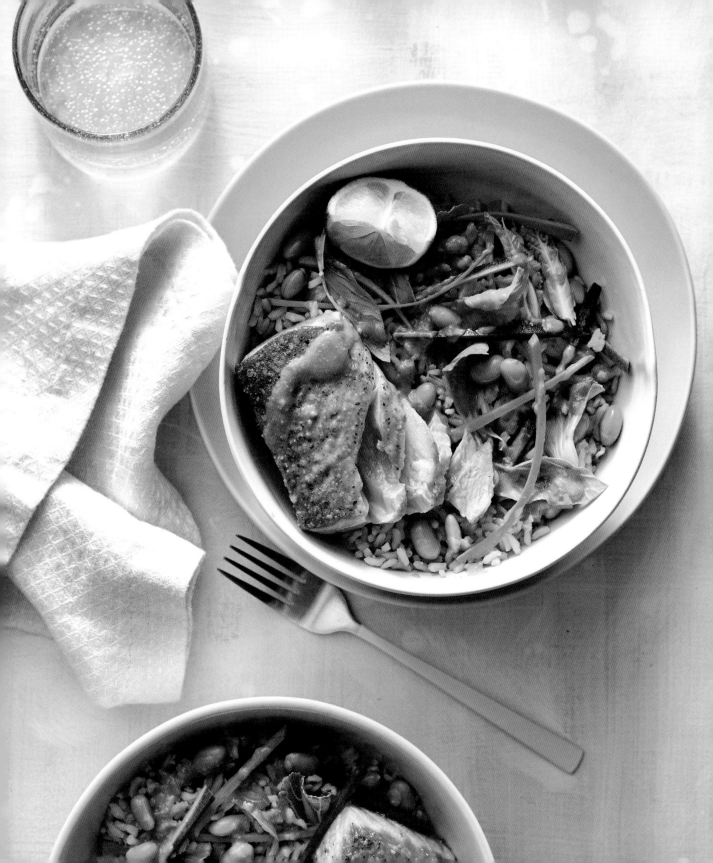

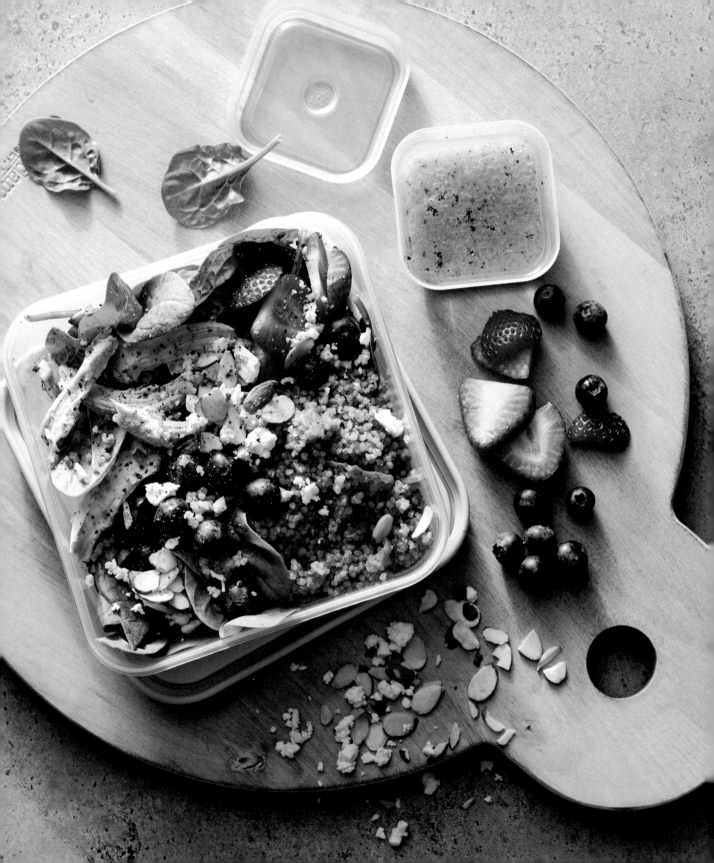

spinach-quinoa bowls with chicken and berries

If you're packing this for work, combine the dressing ingredients in a small container. When you're ready to eat, shake the dressing well, add it to the salad, and toss. No time for a homemade dressing? Use 3 tablespoons of store-bought olive oil vinaigrette (1½ tablespoons for each bowl).

1 Divide the spinach, quinoa, and chicken evenly between two 1-quart airtight containers. Top each salad evenly with the berries, cheese, and almonds. Cover and chill until ready to serve.

2 Just before serving, whisk together the oil, vinegar, mustard, honey, and salt in a small bowl. Divide the dressing evenly between the salads and toss to coat; serve immediately.

(SERVING SIZE: 1 BOWL): CALORIES 396; FAT 20G (SAT 4G, UNSAT 16G); PROTEIN 23G; CARB 31G; FIBER 6G; SUGARS 6G (ADDED SUGARS 1G); SODIUM 688MG; CALC 16% DV; POTASSIUM 7% DV

DAIRY-FREE OPTION: Omit the feta cheese and increase the sliced almonds to 3 tablespoons.

- 3 cups fresh baby spinach or mixed greens
- 1 cup cooked quinoa
- ⅔ cup chopped cooked chicken breast
- ½ cup fresh blueberries or sliced fresh strawberries
- 2 tablespoons crumbled feta cheese
- 1 tablespoon sliced almonds, toasted
- 2 tablespoons extra-virgin olive oil
- 1 tablespoon white wine vinegar
- ¼ teaspoon Dijon mustard
- ½ teaspoon honey
- ½ teaspoon kosher salt

lunch box cheat sheet

No time or energy to figure out a meal for lunch? Then this is an ideal time to throw together a simple snack lunch or quick lunch bowl. The end result can be as nutritious as a cooked meal—or more so—if you pair your food choices well. These two charts walk you through how to create a snack lunch or a pack-and-go lunch bowl for a healthy, filling lunch in 5 minutes or less.

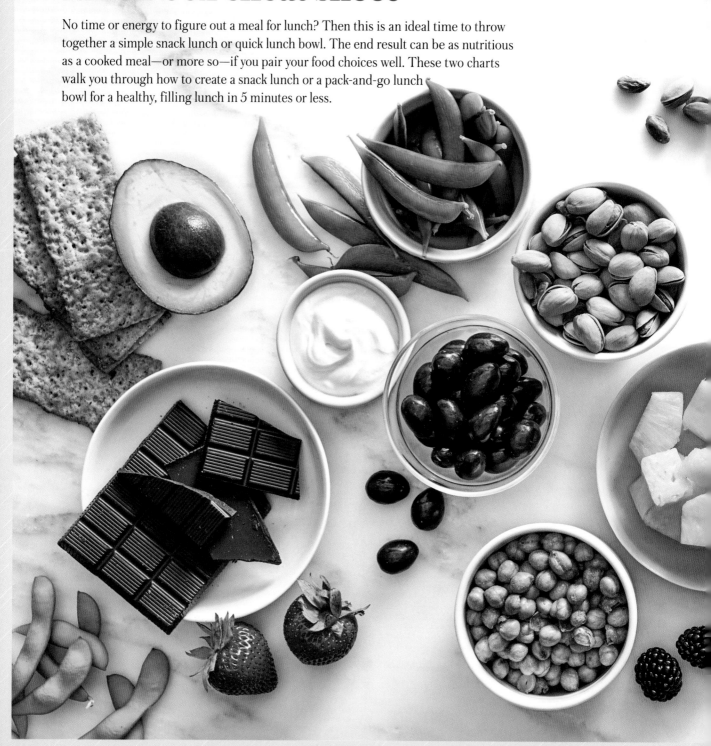

snack lunch ideas

Combine 4 or 5 foods, including at least one from each category.

proteins and carbs

Hard-boiled egg	Rotisserie chicken	Canned tuna	Canned salmon	Chickpea or bean salad	Yogurt	Cheese slices or stick
Cottage cheese	Whole-grain or legume-based crackers	Roasted chickpeas	Popcorn	Edamame	Corn tortilla or whole-grain tortilla	Tortilla chips

veggies and fruit

Cucumber slices	Carrots	Cherry tomatoes	Sugar snap peas	Celery sticks	Roasted green beans	Broccoli florets
Cauliflower florets	Mushrooms	Apple slices	Berries	Fruit salad	Citrus sections	Melon cubes
	Pineapple chunks	Grapes	Peach, nectarine	Clementine	Dried fruits without added sugars	

dips, spreads, and extras

Hummus	Avocado	Guacamole	Salsa	Pico de gallo	Goat cheese	Tzatziki sauce
	Marinara	Vinaigrette or creamy dressing	Peanut butter or other nut butter	Piece of dark chocolate	Chocolate-covered nuts	

pack-and-go lunch bowls

This might be contradictory to say in a cookbook, but you really don't need a recipe to create a pretty amazing lunch. In fact, some of my best tasting (and healthiest) meals are spur-of-the-moment, using whatever ingredients are on hand that day. There's no right or wrong way to create a lunch bowl—just follow the steps and have fun.

① START WITH GREENS
1½ TO 2 CUPS

- ☐ Spring mix
- ☐ Baby spinach
- ☐ Bok choy
- ☐ Romaine
- ☐ Arugula
- ☐ Kale

② PACK IN VEGGIES
AND/OR FRUIT

- ☐ Bell pepper
- ☐ Cucumber
- ☐ Tomatoes
- ☐ Carrot
- ☐ Beets
- ☐ Roasted vegetables
- ☐ Red onion
- ☐ Strawberries
- ☐ Blueberries
- ☐ Grapes
- ☐ Apple
- ☐ Green peas
- ☐ Corn

③ ADD 1 PROTEIN

- ☐ Sautéed tofu
- ☐ Hard-boiled egg
- ☐ Rotisserie chicken
- ☐ Taco meat
- ☐ Steamed or grilled shrimp
- ☐ Baked salmon
- ☐ Shelled edamame
- ☐ Chickpeas
- ☐ Black beans
- ☐ White beans
- ☐ Kidney beans

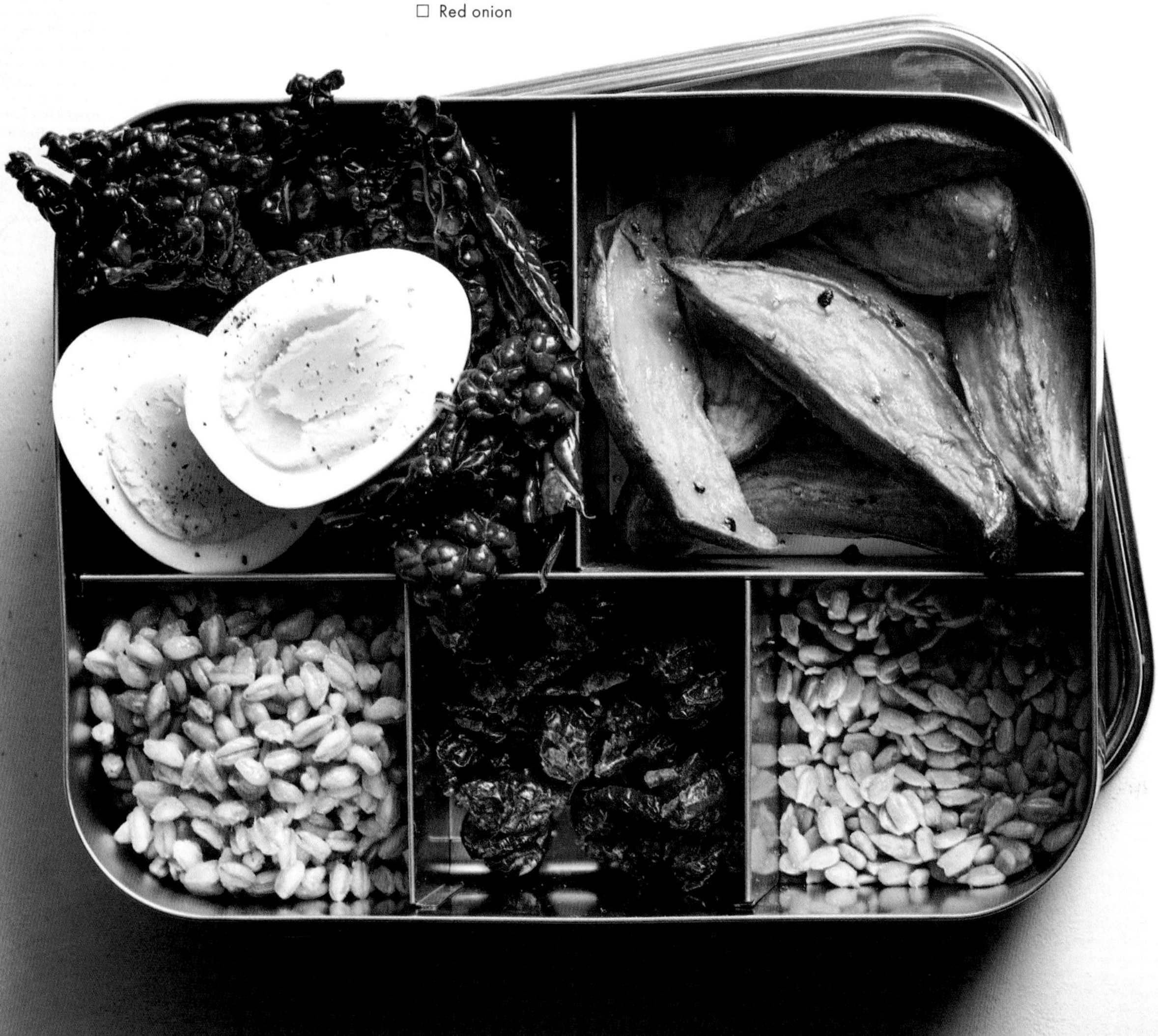

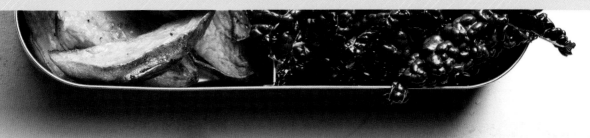

④ ADD 1 OR 2 EXTRAS

- ☐ Feta cheese
- ☐ Goat cheese
- ☐ Parmesan cheese
- ☐ Toasted nuts
- ☐ Dried cranberries
- ☐ Crumbled uncured bacon
- ☐ Olives
- ☐ Diced avocado

⑤ DRESS IT

- ☐ Any homemade or store-bought vinaigrette (see Chapter 2 for recipes; see page 76 for how to buy one)
- ☐ Tzatziki sauce
- ☐ Pesto, thinned with a little vinaigrette
- ☐ Peanut sauce made with nut butter

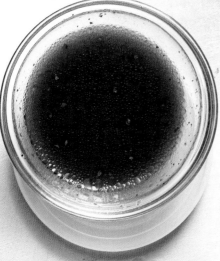

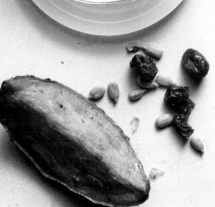

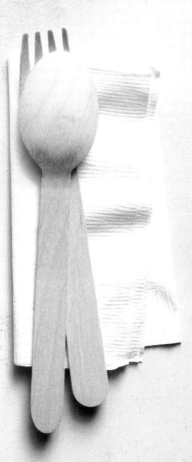

BONUS: ADD A WHOLE GRAIN

Some days call for a lunch that's more substantial than what even a well-planned salad bowl can provide. This is when I like to add a whole grain. Top greens with ½ to ¾ cup of any cooked, slightly warm whole grain, and then proceed with the veggies and fruit, protein, extras, and dressing. Toss well, and enjoy!

LUNCH BOWL IDEAS

Greek Veggie Bowl
Spinach + Tomatoes + Cucumber + Chickpeas + Feta cheese + Tzatziki sauce

Edamame Rice Bowl
Bok choy + Bell pepper + Brown rice + Edamame + Sautéed tofu + Sesame vinaigrette or peanut sauce

Quinoa Spinach Bowl
Spring mix + Blueberries + Quinoa + Goat cheese + Walnuts + Olive oil vinaigrette

Kale–Sweet Potato Bowl
Kale + Roasted sweet potatoes + Farro + Dried cranberries + Sunflower seeds + Balsamic vinaigrette

Vegetarian Tex-Mex Bowl
Romaine + Tomatoes + Red onion + Corn + Black beans + Pumpkin seed kernels + Citrus vinaigrette

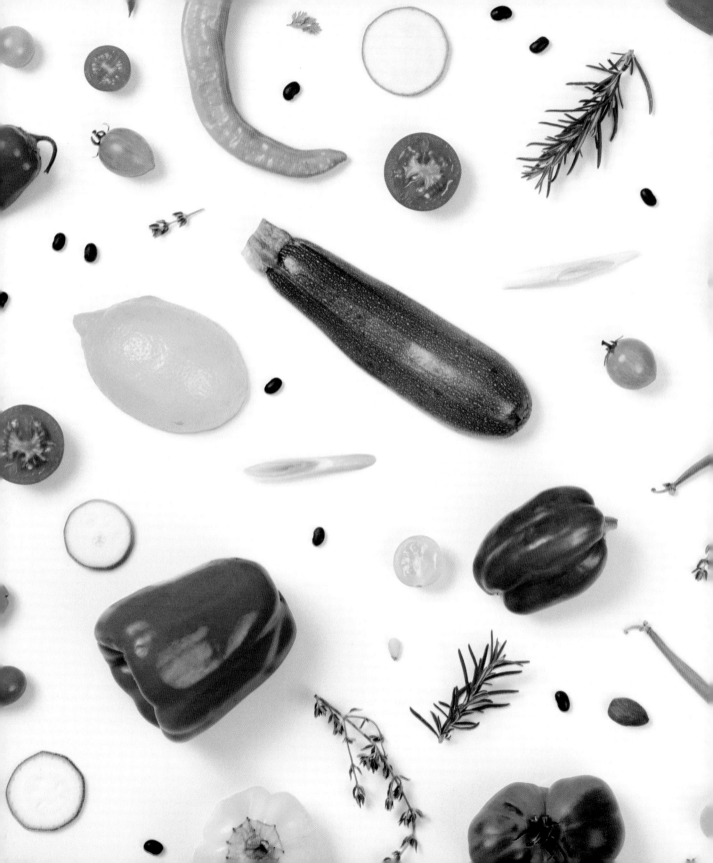

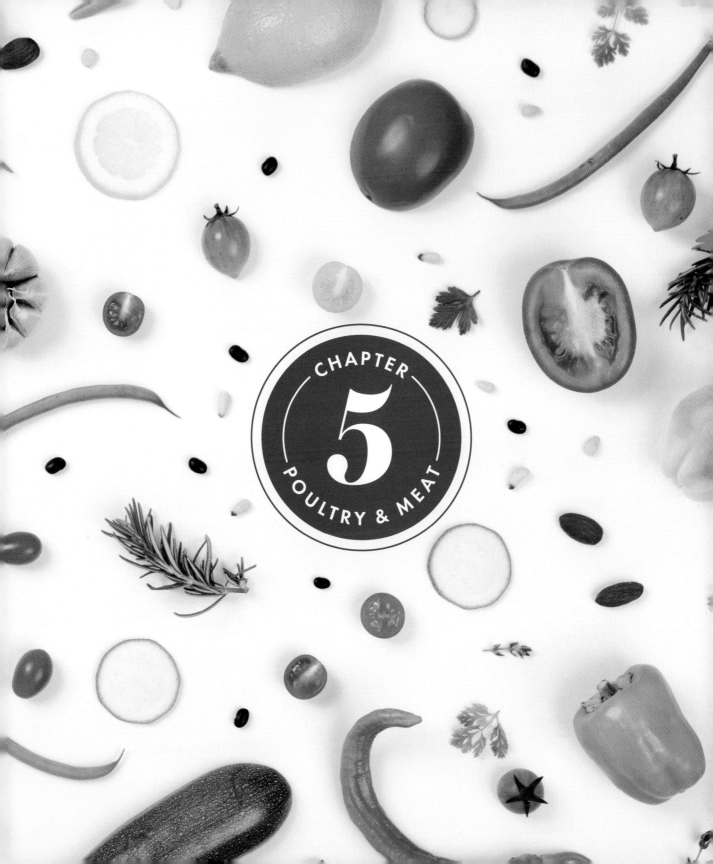

CHAPTER

5

POULTRY & MEAT

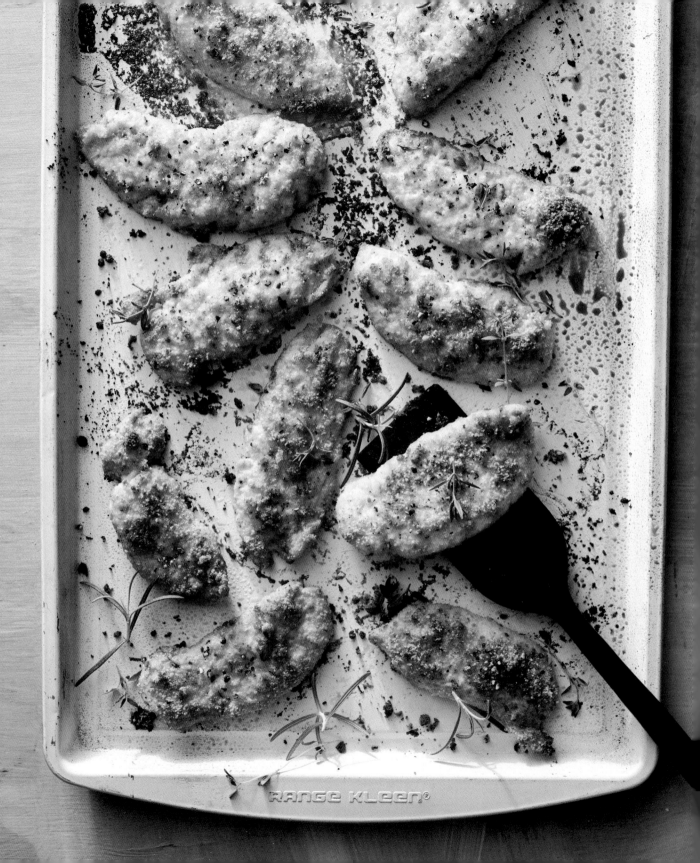

gluten-free chicken tenders

It probably goes without saying that these are a weeknight favorite at my house, which makes me happy since they're a snap to combine and throw in the oven. I also love the fact that using almond flour boosts the nutrients and gives these tenders satiety factor that all-purpose flour can't provide.

1 Preheat the oven to 450°F. Coat a baking sheet with cooking spray.

2 Combine the almond flour, cheese, rosemary, salt, and pepper in a shallow bowl.

3 Place the chicken breast tenders between two sheets of heavy-duty plastic wrap; pound to ¼-inch thickness using a meat mallet or small heavy skillet. Coat both sides of the tenders with cooking spray; dredge the tenders in the almond flour mixture. Place the coated tenders on the prepared baking sheet. Bake for 15 minutes or until browned.

(SERVING SIZE: ABOUT 3 OUNCES): CALORIES 268; FAT 13G (SAT 3G, UNSAT 8G); PROTEIN 32G; CARB 5G; FIBER 1G; SUGARS 0G (ADDED SUGARS 0G); SODIUM 419MG; CALC 14% DV; POTASSIUM 9% DV

Cooking spray

½ cup finely ground almond flour

2 ounces Parmesan cheese, grated (about ½ cup)

1 teaspoon chopped fresh rosemary or thyme

¼ teaspoon kosher salt

¼ teaspoon black pepper

1 pound chicken breast tenders

sodium in chicken

Raw chicken is often injected with a salt solution to add juiciness and increase weight—a process that takes a low-sodium food and adds 4 to 5 times its normal sodium content. To avoid this, look for the percentage of weight that an injected solution makes up on the label (something that raw poultry and most raw meats must state), and choose one with only 1 to 2% solution added—or, even better, none. Also be aware that "solution" equates to added sodium, regardless of whether it is called salt and water or the more wholesome-sounding "broth" and "seasonings."

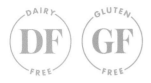

pan-seared chicken with basil–pine nut gremolata

Pounding chicken is one of my favorite weeknight tricks to cut cooking time. It also makes the chicken cook more evenly since each piece is a uniform thickness. If pressed for time, skip the gremolata. Instead, combine ⅓ to ½ cup prepared pesto and 2 tablespoons fresh lemon juice to top the chicken, and sprinkle with scallions.

4 (4-ounce) skinless, boneless chicken breast halves, pounded to ¾-inch thickness

½ teaspoon kosher salt

¼ teaspoon black pepper

3 tablespoons olive oil

⅓ cup pine nuts, toasted

1½ tablespoons fresh lemon juice

⅓ cup fresh basil leaves

2 chopped scallions (green and light green parts only)

1 Heat a large skillet over medium-high. Sprinkle the chicken with ¼ teaspoon of the salt and ⅛ teaspoon of the pepper. Add 1 tablespoon of the oil to the pan; swirl to coat. Add the chicken; cook for 4 minutes on each side or until done. Transfer to a cutting board.

2 Place the pine nuts, lemon juice, basil, scallions, remaining ¼ teaspoon salt, and remaining ⅛ teaspoon pepper in a mini food processor; pulse until finely chopped. Add the remaining 2 tablespoons oil; pulse to combine. Transfer the mixture to a small bowl. Slice the chicken across the grain. Divide the chicken among four plates; top with the gremolata.

(SERVING SIZE: 1 CHICKEN BREAST HALF AND 2½ TABLESPOONS GREMOLATA): CALORIES 305; FAT 21G (SAT 3 G, UNSAT 16 G); PROTEIN 27 G; CARB 2 G; FIBER 1 G; SUGARS 1 G (ADDED SUGARS 0 G); SODIUM 292 MG; CALC 2% DV; POTASSIUM 10% DV

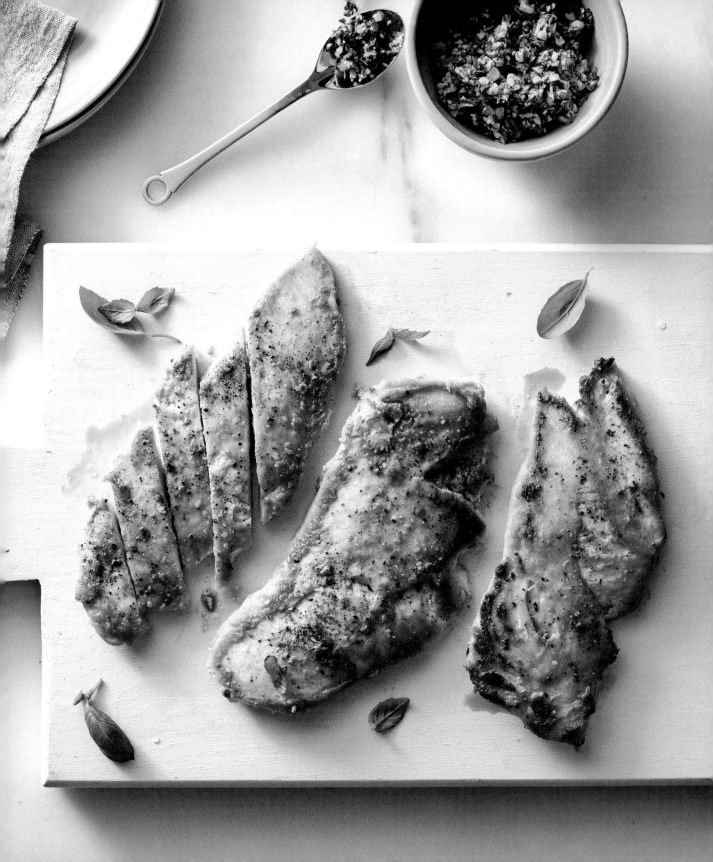

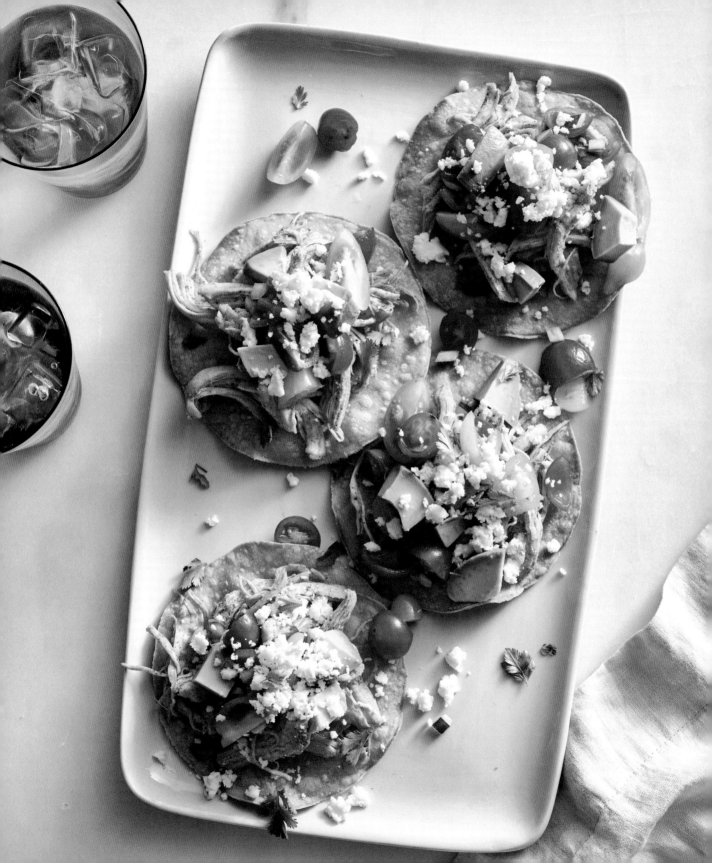

chicken tostadas with avocado salsa

These tostadas can also be served as tacos, if desired. To do this, skip toasting the tortillas in the oven. Instead, wrap the tortillas in a towel and microwave until warm, or lightly coat with cooking spray and cook the tortillas in a skillet until warm and lightly browned, about 1 minute per side.

1 Rub the chicken with the taco seasoning and ¼ teaspoon of the salt and place in a 6-quart multicooker. Pour the broth over the chicken. Close and lock the lid of the cooker; turn the pressure release valve to the sealing position. Program the cooker to cook on manual on high pressure for 9 minutes.

2 Preheat the oven to 375°F. Line a baking sheet with aluminum foil. Combine the tomato, avocado, and onion in a medium bowl. Whisk together the oil, vinegar, and remaining ⅛ teaspoon salt in a small bowl, and pour over the avocado mixture, stirring gently. Let stand until ready to serve (up to 1 hour).

3 Turn the pressure release valve to the venting position to quickly release the pressure (steam) from the cooker until the float valve drops. Carefully remove the lid. Transfer the chicken breasts to a cutting board or plate and let cool for 5 minutes. Meanwhile, lightly coat both sides of each tortilla with cooking spray; place on the prepared baking sheet. Bake the tortillas until lightly browned and crisp, 10 to 15 minutes, turning once. During the last 5 minutes of baking, shred the chicken with two forks. Top each tortilla with ¼ cup of the shredded chicken, about 3 tablespoons of the avocado mixture, and 1½ teaspoons of the cheese. Garnish with cilantro, if desired.

(SERVING SIZE: 2 TOSTADAS): CALORIES 335; FAT 13G (SAT 3G, UNSAT 8G); PROTEIN 29G; CARB 28G; FIBER 6G; SUGARS 2G (ADDED SUGARS 0G); SODIUM 491MG; CALC 10% DV; POTASSIUM 13% DV

STOVETOP OPTION: No multicooker? Simply season the chicken according to the recipe, and combine the chicken and broth in a medium saucepan. Bring the broth to a boil, reduce the heat to maintain a simmer, cover, and cook until the chicken is cooked through, about 15 minutes. Continue as directed.

1 pound skinless, boneless chicken breasts

2 teaspoons All-Purpose Taco Seasoning (page 66) or store-bought organic taco seasoning

⅜ teaspoon kosher salt

½ cup low-sodium chicken broth

1 cup chopped tomato or quartered cherry tomatoes

1 ripe avocado, chopped

2 tablespoons chopped red onion

1 teaspoon olive oil

2 teaspoons red wine vinegar or fresh lime juice

8 (6-inch) corn tortillas

Cooking spray

1 ounce queso fresco (fresh Mexican cheese) or feta cheese, crumbled (about ¼ cup)

Chopped fresh cilantro (optional)

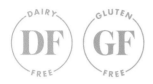

thai chicken noodle soup

This quick soup is a great alternative to traditional chicken noodle soup flavors, but still mild enough that the whole family will eat it. Depending on the width of your pan, you may need to add a little more water or broth before adding the noodles. Turn this into a one-dish meal by adding 1 cup of snow peas with the noodles or stirring in chopped bok choy or greens just before serving.

1 tablespoon olive oil

1½ tablespoons minced fresh ginger

2 teaspoons minced fresh garlic

2 tablespoons green curry paste

3 cups unsalted chicken broth

½ cup water

1 tablespoon fresh lime juice

1 (13.5-ounce) can light coconut milk

¼ cup fresh cilantro stems

3 ounces uncooked brown rice vermicelli noodles

2 cups shredded cooked chicken breast

Fresh cilantro sprigs

Lime wedges (optional)

1 Heat a Dutch oven over medium-high. Add the oil to the pot; swirl to coat. Add the ginger and garlic; sauté for 1 minute. Stir in the curry paste; cook for 1 minute. Add the broth, water, lime juice, coconut milk, and cilantro stems; bring to a simmer and cook for 10 minutes.

2 Stir in the noodles and chicken; cook for 3 minutes or until the noodles are tender. Top with cilantro sprigs, and serve with lime wedges, if desired.

(SERVING SIZE: ABOUT 1½ CUPS): CALORIES 282; FAT 10G (SAT 4G, UNSAT 4G); PROTEIN 27G; CARB 21G; FIBER 2G; SUGARS 0G (ADDED SUGARS 0G); SODIUM 204MG; CALC 1% DV; POTASSIUM 4% DV

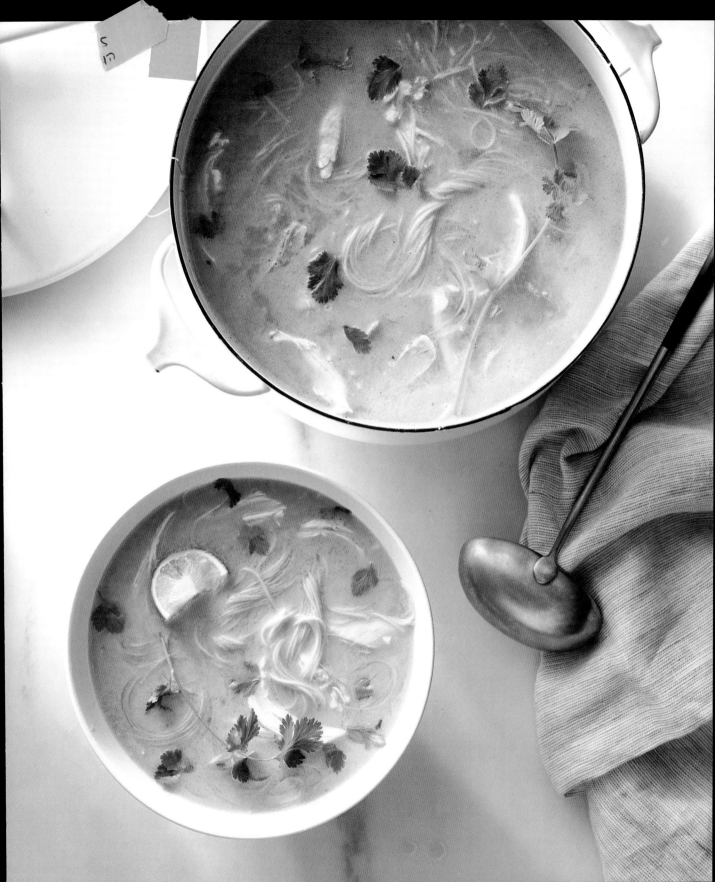

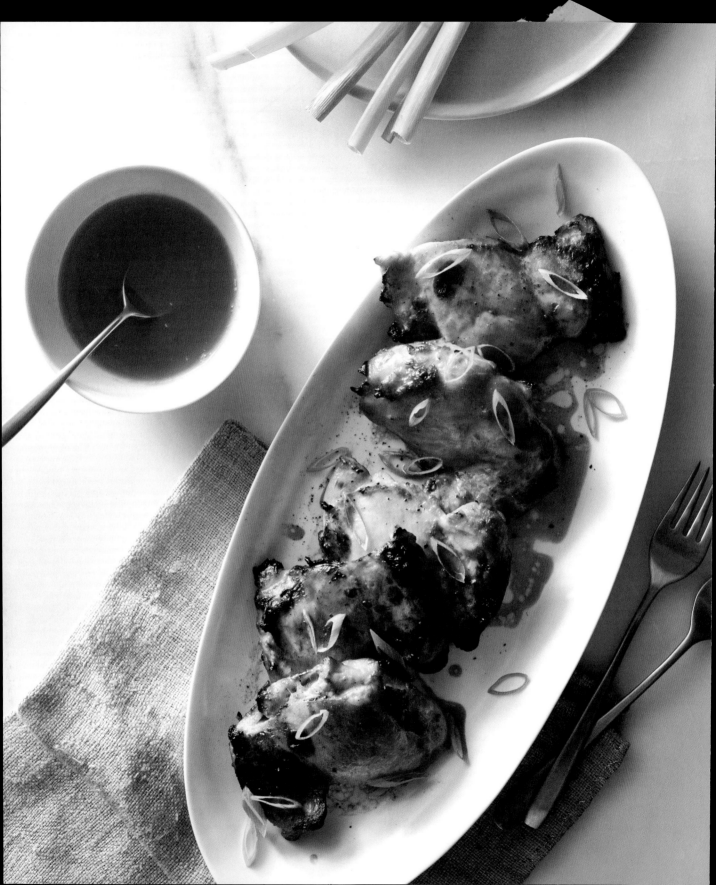

citrus-soy chicken thighs

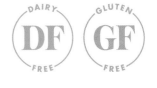

I keep a tube of ginger paste in the refrigerator to use in recipes that call for fresh minced ginger when I don't have a small piece of ginger root on hand. It's okay to let the chicken marinate longer than an hour. In fact, I often combine all the ingredients in a bag before I head to work to marinate in the refrigerator for dinner.

1 Place the orange juice, soy sauce, honey, garlic, and ginger in a large ziplock plastic bag. Add the chicken; seal the bag and marinate in the refrigerator for 1 hour or longer, turning occasionally.

2 Preheat the broiler to high. Line a jelly-roll pan with aluminum foil; coat the foil with cooking spray.

3 Remove the chicken from the bag, reserving the marinade. Place the chicken on the prepared pan; broil for 8 minutes on each side or until done.

4 While the chicken cooks, place the reserved marinade in a small saucepan. Bring to a boil over medium-high. Reduce the heat and cook for 1 minute or until slightly reduced. Serve the sauce with the chicken.

⅔ cup fresh orange juice

2 tablespoons gluten-free lower-sodium soy sauce or tamari

4 teaspoons honey

2 garlic cloves, minced

2 teaspoons finely chopped fresh ginger

8 (2-ounce) skinless, boneless chicken thighs

Cooking spray

(SERVING SIZE: 2 THIGHS AND 2½ TABLESPOONS SAUCE): CALORIES 185; FAT 5G (SAT 1G, UNSAT 3G); PROTEIN 23G; CARB 11G; FIBER 0G; SUGARS 9G (ADDED SUGARS 6G); SODIUM 396MG; CALC 2% DV; POTASSIUM 8% DV

bone broth

Bone broth is made by simmering bones and connective tissue for 6 to 24 hours to create a flavorful stock. The long cooking process allows the nutrients in the bones (such as the proteins, collagen, and gelatin) to leach into the cooking liquid. Consuming bone broth is trendy right now, and many suggest it improves gut health, immunity, wound healing, and joint health, so is it something to make part of your diet?

The bottom line is that we just really don't know much about bone broth and its potential health effects. This doesn't mean to avoid it, but don't feel pressure to incorporate it into your diet just yet. Bone broth is usually a low-calorie source of protein, and homemade stocks and broths add great flavor to soups and recipes. Any other health perks are a bonus and probably don't come exclusively from bone broth. Other ways to reap similar benefits are to opt for protein-rich soups and consume foods rich in vitamins C and A.

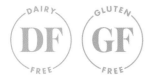

chicken fried quinoa

When making a stir-fry, the actual cooking takes practically zero time, so make sure you have everything prepped before you start. Use two packages of precooked quinoa to get the amount needed for this recipe.

1½ tablespoons sesame oil

½ pound skinless, boneless chicken thighs, cut into ½-inch pieces

½ cup chopped red bell pepper

½ cup chopped scallions

2 garlic cloves, minced

1 teaspoon minced fresh ginger

2½ cups cooled cooked quinoa

¾ cup frozen shelled edamame, thawed

1 large egg, lightly beaten

¼ cup gluten-free lower-sodium soy sauce or tamari

1 Heat a large skillet over medium-high. Add 1 tablespoon of the oil to the pan; swirl to coat. Add the chicken and cook, stirring often, for about 4 minutes. Add the bell pepper, scallions, garlic, and ginger to skillet and cook, stirring often, until the chicken is done and the vegetables are just tender, about 3 minutes. Transfer the chicken mixture to a plate and wipe the skillet clean with a paper towel.

2 Heat the remaining ½ tablespoon oil in the same skillet over medium. Add the quinoa and edamame and cook, stirring constantly, until thoroughly heated, about 2 minutes. Push the quinoa mixture to the side of the skillet. Add the egg to opposite side of the skillet and cook, stirring constantly, until scrambled, about 1 minute; stir in the quinoa mixture. Add the chicken mixture and soy sauce to the skillet and cook, stirring often, until thoroughly heated, about 1 minute.

(SERVING SIZE: 1 CUP): CALORIES 327; FAT 12G (SAT 2G, UNSAT 9G); PROTEIN 22G; CARB 31G; FIBER 5G; SUGARS 2G (ADDED SUGARS 0G); SODIUM 658MG; CALC 5% DV; POTASSIUM 9% DV

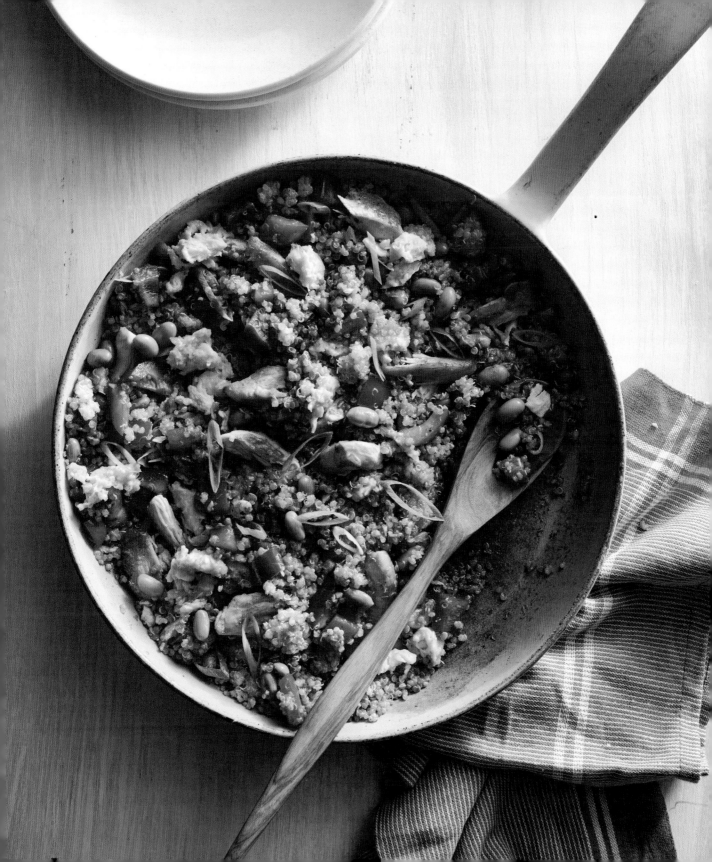

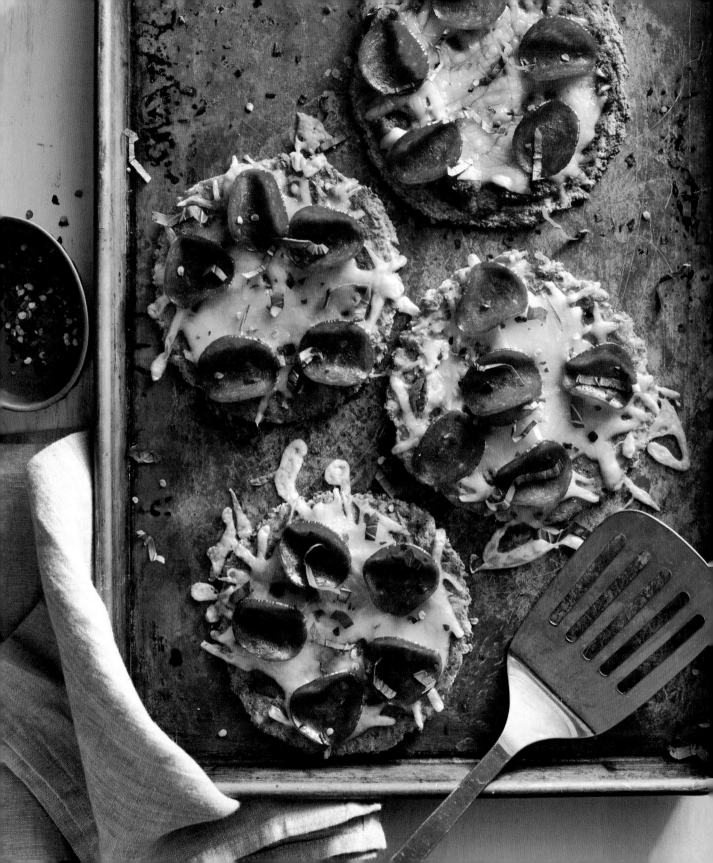

HANDS-ON: 30 MIN. // TOTAL: 55 MIN. // SERVES 4

personal pepperoni cauliflower pizzas

I always loved the idea of a veggie-based pizza crust, but it seemed way too intimidating for dinner. So I decided to start small with personal-size crusts, which seemed more approachable and, as it turns out, make a better pie! Making individual pizzas allows the cauliflower crust to get crispy, creating a solid base for toppings—something that can be hard (or impossible) to do for large crusts whose centers hold on to moisture.

1 Preheat the oven to 400°F. Line a baking sheet with parchment paper and lightly coat with cooking spray.

2 Place the cauliflower and water in a microwavable bowl; cover with plastic wrap and microwave on high until tender, about 4 minutes. Spread the cauliflower over a clean kitchen towel to cool slightly, 5 minutes. Gather the ends of the towel and squeeze the cauliflower to remove the excess moisture.

3 Stir together the cauliflower, almond flour, Parmesan, egg, salt, and baking soda in a medium bowl. Knead until well combined, about 1 minute. Divide the dough into 4 (¼-cup) portions; shape each portion into a ball. Place the dough portions on the prepared baking sheet and shape each into a 5-inch circle. Bake until the crusts are golden brown, about 16 minutes, gently turning the crusts over after 10 minutes.

4 Top each crust with 1 tablespoon of the sauce, leaving a ½-inch border. Sprinkle each with ¼ cup of the mozzarella, and arrange the pepperoni over the pizzas. Bake until the cheese is melted, 5 to 7 minutes.

(SERVING SIZE: 1 PIZZA): CALORIES 268; FAT 18G (SAT 5G, UNSAT 12G); PROTEIN 17G; CARB 12G; FIBER 4G; SUGARS 4G (ADDED SUGARS 0G); SODIUM 334MG; CALC 31% DV; POTASSIUM 7% DV

Canola oil cooking spray
1 (12-ounce) package fresh cauliflower rice or crumbles (about 4 cups)
2 tablespoons water
⅔ cup blanched almond flour (about 2⅜ ounces)
1 ounce Parmesan cheese, grated (about ¼ cup)
1 large egg, lightly beaten
½ teaspoon kosher salt
½ teaspoon baking soda
4 tablespoons prepared tomato-basil pasta sauce
4 ounces preshredded part-skim mozzarella cheese (about 1 cup)
1 ounce uncured turkey pepperoni slices (such as Applegate Naturals), quartered (¼ cup)

cured vs. uncured meats

Processed meats like bacon, hot dogs, pepperoni, and sandwich meat are typically cured with salt and synthetic nitrites to preserve them by slowing bacteria growth and to add color and a salty flavor. Research has linked regular intake of processed meats to an increased risk of some cancers, which many speculate is an effect of nitrites. Until we are sure that the risk is due to nitrites and not processed meats overall, limit your consumption to occasional intake, and choose uncured meats. "Uncured" signifies that no nitrites were used in the curing process, only salt.

OPTIONAL

1 teaspoon olive oil

¾ pound lean ground beef

1½ tablespoons All-Purpose
    Taco Seasoning (page 66)
    or store-bought organic
    taco seasoning

¾ teaspoon kosher salt

1 (14.5-ounce) can no-salt-
    added fire-roasted diced
    tomatoes

1 (14.5-ounce) can no-salt-
    added black beans, rinsed
    and drained

1 cup fresh or frozen corn
    kernels (about 2 ears)

½ cup water

3 cups zucchini spirals

1½ ounces cheddar cheese,
    shredded (about ⅓ cup)

¼ cup chopped scallions

HANDS-ON: 20 MIN. // TOTAL: 20 MIN. // SERVES 4

zucchini taco skillet

How does a one-dish skillet meal in only 20 minutes sound? Pretty good to me—and that's why this is a frequent weeknight dinner on my table. Sometimes store-bought veggie spirals have excess moisture in the container. If this is the case, drain the spirals and place them on a towel to absorb the excess moisture before using them. Or see page 55 for how to make your own veggie noodles.

1 Heat a large skillet over medium. Add the oil to the pan; swirl to coat. Add the beef; cook for 4 minutes, stirring to crumble. Increase the heat to medium-high and add the taco seasoning and salt; cook, stirring often, until the meat is browned, about 2 minutes more. Stir in the tomatoes, beans, corn, and water; bring to a simmer, stirring occasionally. Simmer until slightly thickened, about 5 minutes.

2 Stir in the zucchini spirals. Cover, reduce the heat to medium-low, and cook until the zucchini is just tender, about 3 minutes. Divide evenly among four pasta bowls. Top with the cheese and the scallions.

(SERVING SIZE: 1½ CUPS): CALORIES 352; FAT 12G (SAT 5G, UNSAT 6G); PROTEIN 29G; CARB 32G; FIBER 8G; SUGARS 9G (ADDED SUGARS 0G); SODIUM 763MG; CALC 19% DV; POTASSIUM 13% DV

DAIRY-FREE OPTION: Omit the cheese, and top with ½ diced ripe avocado.

is grass-fed meat healthier?

Grass-fed meat is viewed by many to be a healthier option, often costing $1 to $2 more per pound, so make sure you know what the "grass-fed" labels really mean.

"100% GRASS-FED" or "GRASS-FINISHED" means the animal ate grass for its entire life, other than its mother's milk when it was a baby.

"GRASS-FED" means the animal ate grass and had access to pasture for a portion of its life; the length of this varies greatly by farm.

• None of the grass-fed labels above mean the animal was raised organically and without antibiotics or added growth hormones.

• Most research comparing grass-fed beef to grain-fed (the alternative if grass-fed is not specified) examines beef from cattle that had access to grass their entire life, not just a portion of it. There are no real differences in protein, zinc, or iron content.

• Grass-finished beef tends to be leaner, which means the total amount of fat is slightly lower. The polyunsaturated omega-3 fats are also slightly higher, but when you look at a 3- to 4-ounce serving, the difference isn't really significant enough to suggest that grass-fed is a better source of omega-3s.

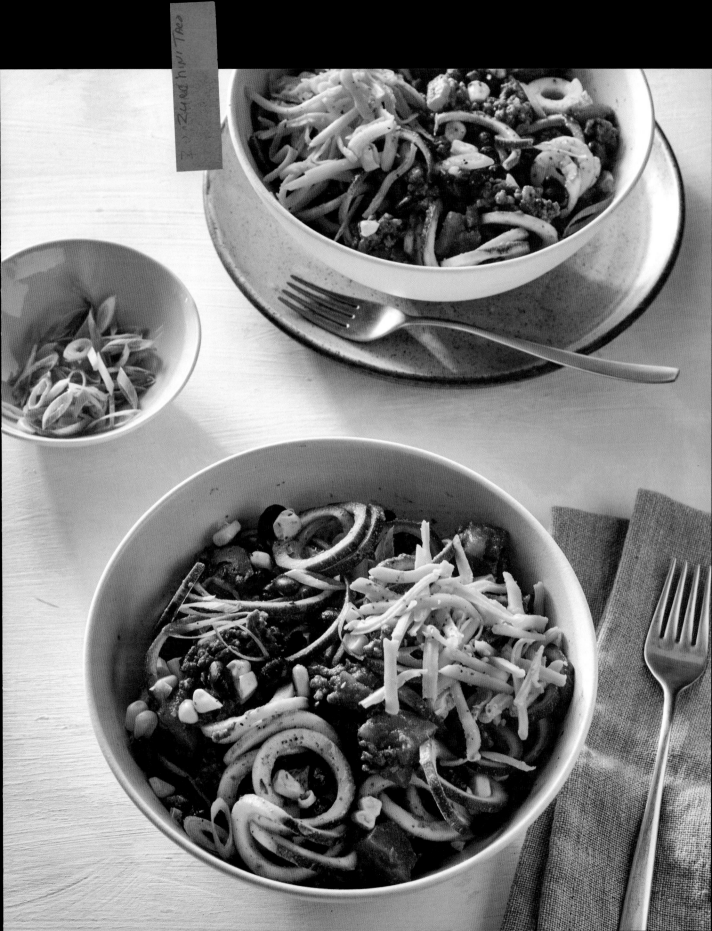

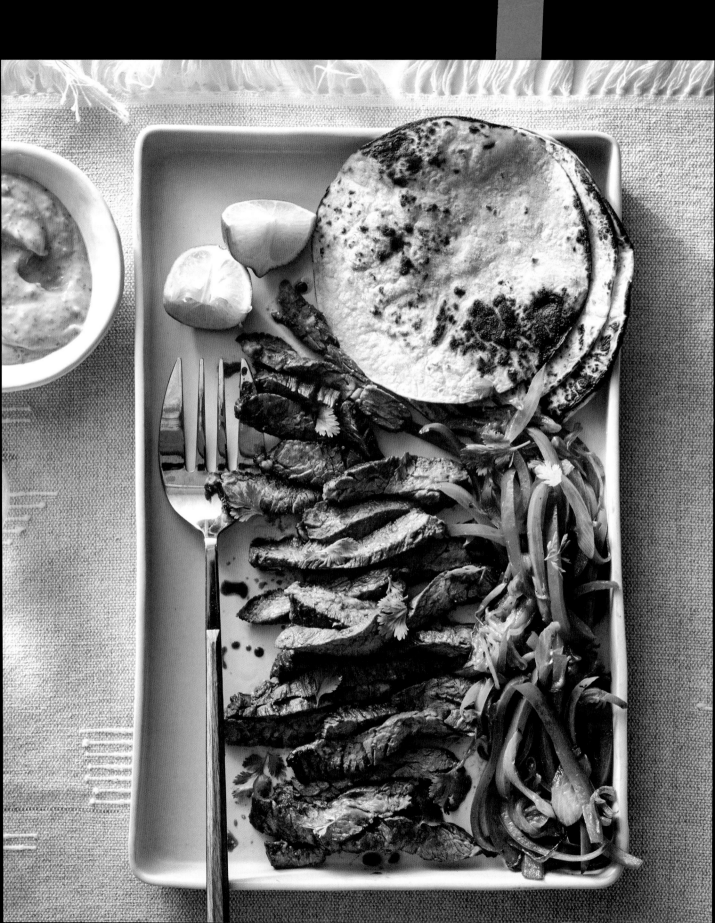

Use bib lettuce instead of tortillas

sheet pan steak fajitas

(DF) DAIRY FREE (GF) GLUTEN FREE

I like to use a red and green bell pepper for color, but any variety of bell pepper—or just green—works equally well. Combine and refrigerate the marinade and steak in the morning before leaving the house, if desired. Also, make sure to line the sheet pan with foil so that cleanup is fast.

1 Preheat the broiler to high with the oven rack 6 inches from the heat source.

2 Combine the lime juice, garlic, and 2 teaspoons of the oil in a large ziplock plastic freezer bag. Add the steak, seal the bag, and shake to coat. Let stand at room temperature, turning occasionally, for 30 minutes. Remove the steak from the marinade, discarding the marinade. Pat the steak dry and rub with the salt and 2 teaspoons of the taco seasoning.

3 Line a large rimmed baking sheet or bottom of a broiler pan with aluminum foil and lightly coat with cooking spray. Combine the bell peppers, onion, remaining 2 teaspoons oil, and remaining 1 teaspoon taco seasoning in a large bowl and toss well to coat. Place the vegetables on half the prepared baking sheet. Place the steak on the other half of the baking sheet. Broil for 6 minutes. Turn the steak over and broil to the desired degree of doneness, about 4 minutes more. Transfer the steak to a cutting board and let rest for 5 minutes; cut the steak diagonally across the grain into thin slices.

4 Add the steak slices to the vegetable mixture and toss to combine. Top the tortillas evenly with the steak-and-vegetable mixture. Top each tortilla with 1 tablespoon of the dressing, yogurt, or diced avocado.

(SERVING SIZE: 2 FAJITAS): CALORIES 422; FAT 20G (SAT 4G, UNSAT 14G); PROTEIN 30G; CARB 32G; FIBER 6G; SUGARS 5G (ADDED SUGARS 0G); SODIUM 716MG; CALC 10% DV; POTASSIUM 15% DV

2 tablespoons fresh lime juice (from 1 lime)

1 garlic clove, grated (about 1 teaspoon)

4 teaspoons avocado oil

1 (1-pound) flank or skirt steak

3/8 teaspoon kosher salt

3 teaspoons All-Purpose Taco Seasoning (page 66) or store-bought organic taco seasoning

Cooking spray

2 medium bell peppers, cut into thin strips

1 medium yellow onion, cut into thin strips

8 (6-inch) yellow corn tortillas, warmed

1/2 cup Avocado-Cilantro Dip and Dressing (page 71), plain Greek yogurt, or diced avocado

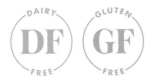

one-pan steak with sweet potatoes and green beans

I'll take cleaning one pan over three any day—especially if messing up fewer dishes makes dinner extra flavorful. This trick of placing the steak on a rack above the vegetables allows the beef juices to drip down on the vegetables as they roast. No special type of rack is required; I usually use a cooling rack.

- 1 (12-ounce) bag trimmed green beans
- 3 (8-ounce) sweet potatoes, peeled, halved lengthwise, and sliced into thin half-moons
- 2 tablespoons olive oil
- 1 teaspoon garlic powder
- 1 teaspoon kosher salt
- 1 (1-pound) flank steak, trimmed
- 2 teaspoons chopped fresh thyme
- ¾ teaspoon black pepper

1 Preheat the broiler to high with the oven rack 6 inches from the heat source. Line a large rimmed baking sheet with aluminum foil.

2 Place the green beans and potatoes on the prepared baking sheet; toss with 1½ tablespoons of the oil, the garlic powder, and ½ teaspoon of the salt. Spread the vegetables in an even layer. Place a wire rack on the pan over the vegetables. Rub the steak with the remaining ½ tablespoon oil; place on the rack in the pan over the vegetables. Sprinkle the steak with 1 teaspoon of the thyme, ¼ teaspoon of the salt, and half the pepper.

3 Broil for 10 minutes. Turn the steak over; sprinkle with the remaining 1 teaspoon thyme, ¼ teaspoon salt, and pepper. Broil for about 5 minutes or to the desired degree of doneness.

4 Remove the steak from the pan and let stand for 5 minutes. Cut it across the grain into thin slices. Place the vegetables in a bowl; pour in the pan juices and toss to coat. Serve with the steak.

(SERVING SIZE: 3 OUNCES STEAK AND ABOUT 1 CUP VEGETABLES): CALORIES 355; FAT 13G (SAT 3G, UNSAT 8G); PROTEIN 29G; CARB 31G; FIBER 6G; SUGARS 8G (ADDED SUGARS 0G); SODIUM 606MG; CALC 9% DV; POTASSIUM 20% DV

one-pan dinner secrets

The thickness of the steak and cut size of the vegetables make a big difference in cooking time, so adjust as needed to get them to your preferred doneness. There's a lot of flexibility for the veggies. Here are some quick substitutions:

- Substitute a (12-ounce) bag broccoli florets or halved Brussels sprouts for the green beans.
- Substitute diced red potatoes for the sweet potatoes.
- Look for bags of ready-to-steam fresh sweet potato cubes to save time.
- Use frozen roasted sweet potato slices. Place them to the side of the beans on the pan. The moisture in the frozen potatoes can prevent the beans from browning.

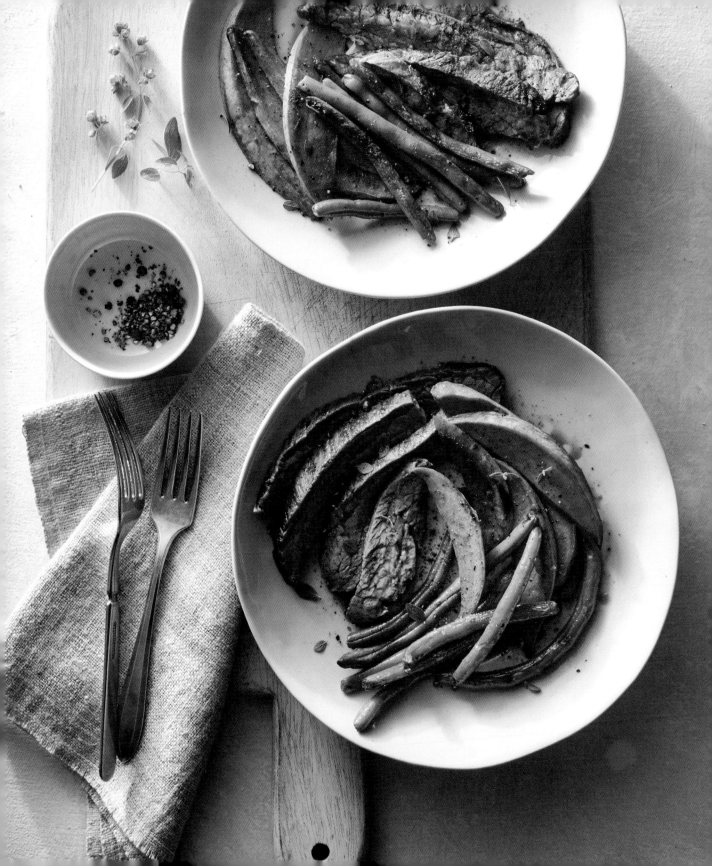

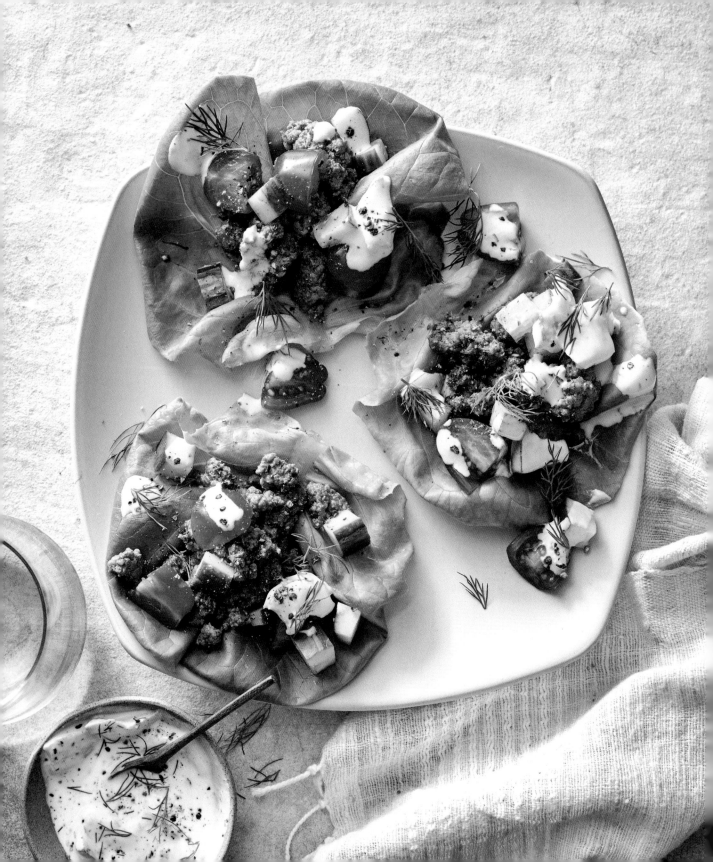

greek lamb lettuce wraps

Crisp lettuce leaves are a refreshing alternative to pita bread or flatbread. When reheating leftovers for lunch the next day, I often assemble them as a salad by spooning the warm lamb mixture over a bed of chopped greens and dolloping with tzatziki sauce.

1 Heat a large skillet over high. Add the oil to the pan; swirl to coat. Add the onion, garlic, cinnamon, salt, pepper, and lamb to the pan; sauté for 5 minutes or until the lamb is done.

2 Combine the tomato and cucumber in a medium bowl. Stir in the lamb mixture. Place about ⅓ cup of the lamb mixture in each lettuce leaf. Top each wrap with 1 tablespoon of the dip.

(SERVING SIZE: 3 WRAPS): CALORIES 337; FAT 23G (SAT 10G, UNSAT 11G); PROTEIN 20G; CARB 15G; FIBER 3G; SUGARS 7G (ADDED SUGARS 0G); SODIUM 636MG; CALC 8% DV; POTASSIUM 8% DV

1 tablespoon olive oil

2 cups finely chopped onion

3 garlic cloves, minced

1 teaspoon ground cinnamon

¾ teaspoon kosher salt

¼ teaspoon black pepper

12 ounces lean ground lamb

1 cup chopped tomato or
 quartered cherry tomatoes

1 cup chopped cucumber

12 Boston lettuce leaves

¾ cup refrigerated Greek
 yogurt tzatziki or
 cucumber-dill dip

lamb perks

Lamb is a red meat that often gets overlooked, but it often leads the pack from a nutrition perspective. Grass is the primary food for lamb, typically regardless of whether it's labeled 100% grass-fed or not, which gives it a slightly higher proportion of CLA (conjugated linoleic acids). These polyunsaturated fatty acids are believed to have an anti-inflammatory effect, reducing risks of heart disease, insulin resistance, and possibly obesity. Anti-inflammatory diet guidelines recommend limiting red meat in one's weekly diet, so when you do indulge, choose lean cuts.

pork scaloppine with white beans

Mediterranean flavors dominate in this quick skillet dinner, and adding just a touch of butter when cooking the pork helps them to mesh perfectly. Pounding thicker pork chops before seasoning and cooking them is another option if you can't find thin cutlets.

4 thin pork cutlets or boneless
   center-cut pork chops
   (about 1 pound), butterflied

½ teaspoon kosher salt

¼ teaspoon black pepper

1 tablespoon Dijon mustard

1½ tablespoons olive oil

½ tablespoon butter

½ cup chopped onion

3 garlic cloves, minced

½ cup chopped tomato

1 (15-ounce) can no-salt-
   added cannellini beans,
   rinsed and drained

1 teaspoon minced fresh sage

½ teaspoon lemon zest

1 Season the pork cutlets lightly with ¼ teaspoon of the salt and the pepper and spread one side of each with mustard. Heat ½ tablespoon of the oil and the butter over medium-high in a large skillet. Add the pork, mustard side down, in a single layer and cook, turning once, until golden brown on both sides, about 4 minutes total. Transfer to a clean plate.

2 Heat the remaining 1 tablespoon oil in the same skillet over medium. Add the onion and cook until translucent, about 5 minutes. Add the garlic and cook for 1 minute more. Stir in the tomato and cook until it has softened slightly and released some juice, about 3 minutes. Stir in the beans, sage, lemon zest, and the remaining ¼ teaspoon salt. Reduce the heat to low. Use the back of a fork to coarsely mash the beans and cook, stirring occasionally, until warm throughout. Serve with the pork.

(SERVING SIZE: 1 CUTLET AND ¼ OF THE MASHED BEANS): CALORIES 367; FAT 20G (SAT 6G, UNSAT 12G); PROTEIN 30G; CARB 18G; FIBER 5G; SUGARS 2G (ADDED SUGARS 0G); SODIUM 455MG; CALC 5% DV; POTASSIUM 13% DV

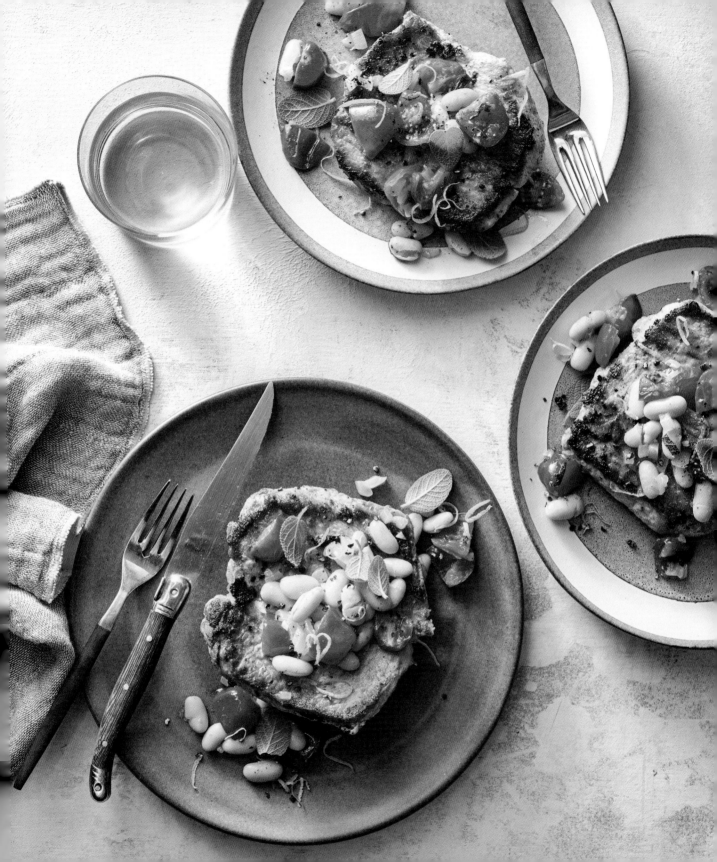

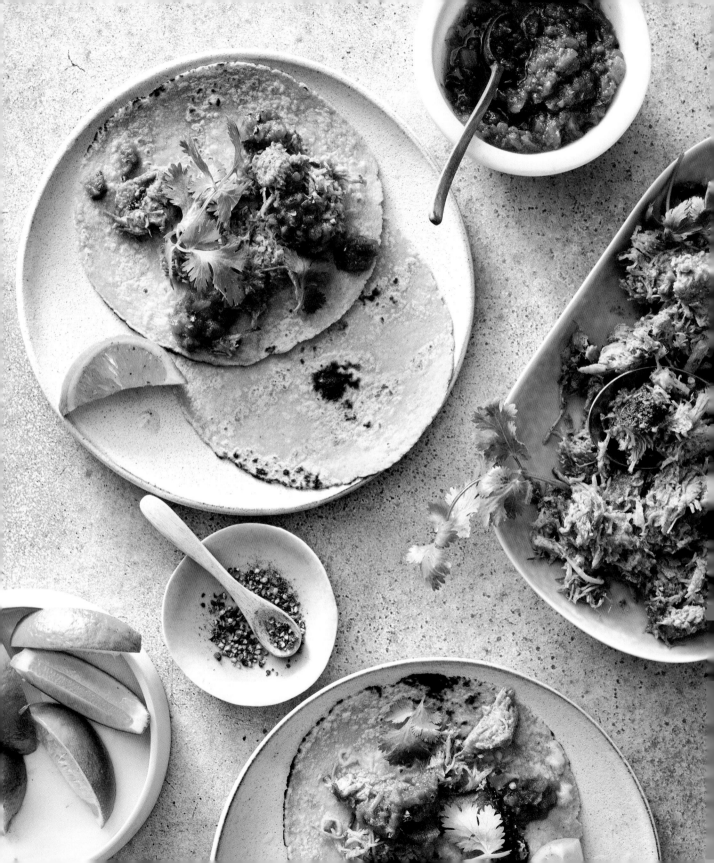

fuss-free pulled pork tacos

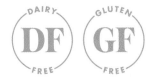

Since this recipe usually makes more than I need, I freeze half to pull out and use for a quick dinner a few weeks down the road. Also, the pulled pork isn't just for tacos—it's great on salads and baked sweet potatoes, as well as by itself!

1 Cut the pork into 12 pieces similar in size. Rub the pork with the taco seasoning and sprinkle with the salt.

2 Place the oil in a multicooker and preheat to sauté. Add the pork and cook, stirring frequently, for 2 to 3 minutes or until the meat is beginning to brown on the outside. Add the salsa. Close and lock the lid on the multicooker, and pressure-cook for 25 to 30 minutes.

3 Meanwhile, preheat the oven to 350°F. Stack the tortillas, wrap them in aluminum foil, and bake until warm, about 15 minutes.

4 Once the multicooker is done, release the steam and open the multicooker as directed by the manufacturer. Let cool slightly; place the pork on a cutting board or plate and shred with two forks. Place approximately 1½ ounces of the pork down the center of each tortilla; sprinkle with the cilantro and serve with the lime wedges and additional salsa. Drizzle with the cooking juices, if desired.

(SERVING SIZE: 2 TACOS): CALORIES 378; FAT 18G (SAT 6G, UNSAT 10G); PROTEIN 27G; CARB 27G; FIBER 4G; SUGARS 5G (ADDED SUGARS 0G); SODIUM 618MG; CALC 11% DV; POTASSIUM 12% DV

SLOW-COOKER OPTION: Follow the directions above, omitting the oil and skipping sautéing. Place the pork in a 4- to 6-quart slow cooker and add the salsa. Cover and cook until the meat is tender and pulls apart easily, 4 to 5 hours on high or 7 to 8 hours on low.

1 (2½-pound) boneless pork butt or shoulder, trimmed of excess fat

2 tablespoons All-Purpose Taco Seasoning (page 66) or store-bought organic taco seasoning

½ teaspoon kosher salt

2 teaspoons olive oil

2 cups refrigerated fresh salsa, plus more for serving

16 (6-inch) corn tortillas

½ cup fresh cilantro sprigs

1 lime, cut into wedges

meat and poultry buying guide

These days the butcher shop can be as confusing as the bread and cereal aisles when it comes to labeling and what terms actually signify a healthier product. Here's a quick overview of what each label term indicates, as well as what some don't indicate, when on meat or poultry.

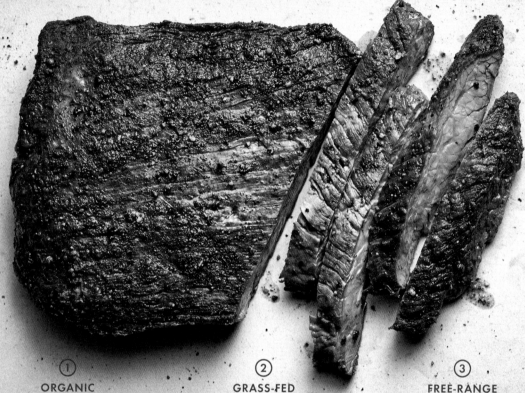

① ORGANIC

If organic is preferred, make sure to choose a product with the label "certified organic," which signifies the animals were fed a 100% organic diet and were given no hormones or antibiotics.

② GRASS-FED

Suggests the animal was fed grass for all or part of its life and that the animal has had some access to the outdoors. However, there is little regulation over the span of time that both of these occur in an animal's life.

"Grass-fed" should not be used as an indicator that the animal was not given antibiotics or hormones and does not mean the animal was fed a 100% organic diet. See page 142 for the nutritional aspects of grass-fed meat.

③ FREE-RANGE

Suggests that the animal had access to the outdoors, but does not necessarily mean the animal was raised outdoors, on farmland (vs. on concrete or in cages), or had space to move around freely.

④ NO ANTIBIOTICS

Exactly what it says: No antibiotics were given to the animal.

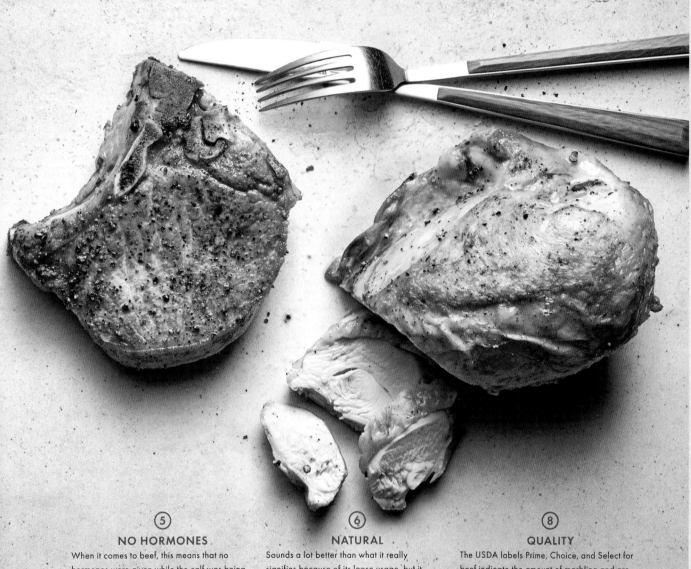

⑤ NO HORMONES

When it comes to beef, this means that no hormones were given while the calf was being raised. However, hormones may have been given to its mother to stimulate ovulation or milk production.

This label signifies nothing on poultry and pork, since it is against federal guidelines to give hormones to those animals being raised for consumption.

⑥ NATURAL

Sounds a lot better than what it really signifies because of its loose usage, but it means the animal product was minimally processed and has had no colorings or artificial ingredients added.

⑦ FRESH

Signifies that the product was never frozen.

⑧ QUALITY

The USDA labels Prime, Choice, and Select for beef indicate the amount of marbling and are a good indication of how tender or juicy a cut will be.

Prime has the highest amount of marbling or fat. It's often from younger cattle and is usually the most tender and juiciest when cooked.

Choice has slightly less marbling and fat. Some cuts will be tender and juicy, but others may require certain cooking methods to make them more tender.

Select has the least amount of marbling and fat, which means it will not be as tender and juicy. However, marinating can help with these aspects, as well as add flavor.

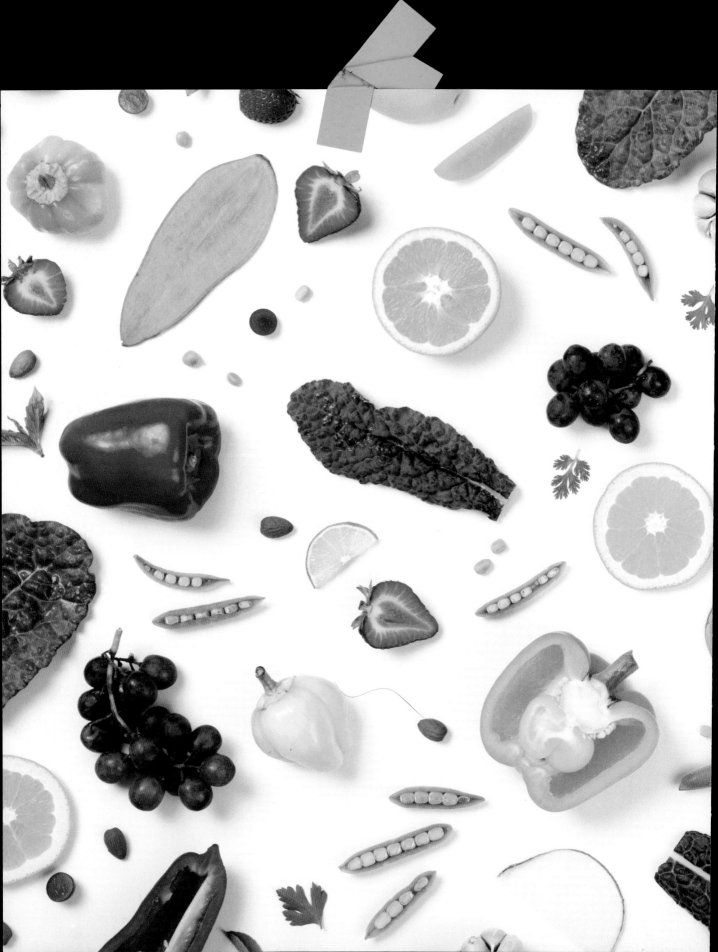

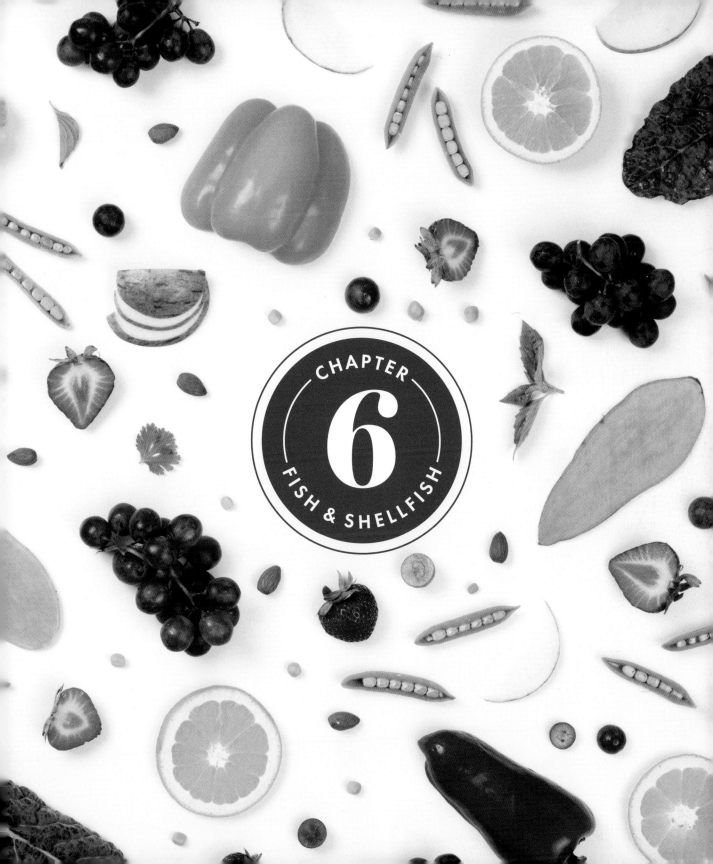

CHAPTER

6

FISH & SHELLFISH

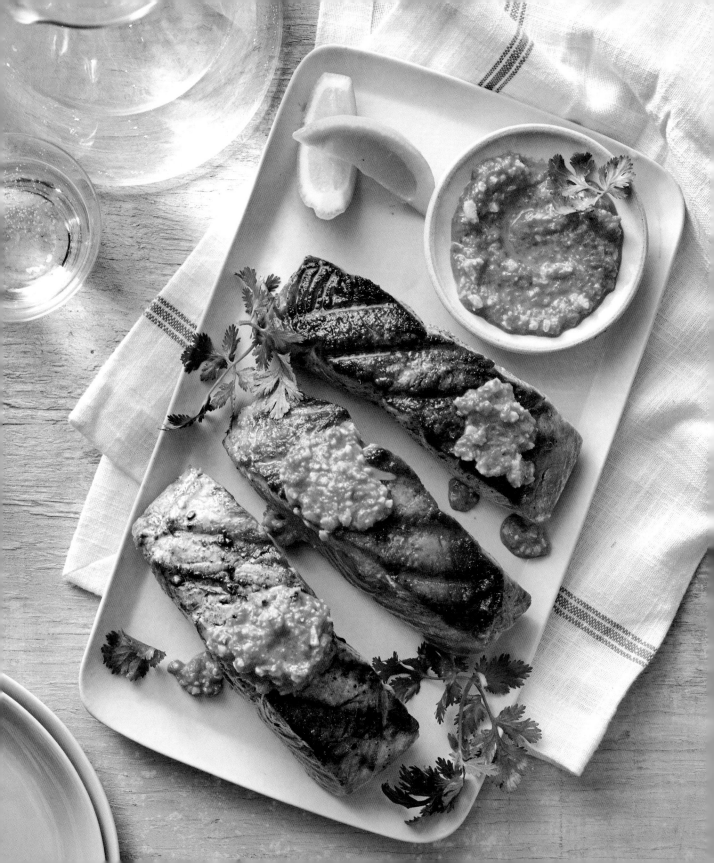

grilled salmon with quick romesco

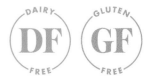

Romesco is a Spanish sauce typically made by pureeing roasted peppers, tomatoes, almonds, and olive oil. The result is a vibrant and creamy—but dairy-free—sauce for meat, fish, and poultry. In this variation, I skip the tomatoes and use jarred roasted peppers to save time. If you don't like the bite of raw garlic, drop the clove in boiling water for 1 minute to blanch it, then proceed with the sauce.

1 Heat a grill pan over medium-high. Coat the pan with cooking spray. Sprinkle the fish evenly with ½ teaspoon of the salt. Arrange the fish in the pan; cook for 4 minutes on each side or until the fish flakes easily when tested with a fork, or to the desired degree of doneness.

2 While the fish cooks, place the remaining ¼ teaspoon salt, the bell peppers, almonds, oil, vinegar, and garlic in a blender or food processor and process until smooth. Serve the romesco over the fish.

(SERVING SIZE: 1 FILLET AND 3 TABLESPOONS SAUCE): CALORIES 340; FAT 18G (SAT 3G, UNSAT 14G); PROTEIN 39G; CARB 3G; FIBER 1G; SUGARS 0G (ADDED SUGARS 0G); SODIUM 498MG; CALC 5% DV; POTASSIUM 21% DV

Cooking spray

4 (6-ounce) skinless salmon fillets

¾ teaspoon kosher salt

½ cup chopped bottled roasted red bell peppers, rinsed and drained

10 whole blanched almonds, or 3 tablespoons slivered almonds

1 tablespoon extra-virgin olive oil

1 teaspoon red wine vinegar

1 garlic clove

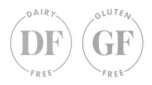

DF — DAIRY FREE

GF — GLUTEN FREE

HANDS-ON: 15 MIN. // TOTAL: 45 MIN. // SERVES 4

sheet pan honey-soy salmon, sweet potatoes, and green beans

While this dinner takes a little longer to cook than others, it requires only 15 minutes of your attention in the kitchen—a practically fuss-free complete dinner. The dish is also packed with omega-3s, as well as vitamins A and C.

Cooking spray

1½ tablespoons gluten-free lower-sodium soy sauce or tamari

3 tablespoons olive oil

1 tablespoon honey

1 tablespoon fresh lime juice (from 1 lime)

2 garlic cloves, minced

4 (5-ounce) skin-on salmon fillets

1 pound sweet potatoes, cut into ¾-inch cubes

½ teaspoon kosher salt

½ teaspoon black pepper

1 (12-ounce) bag trimmed fresh green beans

1 Preheat the oven to 400°F. Line an 18 x 13-inch rimmed baking sheet with aluminum foil; coat with cooking spray.

2 Whisk together the soy sauce, 1 tablespoon of the oil, the honey, lime juice, and half the garlic in a large bowl. Place the salmon in the bowl. Toss to coat.

3 Put the potatoes on the prepared pan. Drizzle with 1 tablespoon of the oil and sprinkle with ¼ teaspoon of the salt and ¼ teaspoon of the pepper; toss to coat. Roast until the potatoes are almost fork-tender, 20 to 25 minutes.

4 A few minutes before the potatoes are done cooking, toss the green beans with the remaining 1 tablespoon oil and remaining garlic, and sprinkle with the remaining ¼ teaspoon salt and ¼ teaspon pepper; toss to coat. Remove the potatoes from the oven; stir and push them toward one end of the pan. Place the marinated salmon in the center of the pan and spread the green beans over the remaining exposed portion of the pan. Roast for 15 minutes.

(SERVING SIZE: 1 FILLET, ¼ OF POTATOES, AND ¼ OF BEANS): CALORIES 444; FAT 21G (SAT 3G, UNSAT 17G); PROTEIN 35G; CARB 28G; FIBER 5G; SUGARS 11G (ADDED SUGARS 4G); SODIUM 697MG; CALC 8% DV; POTASSIUM 27% DV

sweet potatoes

These naturally sweet, bright orange spuds are sometimes called a superfood. This label isn't too far off when you consider that one medium potato contains approximately 25 percent of the RDA for potassium, vitamin C, and vitamin B_6, as well as almost 300 percent of the RDA for vitamin A. Carotenoids like beta-carotene are plant forms of vitamin A that are responsible for the vegetable's deep orange color and help maintain eye health. Higher intakes of carotenoid-rich foods like sweet potatoes, carrots, spinach, and butternut squash have been associated with a lower risk of heart disease and some cancers, thanks to the carotenoids' anti-inflammatory and antioxidant qualities.

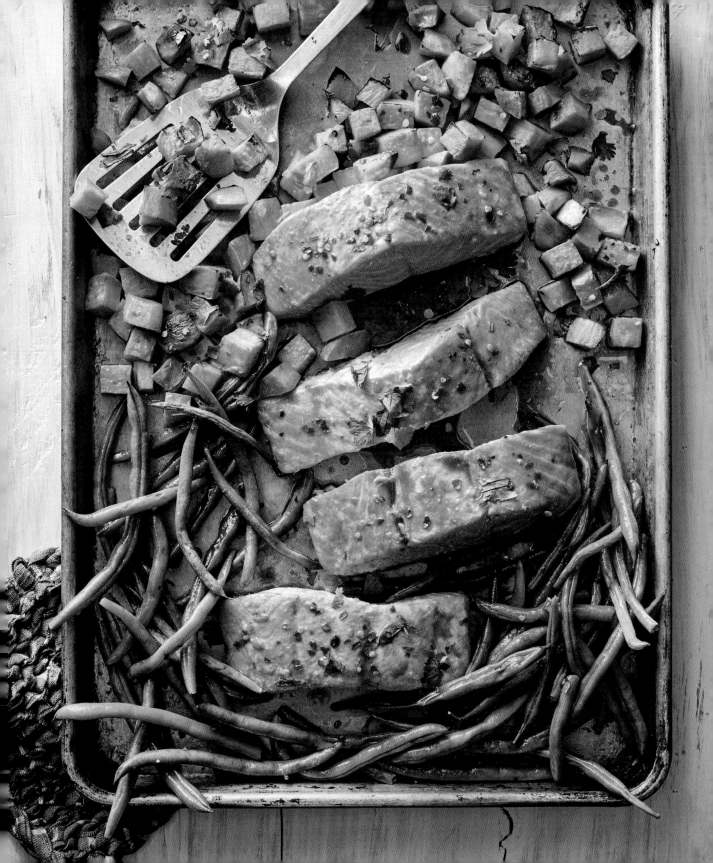

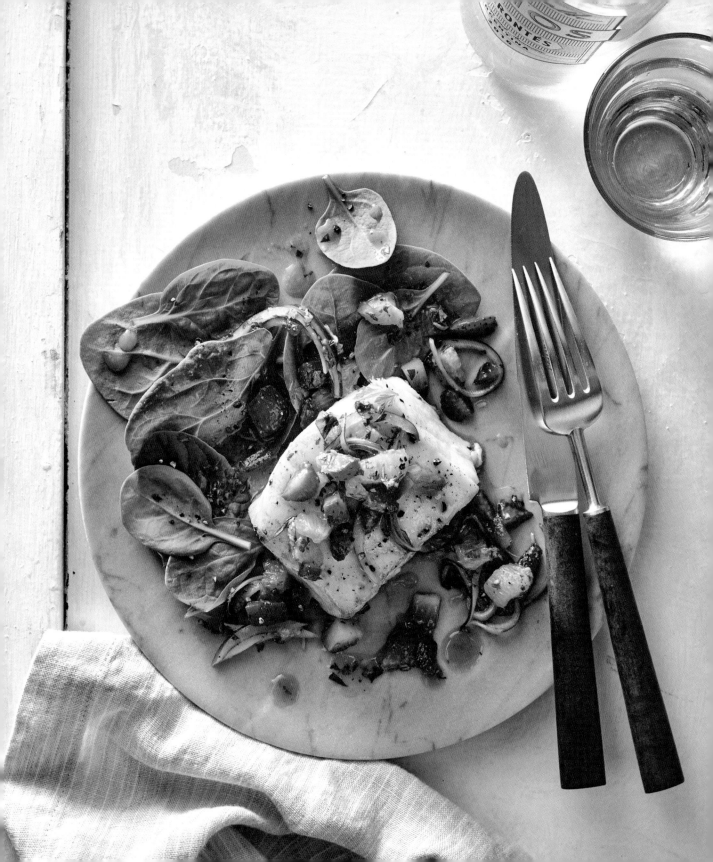

sea bass with strawberry-citrus salsa

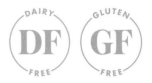

Sustainable and a "best choice" on the FDA and EPA's fish guidelines, black sea bass is a mild, tender fish with a buttery flavor. Other good choices to substitute are cod, sablefish, and barramundi. Use additional orange or grapefruit sections if strawberries aren't in season.

1 Preheat the broiler to high with the oven rack 6 to 8 inches from the heat source.

2 Combine ½ tablespoon of the oil and ½ teaspoon of the salt and ½ teaspoon of pepper in a small bowl. Place the fish on a baking sheet; rub with the oil mixture. Broil the fish until it is beginning to brown and flakes easily with a fork, 10 to 12 minutes. Keep warm.

3 While the fish cooks, peel the orange. Cut the fruit into segments, and coarsely chop. Whisk together the cilantro, lime juice, garlic, the remaining 2 tablespoons oil, and the remaining ¼ teaspoon salt and ¼ teaspoon pepper in a medium bowl; stir in the strawberries, orange segments, and onion. Spoon the salsa over the fish.

(SERVING SIZE: 1 FILLET AND 2 TABLESPOONS SALSA): CALORIES 276; FAT 12G (SAT 2G, UNSAT 9G); PROTEIN 34G; CARB 7G; FIBER 2G; SUGARS 4G (ADDED SUGARS 0G); SODIUM 483MG; CALC 4% DV; POTASSIUM 12% DV

2½ tablespoons olive oil

¾ teaspoon kosher salt

¾ teaspoon black pepper

4 (6-ounce) skinless sea bass fillets

1 small navel orange

3 tablespoons chopped fresh cilantro

1 tablespoon fresh lime juice

1 teaspoon minced garlic

1 cup strawberries, hulled and coarsely chopped

¼ cup thinly vertically sliced red onion

strawberries

Strawberries are loaded with anthocyanins and antioxidants called ellagitannins, both powerful compounds that sweep up harmful free radicals and suppress pro-inflammatory proteins in the body. In fact, research suggests that regularly eating strawberries, as well as most other berries, reduces an individual's risk of heart disease, Alzheimer's, cancer, type 2 diabetes, and other diseases related to chronic inflammation.

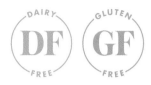

green curry with halibut

Try placing baby spinach in the bottom of the serving bowls before adding the hot rice and curry; the heat slightly wilts the greens. Spinach is a perfect complement to the flavors in this dish—plus, adding a vegetable makes it a complete meal.

1 tablespoon olive oil

3 tablespoons green curry paste

1 (13.5-ounce) can coconut milk

1 cup low-sodium chicken broth

⅛ teaspoon kosher salt

1½ pounds skinless, boneless halibut, cut into 1½-inch pieces

1 tablespoon fresh lime juice

⅓ cup chopped fresh basil

2 cups cooked brown rice

1 Heat a large deep skillet over medium-high. Add the oil to the pan; swirl to coat. Add the curry paste and cook, stirring frequently, for 30 seconds or until fragrant. Add the coconut milk, broth, and half the salt and bring to a simmer. Reduce the heat to low and cook for 3 minutes or until slightly thickened.

2 Sprinkle the halibut with the remaining salt. Add the halibut to the pan, gently stirring to coat the fish with the sauce. Cover and simmer over medium until the fish is opaque throughout, 6 to 8 minutes. Stir in the lime juice and sprinkle with the basil. Divide the rice among four serving bowls. Spoon the curry over the rice.

(SERVING SIZE: ½ CUP RICE AND ¼ OF THE CURRY MIXTURE): CALORIES 347; FAT 10G (SAT 4G, UNSAT 5G); PROTEIN 35G; CARB 27G; FIBER 4G; SUGARS 0G (ADDED SUGARS 0G); SODIUM 783MG; CALC 3% DV; POTASSIUM 18% DV

don't forget selenium

Often overlooked, selenium is an essential mineral that acts as an antioxidant in the body. Playing a key role in protecting brain neurons from oxidative damage, adequate selenium intake may be linked to improved memory and delayed onset or progression of brain diseases such as Alzheimer's and Parkinson's. Fish like halibut, as well as other seafood, and some nuts and seeds such as Brazil nuts and sunflower seeds are all good sources of selenium.

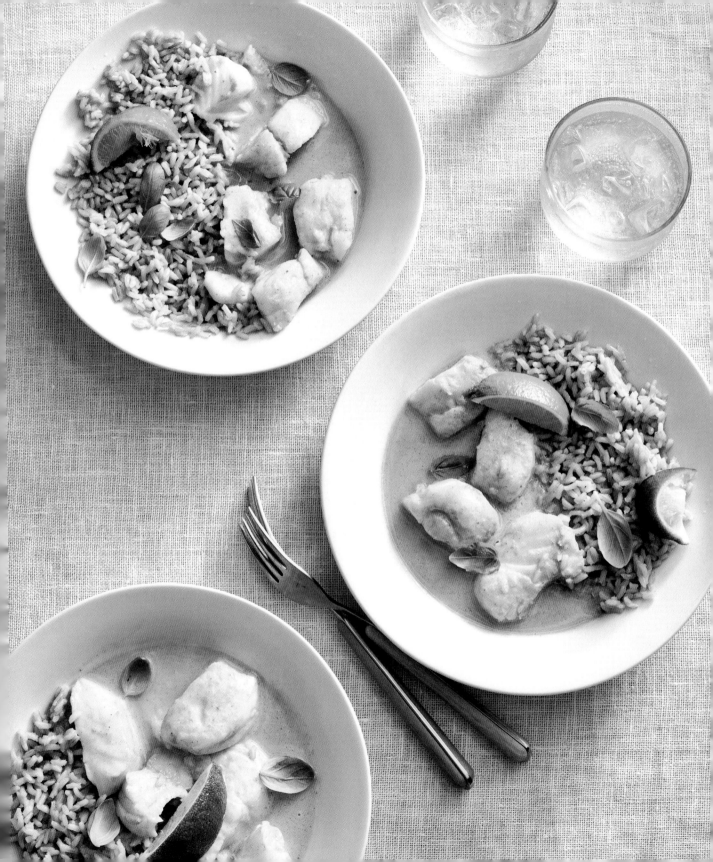

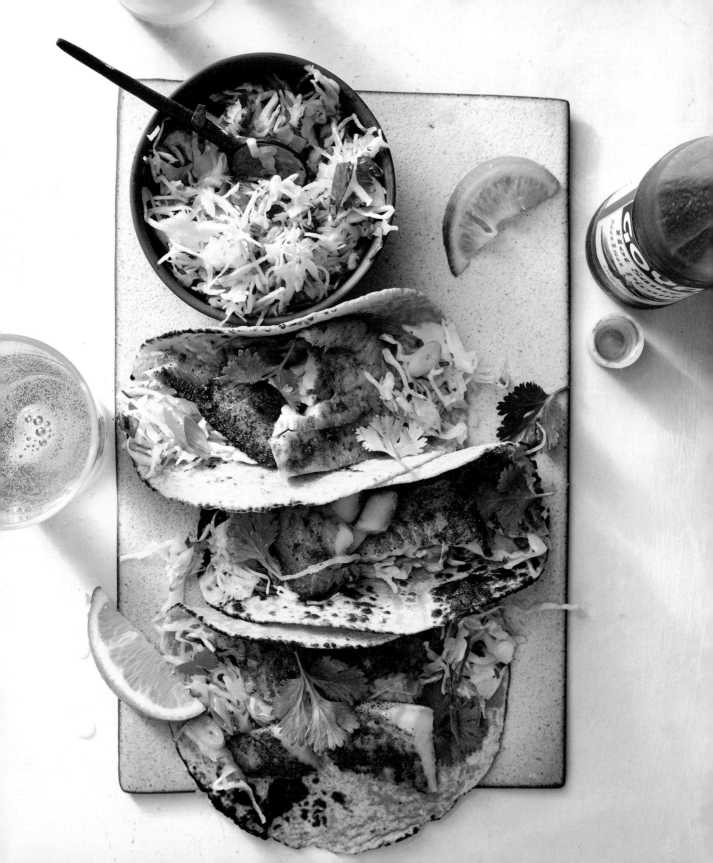

fish tacos with cilantro slaw

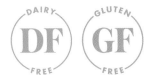

You'll have more slaw than you need for inside the tacos, but I like serving any leftover slaw as a side dish next to the tacos. If you'd prefer, buy a head of green cabbage and cut it into very thin slices to yield 4 cups rather than use bagged coleslaw.

1 Place the coleslaw, scallions, and cilantro in a large bowl. Add the lime juice, 1 tablespoon of the oil, and ¼ teaspoon of the salt; toss well to combine.

2 Heat a large nonstick skillet over medium-high. Add the remaining 2 teaspoons oil to the pan; swirl to coat. Sprinkle the fish evenly with the taco seasoning and remaining ¼ teaspoon salt. Add the fish to the pan; cook for 3 minutes on each side or until the fish flakes easily when tested with a fork, or to the desired degree of doneness. Remove from the heat and cut the fish into bite-size pieces.

3 Warm the tortillas according to the package directions. Spoon about ¼ cup cabbage mixture down the center of each tortilla. Divide the fish evenly among the tortillas; fold in half. Serve the tacos with the remaining cabbage mixture.

(SERVING SIZE: 2 TACOS AND ABOUT 1 CUP CABBAGE MIXTURE): CALORIES 285; FAT 9G (SAT 2G, UNSAT 7G); PROTEIN 26G; CARB 27G; FIBER 5G; SUGARS 3G (ADDED SUGARS 0G); SODIUM 441MG; CALC 8% DV; POTASSIUM 10% DV

1 (10-ounce) bag angel hair coleslaw

⅓ cup thinly sliced scallions

¼ cup chopped fresh cilantro

2 tablespoons fresh lime juice

5 teaspoons olive oil

½ teaspoon kosher salt

1 pound tilapia fillets

1 teaspoon All-Purpose Taco Seasoning (page 66) or store-bought organic taco seasoning

8 (6-inch) corn tortillas

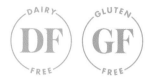

hoisin flounder with sugar snaps

A nice change to the usual stir-fries that use meat or poultry, flounder takes just a few minutes to cook, and sugar snaps give you extra ground to drizzle with hoisin sauce. Look for a 6- to 8-ounce bag of fresh sugar snap peas near the bagged, prewashed produce, or opt for a small frozen bag.

2 tablespoons gluten-free hoisin sauce

1 tablespoon water

2 teaspoons gluten-free lower-sodium soy sauce or tamari

1½ teaspoons minced fresh ginger

1½ teaspoons sesame oil

½ teaspoon black pepper

2½ tablespoons olive oil

4 (6-ounce) founder fillets

1 (6-ounce) bag fresh sugar snap peas

2 scallions, thinly sliced

1 Whisk together the hoisin sauce, water, soy sauce, ginger, sesame oil, and pepper in a small bowl. Transfer 4 teaspoons to a separate small bowl and set aside.

2 Heat a large nonstick skillet over medium-high. Add 1 tablespoon of the olive oil to the pan; swirl to coat. Add two fillets to the pan; cook for 4 minutes. Turn; brush each with 1 teaspoon of the hoisin mixture. Cook for 2 minutes. Remove the fish from the pan. Repeat to cook the remaining fillets, using 1 tablespoon of the olive oil and brushing each fillet with 1 teaspoon of the hoisin mixture. Keep warm.

3 Cook the sugar snaps in the microwave according to the package directions. Drain, if needed. Heat a large nonstick skillet over medium-high. Add the remaining ½ tablespoon olive oil; swirl to coat. Add the peas and scallions; sauté for 3 minutes. Place one fillet on each of four plates; top with the vegetables and drizzle with the reserved hoisin mixture.

(SERVING SIZE: 1 FILLET, ½ CUP VEGETABLES, AND 1 TEASPOON HOISIN MIXTURE): CALORIES 231; FAT 13G (SAT 2G, UNSAT 10G); PROTEIN 20G; CARB 8G; FIBER 2G; SUGARS 4G (ADDED SUGARS 3G); SODIUM 654MG; CALC 6% DV; POTASSIUM 8% DV

fish and autoimmune diseases

A new but promising area of research is the effect that eating fish may have on soothing symptoms or slowing progression of autoimmune diseases like rheumatoid arthritis. Potential benefits center around the fact that inflammation within the body is often involved in either the development or flare-ups of autoimmune conditions, and DHA and EPA happen to have anti-inflammatory effects in the body. In fact, the Arthritis Foundation recommends eating fatty fish two to four times per week. Also, it's important to note that choosing fish with low-mercury levels (see page 183) is even more important since high mercury consumption may also play a role in autoimmune development.

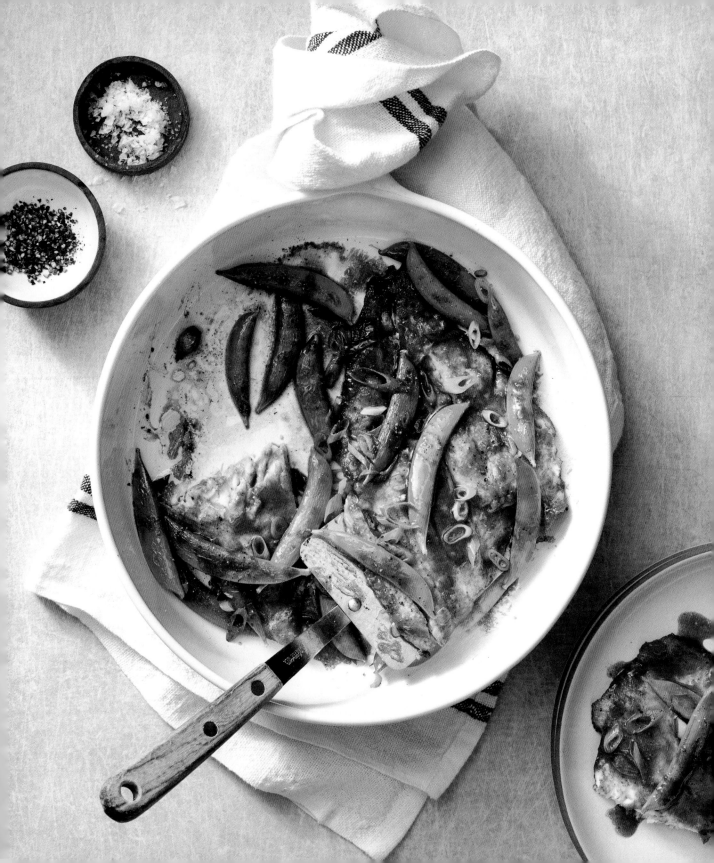

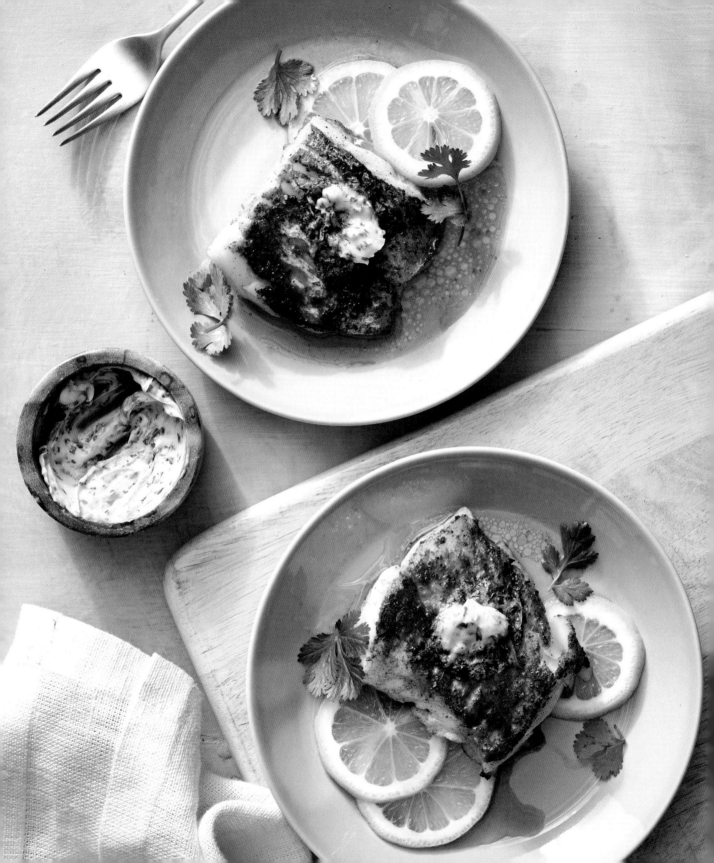

pan-seared cod with cilantro butter

Fresh herbs and lemon butter make it impossible to mess up this quick fish, and the recipe can be prepared a variety of ways. Try omitting the taco seasoning and substituting basil for the cilantro for a Mediterranean spin. Any mild white-fleshed fish such as flounder or orange roughy can be used in place of cod.

1 Sprinkle the taco seasoning over both sides of the fish. Heat a large nonstick skillet over medium-high. Coat the pan with cooking spray. Coat both sides of the fish with cooking spray; place in the pan. Cook for 3 minutes on each side or until the fish flakes easily when tested with a fork, or to the desired degree of doneness. Place the fish on a serving platter; squeeze the lemon quarters over the fish.

2 Place the butter, cilantro, lemon zest, and salt in a small bowl; stir until well blended. Serve the cilantro butter with the fish.

(SERVING SIZE: 1 FILLET AND ABOUT 2 TEASPOONS CILANTRO BUTTER): CALORIES 182; FAT 7G (SAT 4G, UNSAT 2G); PROTEIN 27G; CARB 1G; FIBER 0G; SUGARS 0G (ADDED SUGARS 0G); SODIUM 264MG; CALC 2% DV; POTASSIUM 6% DV

grass-fed butter

The meaning of "grass-fed" in the US varies greatly from livestock living strictly on grass to living only a small portion of their life on grass (see page 142), but there are studies that suggest grass-fed dairy products have some benefits. In countries where grass is the only or predominant source of food for cattle, an individual's intake of high-fat dairy is associated with a reduced cardiovascular risk. This is largely thought to be due to the milk of grass-fed cattle having higher levels of specific omega-3 fatty acids, which have an anti-inflammatory effect.

1 teaspoon All-Purpose
  Taco Seasoning (page 66)
  or store-bought organic
  taco seasoning
4 (6-ounce) cod fillets
Cooking spray
1 lemon, quartered
2 tablespoons butter, softened
2 tablespoons finely chopped
  fresh cilantro
½ teaspoon lemon zest
⅛ teaspoon kosher salt

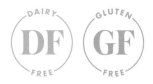

salmon over kale-quinoa salad

The omega-3 fats DHA and EPA in salmon and other oily fish play key roles in suppressing inflammation and boosting production of anti-inflammatory compounds. The American Heart Association recommends eating salmon or other fatty fish twice a week to reap the anti-inflammatory benefits from a cardiovascular standpoint. Choose wild salmon when possible, which has five to ten times fewer contaminants than farm-raised.

Cooking spray

4 (6-ounce) skinless salmon
  fillets

1 tablespoon olive oil

½ teaspoon salt

¼ teaspoon black pepper

6 cups thinly sliced lacinato
  kale

2 cups cooked quinoa

¼ cup Citrus Vinaigrette
  (page 75) or store-bought
  lemon or Greek vinaigrette

⅓ cup seedless red grapes,
  halved

1 Preheat the oven to 425°F. Line a 15 x 11-inch baking sheet with aluminum foil; coat the foil with cooking spray.

2 Place the salmon on the prepared pan. Rub evenly with the oil, ⅜ teaspoon of the salt, and the pepper. Bake for 10 minutes or until the fish flakes easily when tested with a fork.

3 While the fish cooks, place the kale, quinoa, vinaigrette, and grapes in a large bowl; toss to combine. Let stand for 5 minutes. Divide the salad among four plates. Top with the salmon.

(SERVING SIZE: 1¼ CUPS SALAD AND 1 FILLET): CALORIES 550; FAT 26G (SAT 4G, UNSAT 21G); PROTEIN 46G; CARB 33G; FIBER 5G; SUGARS 3G (ADDED SUGARS 0G); SODIUM 514MG; CALC 20% DV; POTASSIUM 24% DV

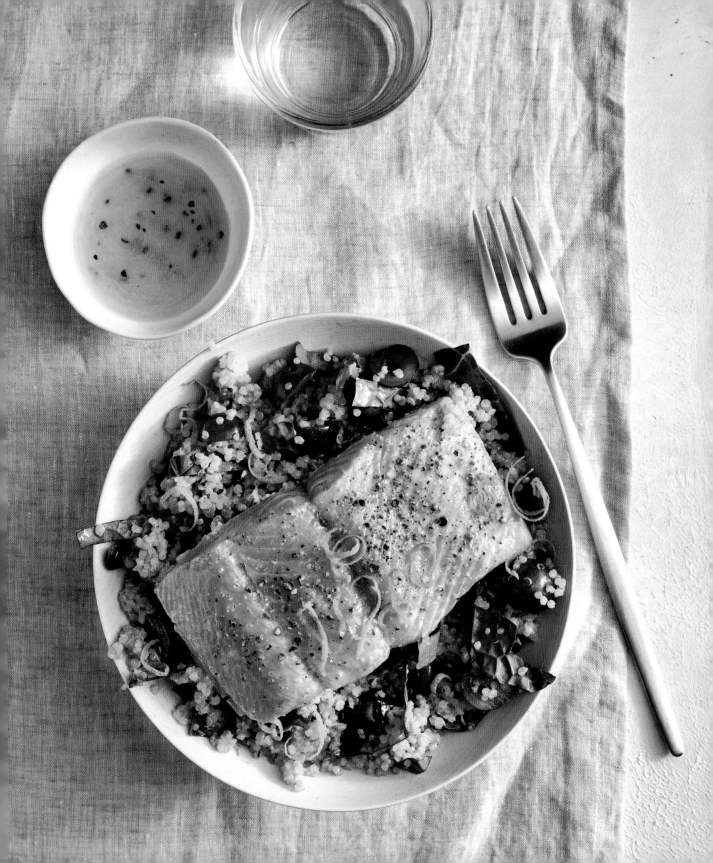

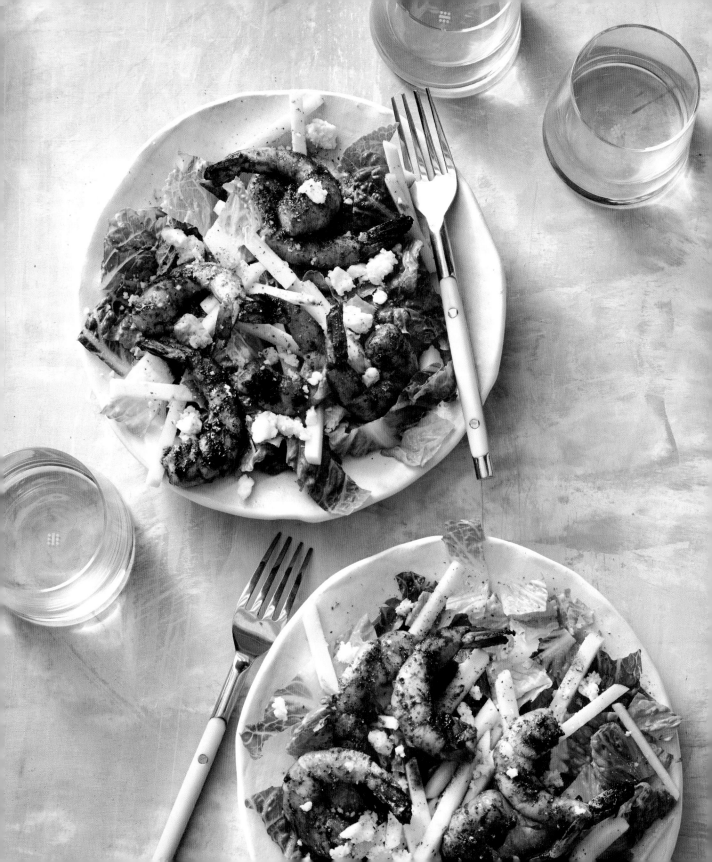

southwestern grilled shrimp salad

─── OPTIONAL ───

For an extra-quick meal, substitute 1¼ pounds of steamed peeled shrimp and skip cooking the shrimp in the skillet; add a little of the seasoning to the dressing instead. Both jicama and Granny Smith apples offer a slightly sweet crunch that complements the salad's other ingredients and textures.

1 Combine the shrimp, 1 tablespoon of the oil, the taco seasoning, and ⅛ teaspoon of the salt in a large bowl. Heat a grill or grill pan to medium-high and cook the shrimp for 2 to 3 minutes per side or until opaque throughout.

2 Place the lettuce and apple in a large bowl. Whisk together the remaining 2½ tablespoons oil, the lime juice, honey, vinegar, and remaining ⅛ teaspoon salt. Pour over the lettuce mixture and toss well to coat the greens. Divide the salad evenly among four plates, and top evenly with the shrimp. Sprinkle each salad with 1 tablespoon of the cheese.

(SERVING SIZE: 1 SALAD): CALORIES 324; FAT 15G (SAT 3G, UNSAT 11G); PROTEIN 37G; CARB 12G; FIBER 4G; SUGARS 7G (ADDED SUGARS 4G); SODIUM 493MG; CALC 19% DV; POTASSIUM 15% DV

DAIRY-FREE OPTION: Omit the cheese, and sprinkle the salad with 2 tablespoons toasted pumpkin seed kernels (pepitas).

- 1½ pounds peeled and deveined large shrimp
- 3½ tablespoons extra-virgin olive oil
- 2 teaspoons All-Purpose Taco Seasoning (page 66) or store-bought organic taco seasoning
- ¼ teaspoon kosher salt
- 6 cups chopped romaine lettuce
- ½ small jicama, or 1 Granny Smith apple, peeled and cut into matchsticks
- 1½ tablespoons fresh lime juice
- 1 tablespoon honey
- 2 teaspoons balsamic or red wine vinegar
- 4 tablespoons crumbled cotija cheese, queso fresco, or feta cheese

lemony shrimp and spinach with feta

Spinach is one of my favorite leafy greens to keep on hand because of its versatility in quick meal prep. While all leafy greens are recommended, spinach offers a mix of antioxidants that boost the immune system and suppress inflammation. Serve this over sautéed spaghetti squash strands, zucchini noodles, or a whole-grain pasta.

2 tablespoons olive oil

1½ pounds large shrimp, peeled and deveined

3 garlic cloves, minced

1½ cup unsalted chicken broth or vegetable broth

1 teaspoon lemon zest

3 tablespoons fresh lemon juice

1 (6-ounce) package fresh baby spinach

¼ teaspoon kosher salt

⅛ teaspoon black pepper

¼ cup crumbled feta cheese

1 Heat a large skillet over medium-high. Add the oil to the pan; swirl to coat. Add the shrimp and garlic to the pan; sauté for 3 to 4 minutes or until the shrimp just turn pink. Remove the shrimp mixture from the pan; keep warm.

2 Add the broth, lemon zest, and lemon juice to the skillet, stirring to loosen the particles from the bottom of the skillet. Cook for 4 to 5 minutes or until the liquid is reduced by half. Add the spinach, salt, and pepper; cook for 2 minutes or until the spinach is just wilted. Stir in the shrimp and sprinkle with the cheese. Serve immediately.

(SERVING SIZE: ¼ OF THE SHRIMP AND SPINACH): CALORIES 248; FAT 10G (SAT 3G, UNSAT 7G); PROTEIN 37G; CARB 4G; FIBER 1G; SUGARS 1G (ADDED SUGARS 0G); SODIUM 460MG; CALC 20% DV; POTASSIUM 10% DV

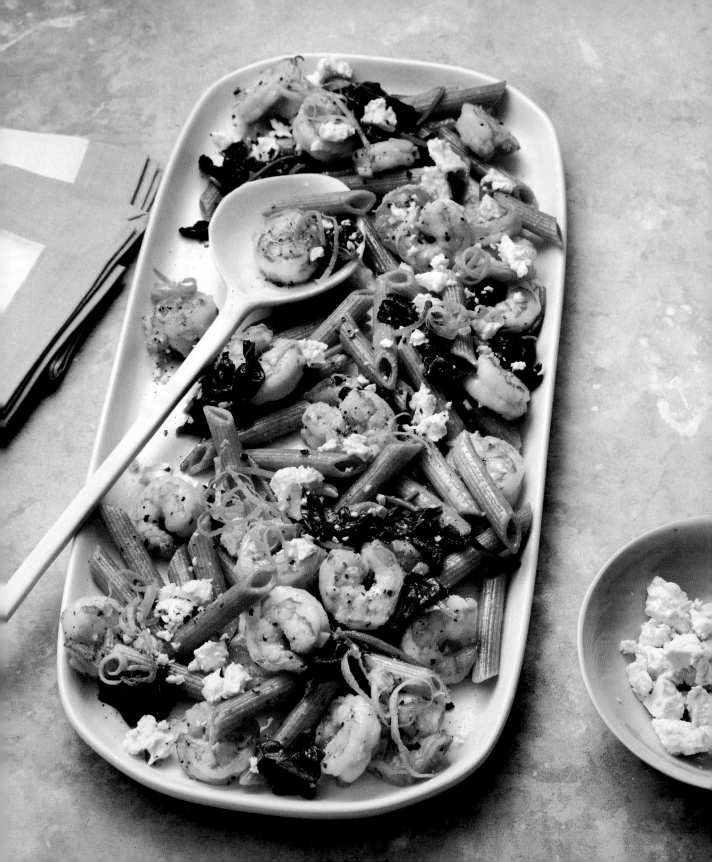

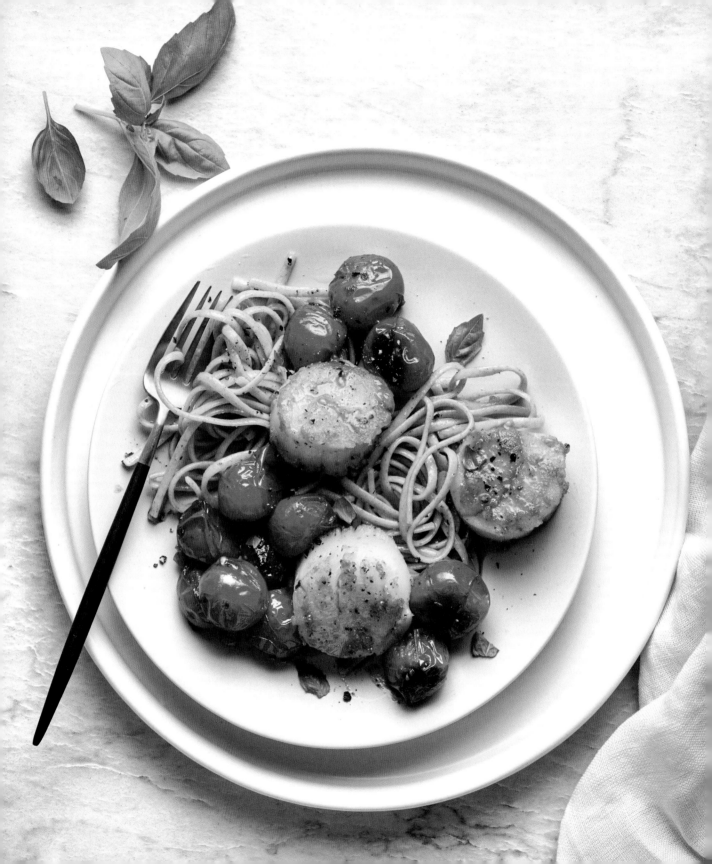

seared scallops with roasted tomatoes

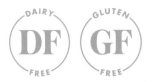

This recipe is a perfect example of how some of the best dishes are those with super-simple ingredients. Serve over chickpea or brown rice pasta, spaghetti squash strands, or zucchini noodles that have been tossed with a little olive oil and lemon zest.

1 Preheat the oven to 450°F. Line a 15 x 11-inch baking sheet with aluminum foil.

2 Combine the tomatoes, 1 tablespoon of the oil, the vinegar, ¼ teaspoon of the pepper, and ⅛ teaspoon of the salt in a medium bowl; toss well to coat. Spread the tomatoes on the prepared baking sheet. Roast for 10 minutes or until the tomatoes are soft and lightly charred in places.

3 While the tomatoes cook, heat a large cast-iron skillet over medium-high. Add the remaining 1 tablespoon oil to the skillet; swirl to coat. Pat the scallops dry; sprinkle both sides of the scallops with the remaining ¼ teaspoon pepper and remaining ⅛ teaspoon salt. Add the scallops to the skillet; cook for 2 minutes on each side or to the desired degree of doneness. Serve the scallops with the tomatoes; sprinkle evenly with the basil.

3 cups cherry tomatoes
2 tablespoons olive oil
1 teaspoon red wine vinegar
½ teaspoon black pepper
¼ teaspoon kosher salt
1½ pounds sea scallops
¼ cup thinly sliced fresh basil

(SERVING SIZE: ABOUT 4½ OUNCES SCALLOPS AND ABOUT ⅓ CUP TOMATOES): CALORIES 199; FAT 8G (SAT 1G, UNSAT 6G); PROTEIN 22G; CARB 10G; FIBER 1G; SUGARS 3G (ADDED SUGARS 0G); SODIUM 793MG; CALC 3% DV; POTASSIUM 13% DV

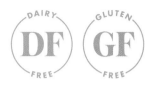

no-cook asian shrimp salad

Served chilled or slightly warm, this bright salad is ideal for summer dinners or weekday lunches. I like to top servings with a sprinkle of extra scallions, sesame seeds, or chopped peanuts or cashews. For a heartier salad, add slightly steamed shelled edamame.

1 (6-ounce) package snow peas

3 cups cooked brown rice

½ cup shredded carrot

⅓ cup sliced scallions (sliced on an angle)

1 pound cooked peeled fresh medium shrimp

2 tablespoons rice vinegar

2 tablespoons gluten-free lower-sodium soy sauce or tamari

1½ tablespoons sesame oil

1 teaspoon grated fresh ginger

1 Steam the peas according to the package directions and let cool.

2 Place the rice, carrot, scallions, shrimp, and cooled peas in a large bowl; toss well. Whisk together the vinegar, soy sauce, oil, and ginger in a small bowl. Pour over the rice mixture; toss well. Cover and chill until ready to serve.

(SERVING SIZE: 1¼ CUPS): CALORIES 349; FAT 7G (SAT 1G, UNSAT 5G); PROTEIN 32G; CARB 39G; FIBER 4G; SUGARS 2G (ADDED SUGARS 0G); SODIUM 422MG; CALC 11% DV; POTASSIUM 11% DV

types of peas

You'll see at least three types of peas used in this cookbook—green, snow, and snap. All three legumes are similar in nutrients, offering a healthy balance of carbs, fiber, and protein, as well as phytochemical compounds with anti-inflammatory and antioxidant effects. Each differs slightly in texture, flavor, and usage.

	GREEN (PER ½ CUP)	SNOW (PER 1 CUP)	SNAP (PER 1 CUP)
OTHER NAME(S)	Garden or sweet peas	Chinese pea pods	Sugar snap peas
TYPICALLY EATEN	Shelled	Shelled	Whole pod
CHARACTERISTICS	Round, sweet	Flat, dense	Sweet, plump, crisp
CALORIES	60	30	30
CARB	10g	5g	5g
FIBER	4g	2g	2g
SUGAR	4g	3g	3g
PROTEIN	4g	2g	2g
VITAMIN C	38% DV	50% DV	50% DV

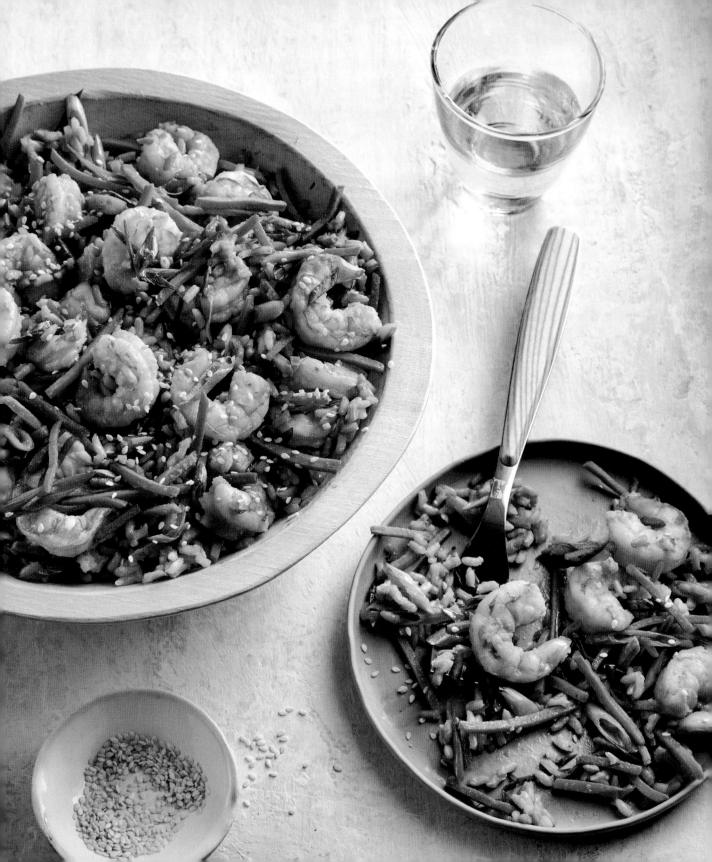

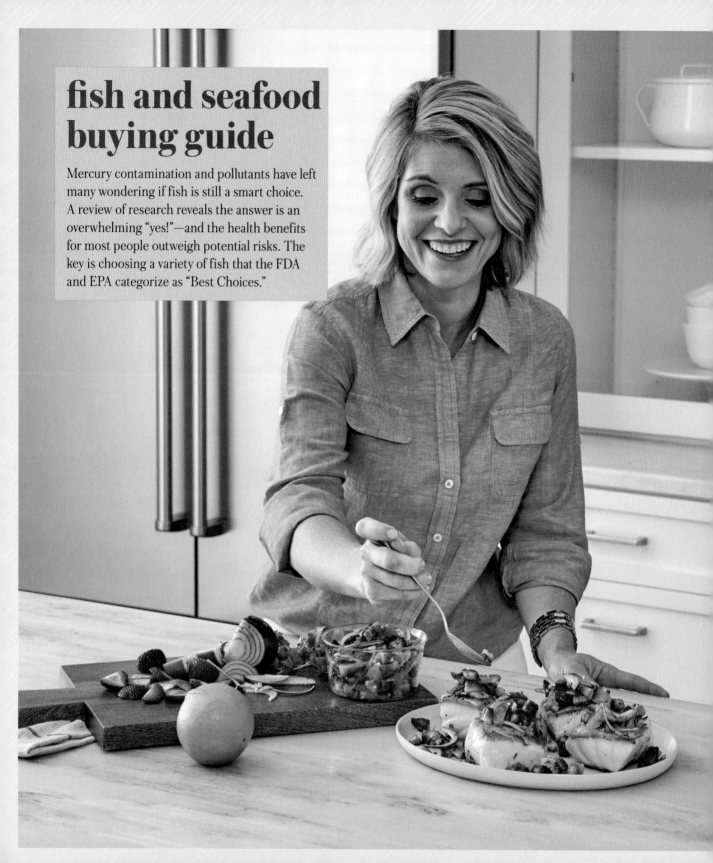

fish and seafood buying guide

Mercury contamination and pollutants have left many wondering if fish is still a smart choice. A review of research reveals the answer is an overwhelming "yes!"—and the health benefits for most people outweigh potential risks. The key is choosing a variety of fish that the FDA and EPA categorize as "Best Choices."

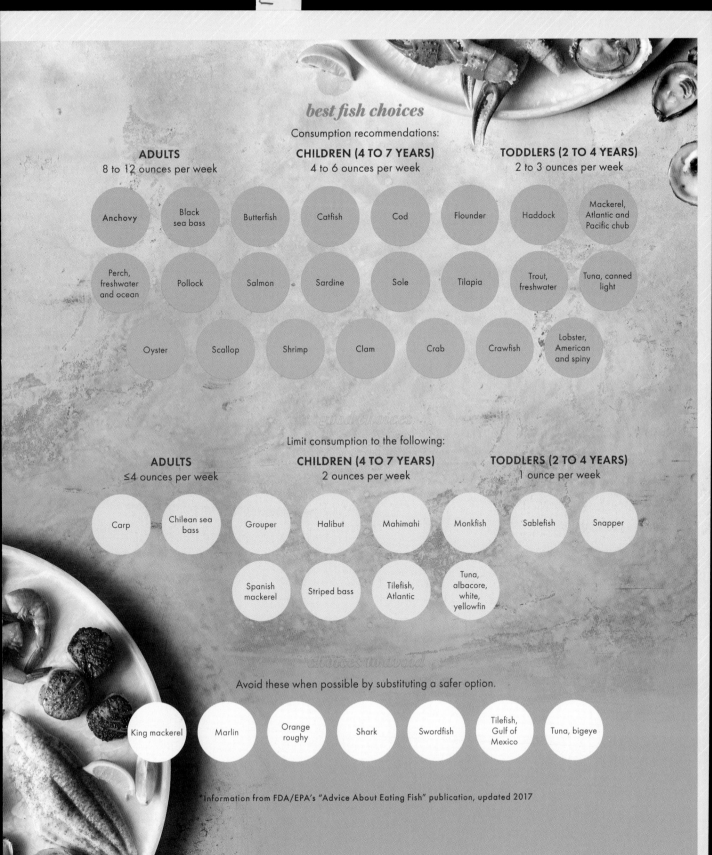

Meatless Meals

best fish choices

Consumption recommendations:

ADULTS
8 to 12 ounces per week

CHILDREN (4 TO 7 YEARS)
4 to 6 ounces per week

TODDLERS (2 TO 4 YEARS)
2 to 3 ounces per week

Anchovy · Black sea bass · Butterfish · Catfish · Cod · Flounder · Haddock · Mackerel, Atlantic and Pacific chub

Perch, freshwater and ocean · Pollock · Salmon · Sardine · Sole · Tilapia · Trout, freshwater · Tuna, canned light

Oyster · Scallop · Shrimp · Clam · Crab · Crawfish · Lobster, American and spiny

Limit consumption to the following:

ADULTS
≤4 ounces per week

CHILDREN (4 TO 7 YEARS)
2 ounces per week

TODDLERS (2 TO 4 YEARS)
1 ounce per week

Carp · Chilean sea bass · Grouper · Halibut · Mahimahi · Monkfish · Sablefish · Snapper

Spanish mackerel · Striped bass · Tilefish, Atlantic · Tuna, albacore, white, yellowfin

Avoid these when possible by substituting a safer option.

King mackerel · Marlin · Orange roughy · Shark · Swordfish · Tilefish, Gulf of Mexico · Tuna, bigeye

*Information from FDA/EPA's "Advice About Eating Fish" publication, updated 2017

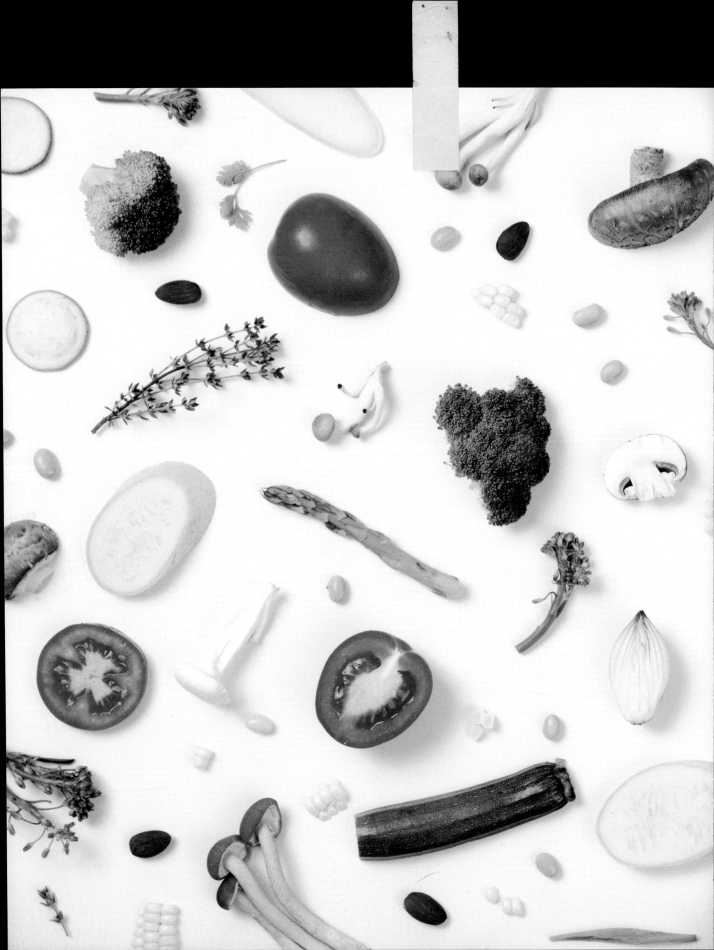

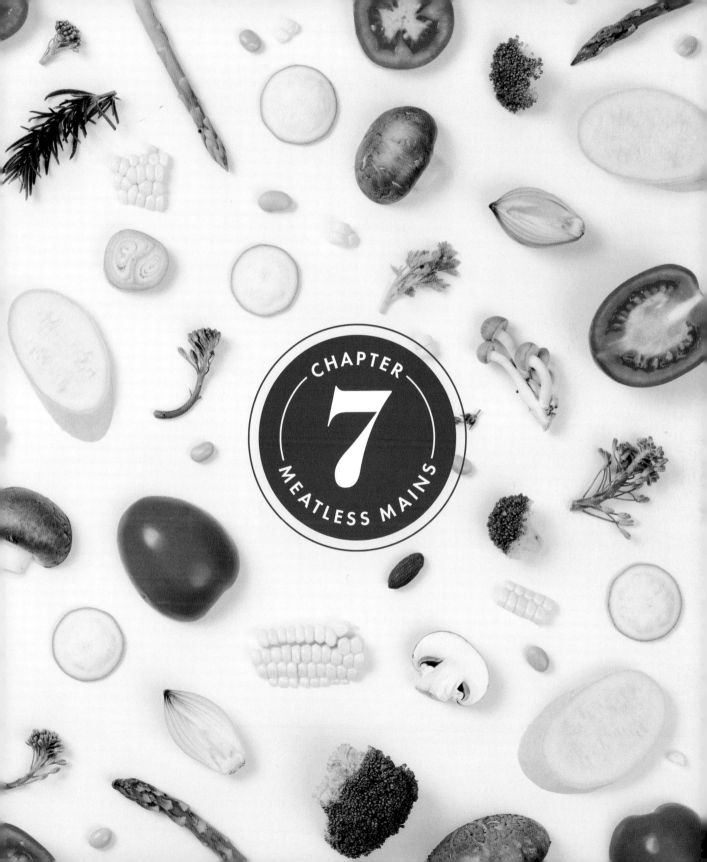

CHAPTER

7

MEATLESS MAINS

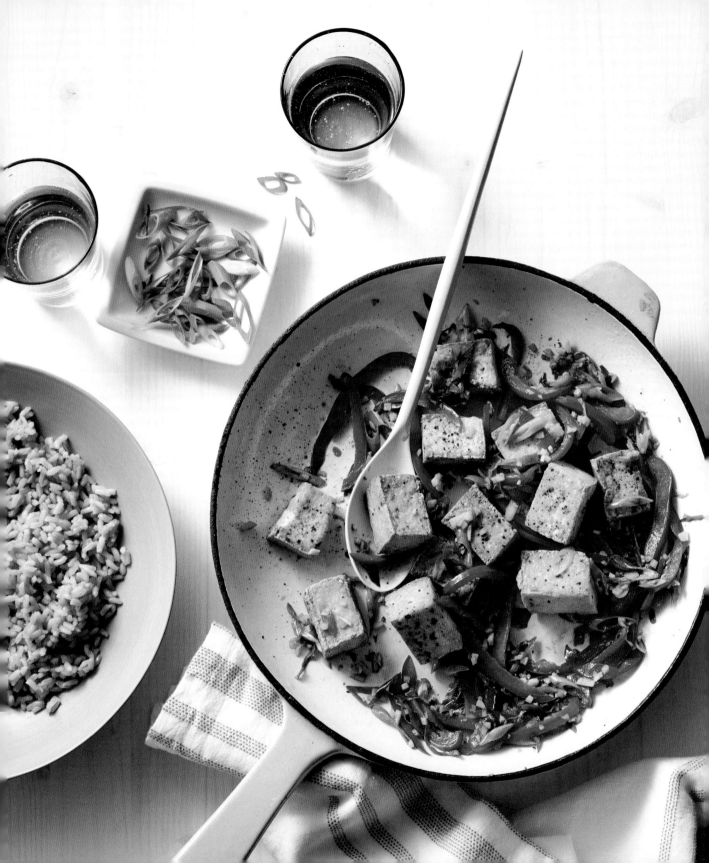

seared tofu with gingered vegetables

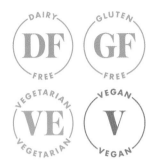

Letting the tofu stand while you're prepping the vegetables allows the liquid to drain so that the tofu will brown nicely in the skillet. Feel free to toss other veggies into the stir-fry to add additional color and nutrients. One package of ready-to-heat brown rice will give you 2 cups of hot cooked rice in less than two minutes.

1 Place the tofu on several layers of paper towels; let stand for 10 minutes. Cut the tofu into 1-inch cubes.

2 While the tofu stands, heat a large skillet over medium-high. Add 2 teaspoons of the oil to the pan; swirl to coat. Add the garlic, ginger, and bell pepper to the pan; sauté for 3 minutes. Stir in ¾ cup of the scallions, the vinegar, and soy sauce; cook for 30 seconds. Remove from the pan. Wipe the skillet with paper towels.

3 Heat the same skillet over medium-high. Add the remaining 1 teaspoon oil to the pan and swirl to coat. Sprinkle the tofu with the salt and black pepper. Add the tofu to the pan; cook for 8 minutes or until golden, turning to brown on all sides. Return the bell pepper mixture to the pan and cook for 1 minute or until thoroughly heated. Divide the rice among four bowls; top with the tofu mixture and sprinkle evenly with the remaining ¼ cup scallions.

(SERVING SIZE: ABOUT ½ CUP RICE AND 1 CUP TOFU MIXTURE): CALORIES 277; FAT 10G (SAT 1G, UNSAT 8G); PROTEIN 15G; CARB 31G; FIBER 4G; SUGARS 3G (ADDED SUGARS 0G); SODIUM 590MG; CALC 10% DV; POTASSIUM 4% DV

- 1 pound extra-firm tofu
- 3 teaspoons sesame oil
- 3 garlic cloves, minced
- 1 tablespoon minced fresh ginger
- 1 large red bell pepper, thinly sliced
- 1 cup sliced scallions
- 2 tablespoons rice vinegar
- 2 tablespoons gluten-free lower-sodium soy sauce or tamari
- ½ teaspoon kosher salt
- ¼ teaspoon black pepper
- 2 cups hot cooked brown rice

ginger

Adding a fresh, lemon-like spice to recipes, ginger comes from the roots of an Asian plant and has been used in complementary medicine for thousands of years. Many of the same compounds responsible for ginger's strong flavor also appear to be responsible for its documented anti-inflammatory effects, including pain relief for some with arthritis and joint pain. Its protective role against free radicals suggests it may even play a therapeutic role in preventing cancer development or growth.

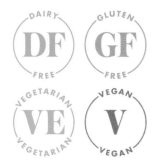

(DF) DAIRY FREE (GF) GLUTEN FREE (VE) VEGETARIAN (V) VEGAN

thai zoodle bowls

Zucchini noodles (or "zoodles"), my favorite veggie noodle to use, have a mild flavor that pairs well with most any sauce. With a softer texture than sweet potatoes and beets, zucchini are easier to spiralize and quicker to cook.

2 tablespoons sesame oil

1 cup thinly sliced red bell pepper

4 medium zucchini, spiralized into thick noodles (about 6 cups)

½ teaspoon kosher salt

3 cups fresh baby spinach

8 ounces extra-firm tofu, cut into ½-inch cubes

½ cup canned light coconut milk

¼ cup water

3 tablespoons almond butter

2 tablespoons yellow curry paste

¼ cup chopped unsalted cashews

4 lime wedges

1 Heat a large nonstick skillet over medium-high. Add 1 tablespoon of the oil to the pan; swirl to coat. Add the bell pepper and sauté for 4 minutes. Add the zucchini spirals; sprinkle with ¼ teaspoon of the salt. Cover and cook for 2 minutes. Stir in the spinach and cook until wilted. Place the zucchini mixture in a large bowl.

2 Add the remaining 1 tablespoon oil to the pan; swirl to coat. Add the tofu; cook, stirring occasionally, for 4 minutes.

3 Combine the coconut milk, water, almond butter, curry paste, and remaining ¼ teaspoon salt in a medium bowl. Add ½ cup of the sauce to the zucchini mixture; toss to combine. Divide the zucchini mixture among four bowls; top evenly with the tofu, remaining ½ cup sauce, and the cashews. Serve with the lime wedges.

(SERVING SIZE: 1 BOWL): CALORIES 316; FAT 23G (SAT 5G, UNSAT 17G); PROTEIN 13G; CARB 18G; FIBER 5G; SUGARS 7G (ADDED SUGARS 0G); SODIUM 670MG; CALC 16% DV; POTASSIUM 15% DV

coconut milk

There's a big difference between canned coconut milk and the coconut milk sold in cartons in the dairy case when it comes to consistency, nutrition, and best usage. Here are the differences:

CANNED COCONUT MILK is made from coconut flesh that's been simmered and strained to create a thick, creamy liquid. Canned coconut milk often serves as the base for Thai and Asian dishes and has a slightly sweet aroma, but no added sugars. It's a calorie-dense liquid, though, with 1 cup having approximately 400 calories and 36 grams of primarily saturated fats.

COCONUT MILK IN THE DAIRY CASE is essentially a very watered-down version of canned coconut milk. It's grown in popularity as an alternative to dairy milk for vegetarians and vegans and for those who want a dairy-free milk that's not made from nuts or soy. To avoid added sugars, purchase "unsweetened" versions. One cup of coconut milk from a carton has approximately 60 calories and 5 grams of saturated fat.

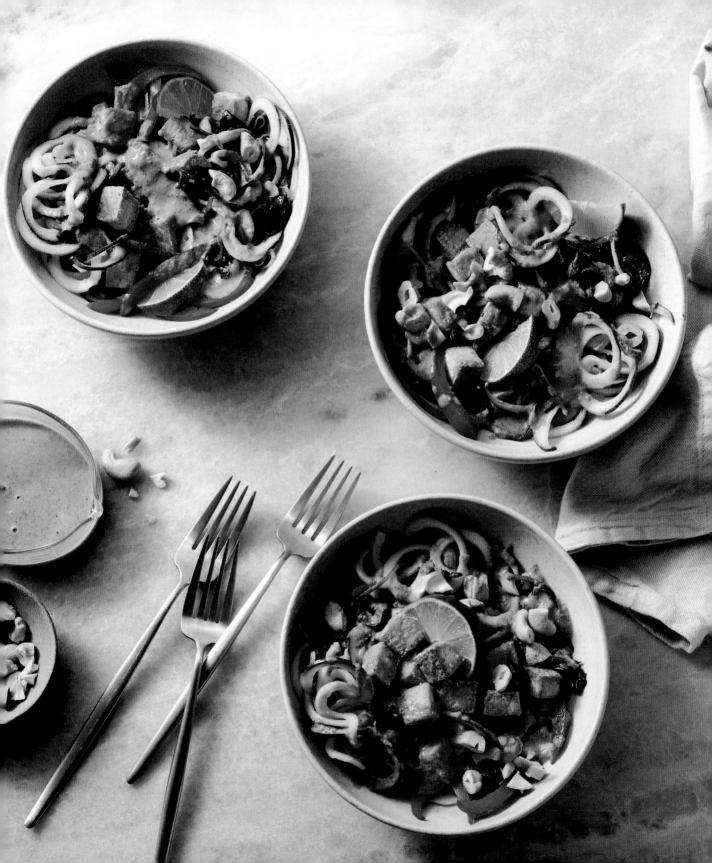

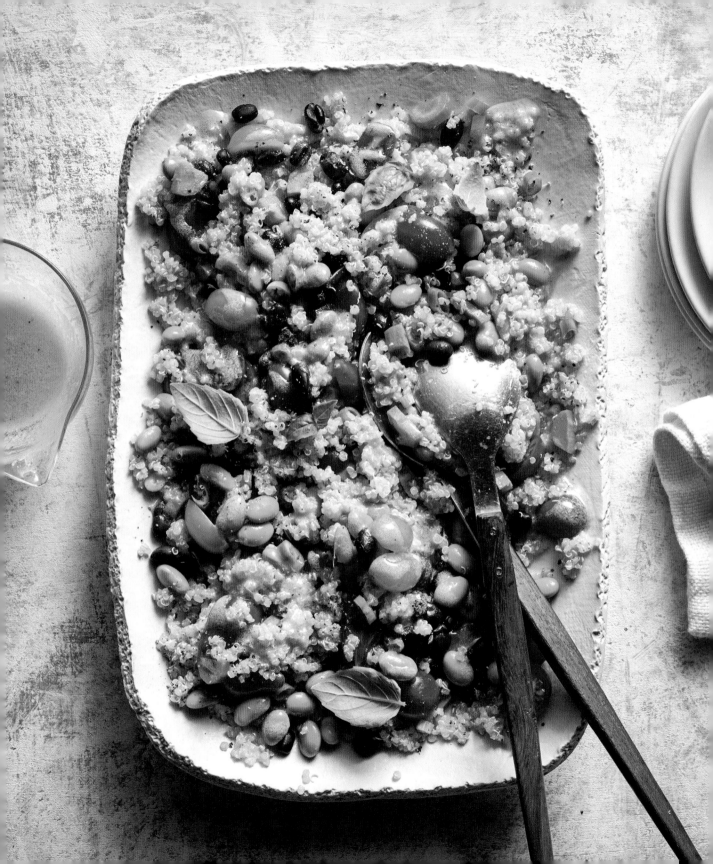

lemony black bean–quinoa salad

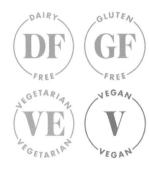

Delicious and filling, this grain-and-bean salad was created as a meatless dinner option, but it's also good topped with cooked tofu, chicken, or shrimp, or served as a side dish. There's no pressure to make the dressing. When short on time, I like using Tessemae's Lemon Garlic Dressing. Another option is to add 1 to 2 teaspoons of fresh lemon juice to a basic olive oil vinaigrette.

1 Cook the edamame in the microwave according to the package directions. Let cool for 10 minutes.

2 Combine the quinoa, tomato, scallions, carrot, black beans, basil, salt, pepper, and 1 cup of the cooled edamame in a large bowl; reserve the remaining edamame for another use. Add the dressing and stir gently to combine. Store, covered, in the refrigerator until ready to serve.

(SERVING SIZE: 1¼ CUPS): CALORIES 340; FAT 14G (SAT 2G, UNSAT 11G); PROTEIN 14G; CARB 40G; FIBER 9G; SUGARS 3G (ADDED SUGARS 0G); SODIUM 307MG; CALC 9% DV; POTASSIUM 9% DV

canned food sodium hacks

While fresh is ideal, canned is more realistic at times. However, the sodium in canned items is always higher than fresh due to the need for preservatives. Try these two tricks to significantly reduce sodium when using canned goods:

- Buy canned products that say "reduced sodium" or "no salt added." You can always add salt or seasoning, but this allows you to control the amount of sodium added.
- Drain and rinse canned items to reduce the sodium by up to 40 percent. For beans, this often means ditching 200mg of sodium per ½ cup.

1 (10-ounce) package frozen shelled edamame

3 cups cooked quinoa

1 cup chopped tomato or halved cherry tomatoes

¼ cup sliced scallions

⅓ cup chopped carrot

1 cup canned black beans, rinsed and drained

½ cup chopped fresh basil

½ teaspoon kosher salt

¼ teaspoon black pepper

⅓ cup Citrus Vinaigrette (page 75) or store-bought lemon or Greek vinaigrette

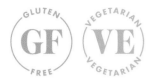

gluten-free margherita flatbread

No yeast required, hard to mess up, and worth the work: These are my qualifications for any dough at my house, and this one meets them all! Almond flour gives the crust a golden color and rich flavor thanks to the almonds' healthy fats, which replace the refined carbs used in other pizza crusts. Don't let the total amount of fat scare you away—the fats are primarily heart-healthy and packed with omega-3s. Pair these flatbreads with a salad and glass of wine, or serve as an appetizer or snack.

1½ cups blanched almond flour (about 5¼ ounces)

1 ounce Parmesan cheese, grated (about ¼ cup)

½ teaspoon baking soda

½ teaspoon plus ⅛ teaspoon kosher salt

2 tablespoons 1% milk or unsweetened nondairy milk

1 large egg, lightly beaten

2 teaspoons olive oil or jarred basil pesto

2 medium plum tomatoes, cut into ¼-inch-thick rounds and quartered

4 ounces fresh part-skim mozzarella cheese, cut into 1-inch cubes

⅓ cup roughly torn fresh basil

Store-bought balsamic glaze (such as Gia Russa; optional)

1 Whisk together the almond flour, Parmesan, baking soda, and the ½ teaspoon salt in a medium bowl. Stir in the milk and egg, and knead until the dough is smooth. Shape into 2 equal (4½-ounce) ovals; wrap in plastic wrap and refrigerate until slightly firm, about 30 minutes.

2 Preheat the oven to 350°F.

3 Place 1 dough oval in the center of a large piece of parchment paper and place another piece of parchment on top. Roll the dough into a 13½-inch oblong shape, approximately ¼ inch thick. Slide the dough, with the parchment, onto a large rimmed baking sheet. Repeat the procedure with the remaining dough. Remove and discard the top sheets of parchment. Bake until golden and crisp on the edges, about 13 minutes.

4 Remove from the oven and brush the crusts with oil. Arrange the tomatoes and cheese evenly over the crusts, leaving a ½-inch border. Bake until the cheese is melted, 4 to 6 minutes. Top with the basil and sprinkle evenly with the ⅛ teaspoon salt. Drizzle with balsamic glaze, if desired, and cut each pizza in half before serving.

(SERVING SIZE: ½ OF 1 PIZZA): CALORIES 259; FAT 21G (SAT 4G, UNSAT 15G); PROTEIN 13G; CARB 8G; FIBER 3G; SUGARS 2G (ADDED SUGARS 0G); SODIUM 530MG; CALC 26% DV; POTASSIUM 7% DV

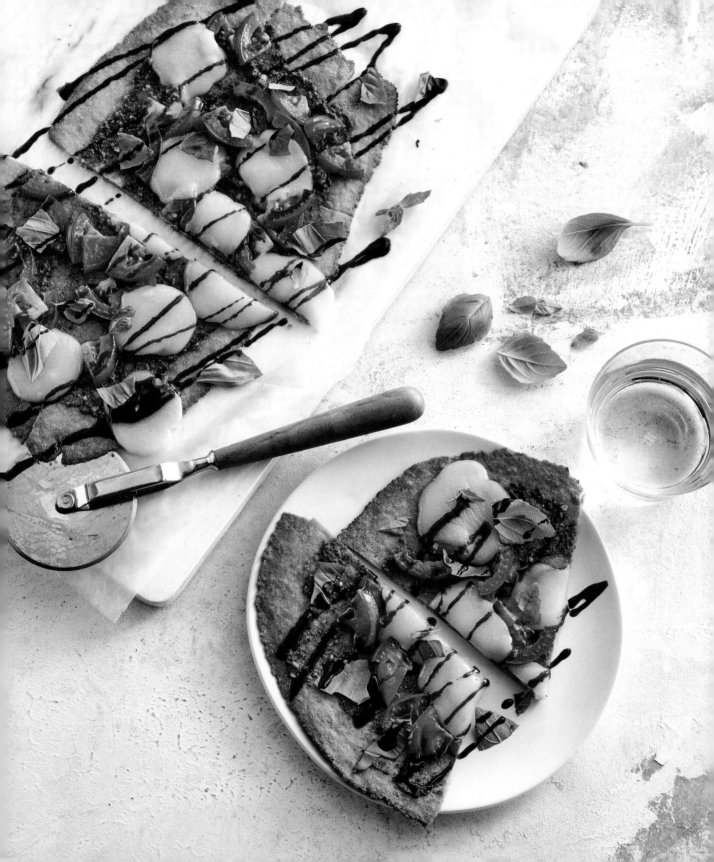

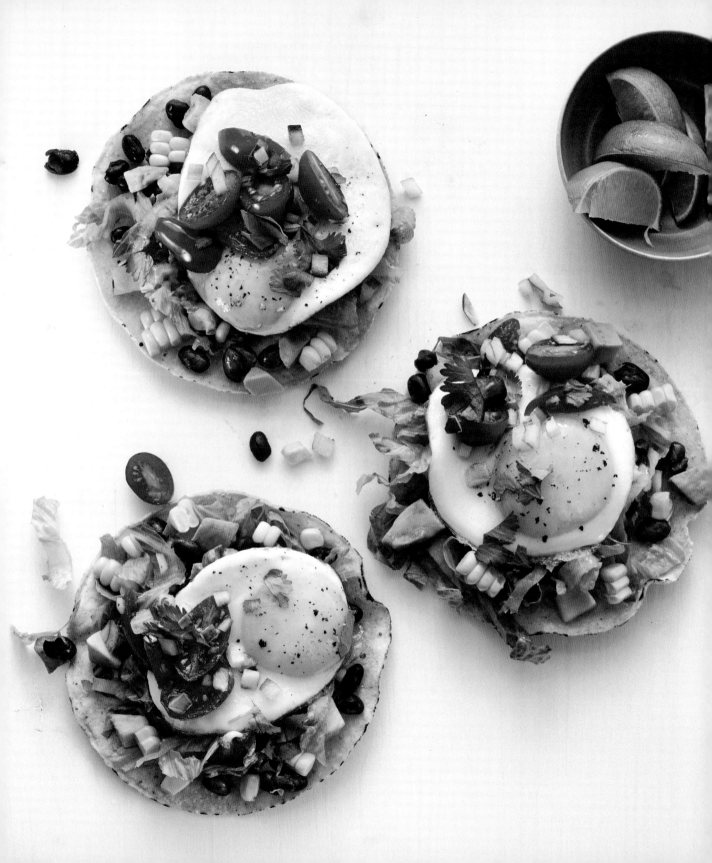

huevos rancheros tostadas

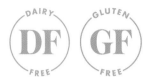

It's easy to get a head start on this recipe since you can be make the tostada shells up to three days in advance and store them in an airtight container at room temp. And you can stir together the bean salad up to two days in advance—just don't add the lettuce until right before serving.

1 Preheat the oven to 375°F. Line a baking sheet with aluminum foil. Lightly coat both sides of each tortilla with cooking spray; place on the prepared baking sheet. Bake until browned and crisp, 13 to 14 minutes, turning once.

2 Meanwhile, stir together the tomatoes, cilantro, onion, 2 tablespoons of the lime juice, and ⅛ teaspoon of the salt in a small bowl. Let stand until ready to serve.

3 Combine the beans, corn, and avocado in a medium bowl. In a small bowl, whisk together the oil, ¼ teaspoon of the salt, and the remaining 2 tablespoons lime juice. Pour over the bean mixture and stir to combine. Add the lettuce and toss gently to coat.

4 Lightly coat a large nonstick skillet with cooking spray and heat over medium. Gently break the eggs into the hot skillet and sprinkle with the remaining ⅛ teaspoon salt; cook for 2 minutes. Cover and cook until the desired degree of doneness, about 2 minutes more. To serve, place one toasted tortilla on each of 4 plates. Top the tortillas evenly with the bean mixture, cooked eggs, and salsa. Garnish with cilantro, if desired.

(SERVING SIZE: 1 TORTILLA, 1 CUP BEAN SALAD, 1 EGG, AND ¼ CUP SALSA): CALORIES 340; FAT 16G (SAT 3G, UNSAT 11G); PROTEIN 16G; CARB 37G; FIBER 10G; SUGARS 4G (ADDED SUGARS 0G); SODIUM 346MG; CALC 12% DV; POTASSIUM 16% DV

4 (6-inch) corn tortillas

Cooking spray

1 cup cherry tomatoes, quartered

3 tablespoons chopped fresh cilantro, plus more for garnish

2 tablespoons finely chopped red onion or shallot

4 tablespoons fresh lime juice

½ teaspoon kosher salt

1 (15-ounce) can no-salt-added black beans, rinsed and drained

½ cup fresh corn kernels (about 1 ear)

1 ripe avocado, chopped

1 tablespoon extra-virgin olive oil

2 to 3 cups chopped romaine lettuce

4 large eggs

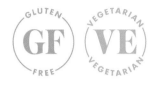

roasted veggie–polenta bowl

This recipe is so satisfying and filling, I promise you won't miss the meat! Homemade lemon pepper—just a quick mix of freshly ground black pepper and lemon zest—gives the roasted vegetables a savory, tangy kick that complements the creamy polenta.

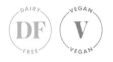

1 pound zucchini (about 2 medium), halved lengthwise and cut into ⅓-inch-thick slices

2 cups fresh broccoli florets

1 medium red onion, chopped

1 cup cherry tomatoes

5 teaspoons olive oil

1½ teaspoons garlic powder

¾ teaspoon kosher salt

1 teaspoon lemon zest

½ teaspoon black pepper

1¼ cups stone-ground yellow cornmeal

2 cups low-sodium vegetable broth or chicken broth

3 cups 1% milk

1½ teaspoons minced fresh thyme

½ ounce Parmesan cheese, grated (about ⅓ cup)

1 Preheat the oven to 425°F. Line a rimmed baking sheet with aluminum foil.

2 Combine the zucchini, broccoli, onion, tomatoes, oil, garlic powder, and ¼ teaspoon of the salt in a large bowl; toss to combine. Arrange in an even layer on the prepared baking sheet, and roast until the vegetables are tender and browned and the tomatoes have burst, 15 to 20 minutes. Whisk together the lemon zest and pepper in a small bowl; sprinkle over the vegetables.

3 Meanwhile, combine the cornmeal, broth, milk, and thyme in a microwavable 2-quart baking dish or large glass measuring cup and whisk until blended. Microwave on high in 5-minute intervals, whisking after each interval, until the polenta is creamy and tender, about 15 minutes. Gently whisk the polenta until smooth. Add the Parmesan and remaining ½ teaspoon salt, and whisk well. Spoon the polenta into four bowls and top with the roasted vegetables.

(SERVING SIZE: ABOUT 1¼ CUPS POLENTA AND 1 CUP VEGETABLES): CALORIES 336; FAT 10G (SAT 3G, UNSAT 6G); PROTEIN 13G; CARB 50G; FIBER 10G; SUGARS 15G (ADDED SUGARS 0G); SODIUM 608MG; CALC 33% DV; POTASSIUM 17% DV

DAIRY-FREE AND VEGAN OPTION: Prepare the recipe as directed, substituting unsweetened nondairy milk (such as almond or soy) for the 1% milk and omitting the Parmesan cheese. Sprinkle each serving with ½ tablespoon toasted pine nuts.

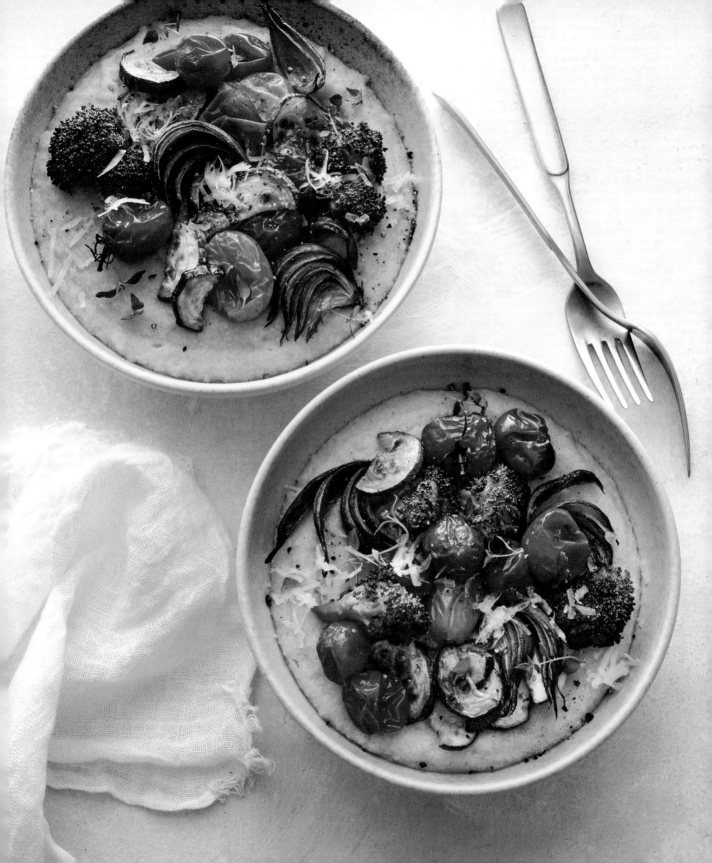

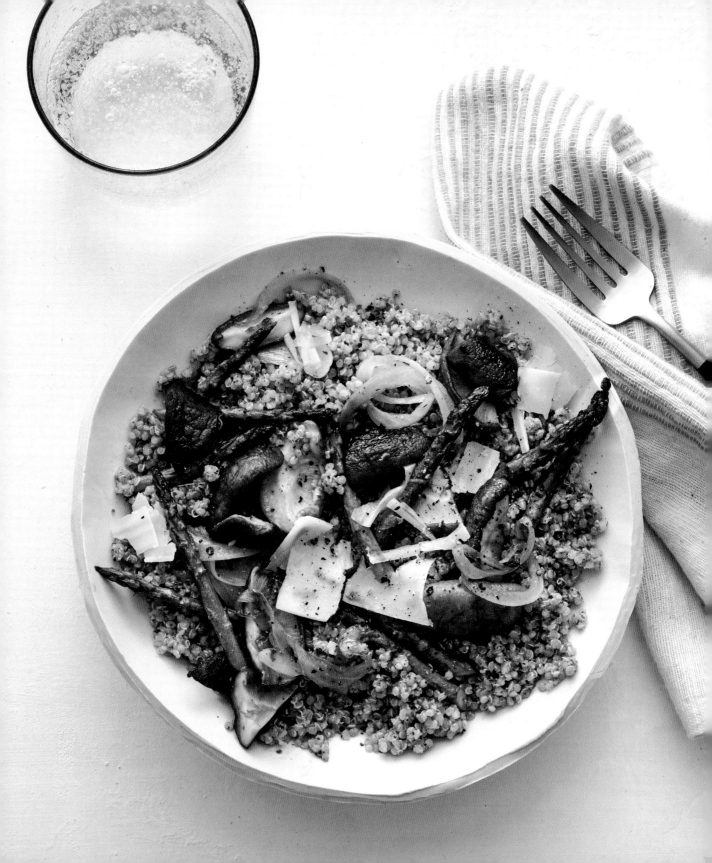

pesto spring grain bowl

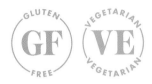

Grain bowls can be made ahead or prepared in just a few minutes using any cooked or ready-to-heat grain you have on hand. Leftovers make a hearty lunch, so prepare an extra serving to pack for the next day. Top with shredded rotisserie chicken, sautéed tofu, or grilled shrimp for a protein boost.

1 Heat a large skillet over medium-high. Add 1 teaspoon of the oil to the pan; swirl to coat. Add the mushrooms; cook, stirring occasionally, until the mushrooms are browned and the liquid they release has evaporated, about 6 minutes. Sprinkle with ⅛ teaspoon of the salt; transfer to a plate.

2 Reduce the heat to medium; add 2 teaspoons of the oil to the skillet and swirl to coat. Add the onion and asparagus; cook, stirring occasionally, until just tender, about 6 minutes. Sprinkle with ⅛ teaspoon of the salt; transfer to the plate with the mushrooms.

3 Place the farro in a large bowl. Combine the remaining 1 tablespoon oil, remaining ¼ teaspoon salt, the pesto, and vinegar in a small bowl; pour over the farro and toss to coat. Divide the farro evenly among four serving bowls. Top evenly with the asparagus mixture and the mushrooms. Sprinkle each bowl evenly with the Parmesan.

(SERVING SIZE: 1 BOWL): CALORIES 329; FAT 11G (SAT 2G, UNSAT 8G); PROTEIN 13G; CARB 48G; FIBER 6G; SUGARS 3G (ADDED SUGARS 0G); SODIUM 435MG; CALC 15% DV; POTASSIUM 6% DV

- 2 tablespoons olive oil
- 2 cups shiitake mushrooms, trimmed and sliced
- ½ teaspoon kosher salt
- 1 sweet onion, thinly sliced
- 8 ounces fresh asparagus, cut into 2-inch pieces
- 4 cups hot cooked farro, quinoa, or brown rice
- 1 tablespoon Simple Green Pesto (page 67) or store-bought pesto
- 2 teaspoons sherry vinegar or fresh lemon juice
- 1 ounce Parmesan cheese, shaved (about ¼ cup)

shiitake mushrooms

Research suggests that eating shiitake mushrooms daily lowers inflammatory markers and improves immune system function. This isn't limited to shiitakes, though. Oyster and enoki mushrooms also have anti-inflammatory powers. Make sure you eat them raw or cooked at low to moderate temps for the most anti-inflammatory impact.

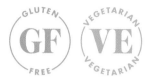

GF — GLUTEN FREE

VE — VEGETARIAN

quick roasted tomato pasta

Think a homemade tomato sauce in 15 minutes is impossible? This recipe offers up a quick, flavorful sauce. I'm partial to a chickpea or other legume-based pasta for the health perks, but you can use any whole-grain pasta.

8 ounces uncooked chickpea spaghetti

3 cups cherry tomatoes

2 tablespoons olive oil

2 teaspoons red wine vinegar

½ teaspoon kosher salt

⅛ teaspoon crushed red pepper

⅓ cup chopped or torn fresh basil leaves

½ cup crumbled semisoft goat cheese (2 ounces)

1 Preheat the oven to 450°F.

2 Cook the pasta according to the package directions in a large Dutch oven. Drain, reserving ⅓ cup of the cooking water. Return the spaghetti to the pot; keep warm.

3 Meanwhile, combine the tomatoes, 1 tablespoon of the oil, the vinegar, ½ teaspoon of the salt, and the pepper on a jelly-roll pan and toss well to coat. Bake for 10 minutes or until soft and lightly charred in places.

4 Add the tomatoes and any juices from the pan to the spaghetti in the Dutch oven. Add 3 tablespoons of the reserved cooking water to the jelly-roll pan, scraping to loosen any browned bits; pour the water and remaining 1 tablespoon oil into the pot. Place the Dutch oven over medium heat. Add the remaining reserved cooking water, 1 tablespoon at a time, until the pasta mixture is moist, tossing frequently. Stir in the basil. Sprinkle with the cheese. Serve immediately.

(SERVING SIZE: ABOUT 1⅓ CUPS): CALORIES 322; FAT 15G (SAT 4G, UNSAT 9G); PROTEIN 18G; CARB 36G; FIBER 9G; SUGARS 8G (ADDED SUGARS 0G); SODIUM 365MG; CALC 11% DV; POTASSIUM 6% DV

legume-based pastas

Whole-grain pastas provide more nutrients than refined types, but they still impact your blood sugar—sometimes not much differently than refined types. A legume-based pasta made from chickpeas or lentils has a lower glycemic effect, as well as more fiber and protein. Make sure to watch the cooking time. Legume-based pastas get gummy quickly if overcooked. Use the lower end of the cooking time range listed on the package.

PASTA TYPE (2 OUNCES DRY/ APPROX. 1 CUP COOKED)	CALORIES	CARBS	FIBER	PROTEIN
Whole wheat	230	47g	6g	9g
Brown rice	190	42g	4g	4g
Chickpea	190	32g	8g	14g
Green lentil	200	35g	7g	14g

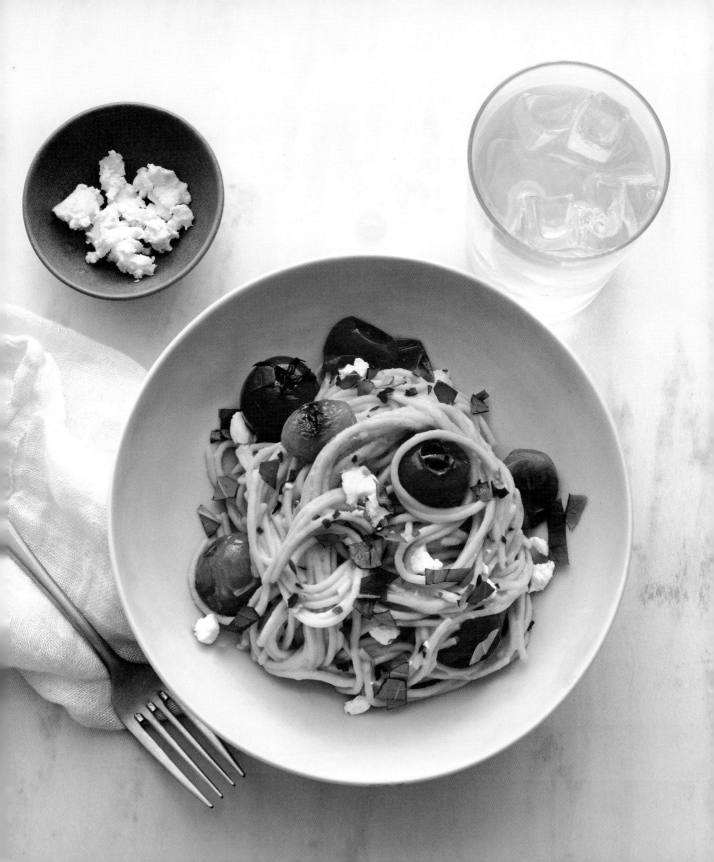

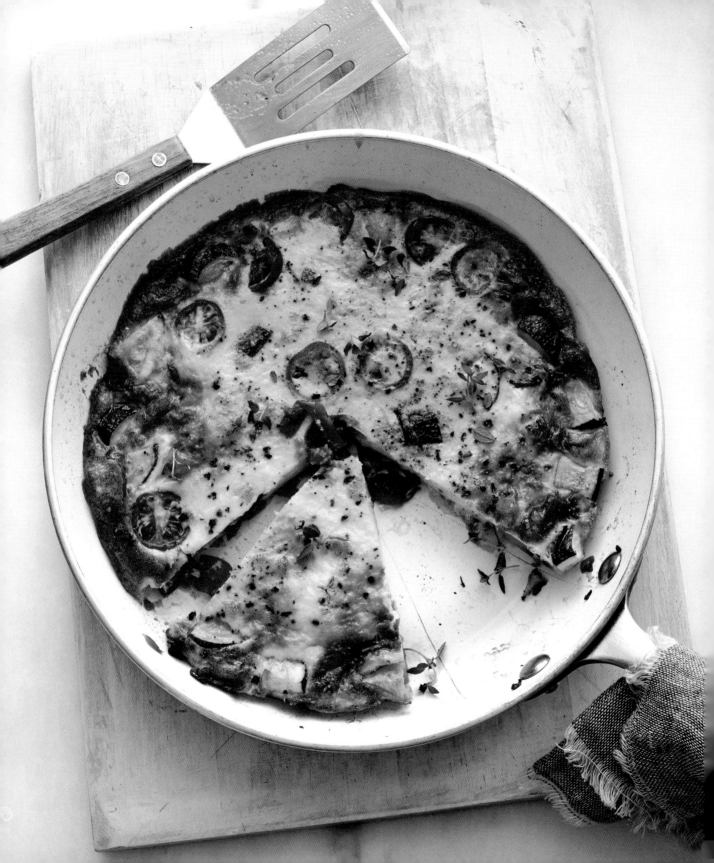

zucchini frittata with goat cheese

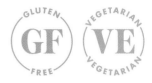

No dinner plans? No problem. Eggs are always a hit for dinner, and frittatas are easy to throw together—not to mention way less complicated than an omelet. Change up your frittata ingredients based on what vegetables, herbs, and cheeses you have on hand. I've never had a bad combo!

1 Preheat the broiler to high.

2 Whisk together the half-and-half, thyme, salt, pepper, and eggs in a large bowl.

3 Heat a medium ovenproof skillet over medium. Add the oil to the pan; swirl to coat. Add the shallots and zucchini; sauté for 5 minutes or until the zucchini begins to soften. Add the tomatoes and the egg mixture to the pan; sprinkle with the cheese. Cook for 5 minutes or until the eggs are partially set. Place the pan in the oven; broil for 2 to 3 minutes or until the top is lightly browned and the eggs are set. Remove the pan from the oven. Cut the frittata into 8 wedges. Garnish with thyme sprigs, if desired.

(SERVING SIZE: 2 WEDGES): CALORIES 216; FAT 15G (SAT 6G, UNSAT 8G); PROTEIN 14G; CARB 7G; FIBER 2G; SUGARS 4G (ADDED SUGARS 0G); SODIUM 417MG; CALC 11% DV; POTASSIUM 8% DV

- 2 tablespoons half-and-half
- 2 teaspoons chopped fresh thyme, plus sprigs for garnish (optional)
- ½ teaspoon kosher salt
- ¼ teaspoon black pepper
- 6 large eggs
- 2 teaspoons olive oil
- ½ cup thinly sliced shallots
- 1 cup diced zucchini
- 1 cup halved cherry or grape tomatoes
- ½ cup crumbled goat cheese (2 ounces)

eggs and brain health

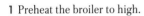

Packed with protein and low in calories, eggs are also a good source of vitamin D. It's estimated that up to 75 percent of us don't get enough vitamin D—a scary fact in light of a recent study that found that older adults who were moderately deficient in vitamin D had a 53 percent increased risk of developing Alzheimer's. Adequate intake of vitamin D appears to have an anti-inflammatory effect on the brain, as well as other positive effects on memory, depression, and preventing brain deterioration that are being investigated.

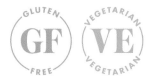

greek spaghetti squash toss

If you don't have spaghetti squash already cooked, follow the directions on page 53 to quickly cook one in the microwave. Make sure to toss well to coat every strand of this simple skillet dinner. The end result is a quick, veggie-based meal—a nice alternative to salads when you want to fill up on vegetables.

1 tablespoon olive oil
1 cup thinly sliced red onion
2 garlic cloves, minced
1 (15-ounce) can no-salt-added chickpeas, rinsed and drained
2 teaspoons chopped fresh thyme
1 cup cherry tomatoes, halved
6 cups cooked spaghetti squash strands
4 cups torn fresh baby spinach leaves
½ teaspoon kosher salt
6 tablespoons crumbled feta cheese

Heat a large nonstick skillet over medium-high. Add the oil to the pan; swirl to coat. Add the onion and garlic; sauté for 4 minutes. Add the chickpeas, thyme, and tomatoes; cook for 1 minute. Add the spaghetti squash, spinach, and salt; toss gently to combine. Cook for 2 minutes or until the spinach is just wilted. Divide the squash mixture among four bowls, and sprinkle each with 1½ tablespoons of the cheese.

(SERVING SIZE: ABOUT 2 CUPS): CALORIES 270; FAT 8G (SAT 3G, UNSAT 4G); PROTEIN 11G; CARB 40G; FIBER 10G; SUGARS 9G (ADDED SUGARS 0G); SODIUM 482MG; CALC 24% DV; POTASSIUM 13% DV

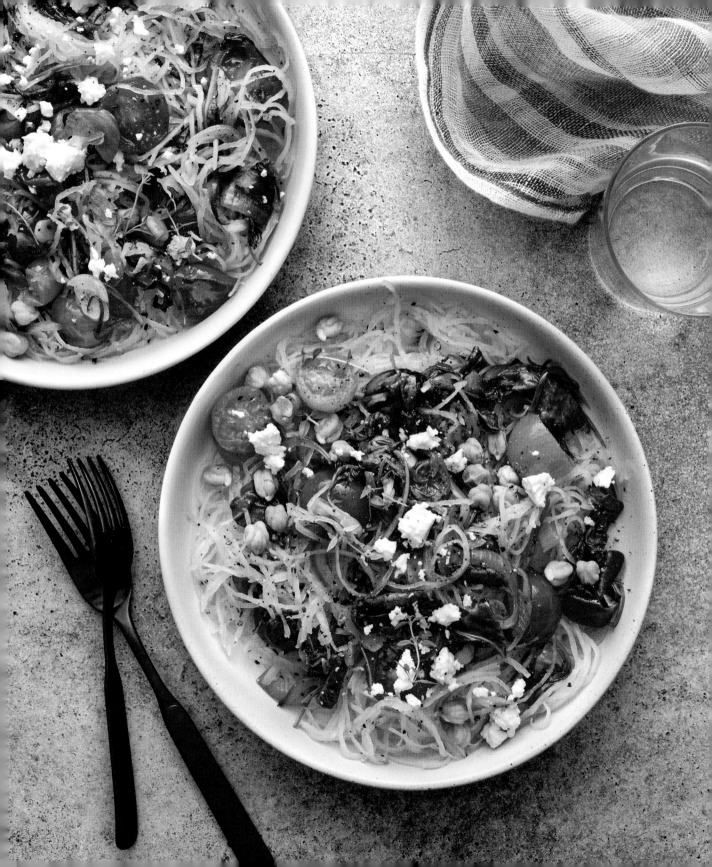

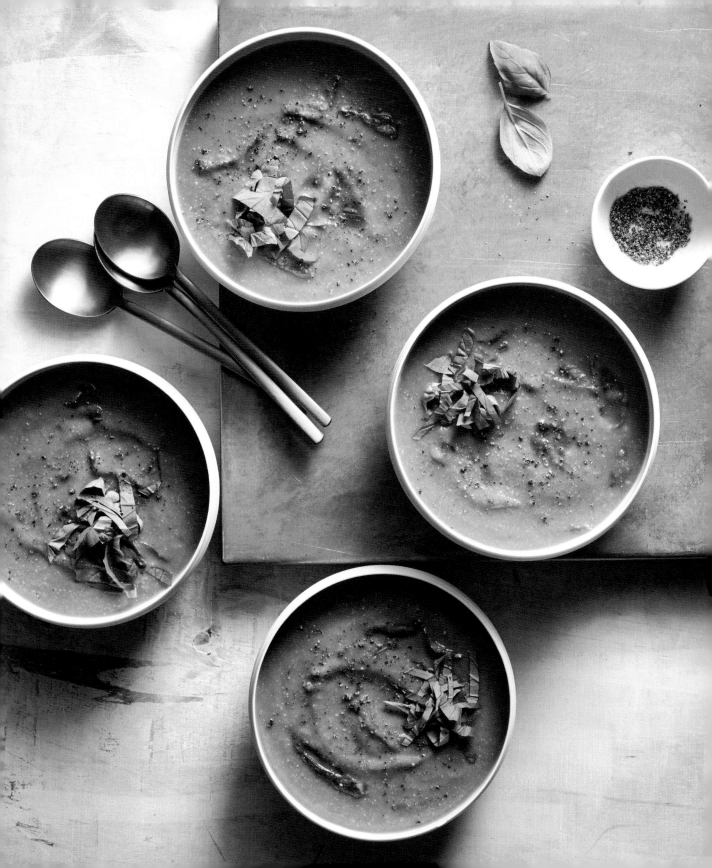

creamy tomato soup with spinach

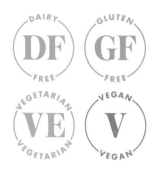

Creating a dairy-free soup that has a truly creamy consistency took several recipe tests. I finally found the trick using a combination of pureed cashews and white beans, ingredients that also make a bowl of soup super filling and satisfying. And even though it contains two cans of beans, the soup truly tastes like a rich tomato soup.

1 Heat a large saucepan over medium. Add the oil to the pan; swirl to coat. Add the onion and cook, stirring occasionally, until the onion is tender, about 4 minutes. Add the garlic, tomatoes, tomato paste, beans, rosemary, broth, and ½ teaspoon of the salt. Bring to a boil, stirring occasionally. Reduce the heat to low and simmer, stirring occasionally, for 15 minutes.

2 Place the cashews and water in a microwavable bowl. Microwave on high for 3 minutes; drain. Add the cashews to the saucepan.

3 Remove and discard the rosemary. Working in batches, transfer the tomato mixture to a blender. Remove the center piece of the blender lid to allow steam to escape; secure the lid on the blender. Place a clean dish towel over the opening in the lid to avoid splatters and blend until smooth. Transfer to a large bowl. Return the pureed soup to the saucepan and stir in the spinach, basil, vinegar, and remaining ¼ teaspoon salt. Cook over low, stirring occasionally, until the spinach is wilted, about 2 minutes.

(SERVING SIZE: ABOUT 2 CUPS): CALORIES 257; FAT 7G (SAT 1G, UNSAT 5G); PROTEIN 10G; CARB 38G; FIBER 9G; SUGARS 11G (ADDED SUGARS 0G); SODIUM 525MG; CALC 8% DV; POTASSIUM 8% DV

kitchen hack

Normally, cashews are soaked overnight before being blended into nondairy sauces. Microwaving the cashews in water for a few minutes is a genius time-saving hack!

1 tablespoon olive oil

1 cup finely chopped white onion

3 garlic cloves, minced

1 (26.5-ounce) package chopped tomatoes (such as Pomi)

1 tablespoon tomato paste

2 (15-ounce) cans no-salt-added cannellini or other white beans, rinsed and drained

1 (3-inch) fresh rosemary sprig

6 cups unsalted vegetable broth

¾ teaspoon kosher salt

½ cup whole raw cashews

½ cup water

2 cups chopped fresh baby spinach

⅓ cup thinly sliced fresh basil

2 tablespoons red wine vinegar

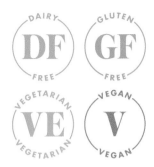

creamy black bean and cilantro soup

Pumpkin is the secret ingredient here, but you'll never taste it! It provides a creamy texture and balances ingredient flavors, as well as adding an extra dose of beta-carotene, vitamin E, and B vitamins. Using store-bought salsa is a great way to get a lot of flavor with just one ingredient. The hard part with this soup is deciding what toppings to sprinkle it with.

1 tablespoon olive oil

1 cup finely chopped white onion

2 garlic cloves, minced

1 teaspoon ground cumin

2 (15-ounce) cans no-salt-added black beans, rinsed and drained

¾ cup refrigerated fresh salsa

3 cups unsalted vegetable broth

½ teaspoon kosher salt

½ cup canned pure pumpkin

2 tablespoons chopped fresh cilantro

1 tablespoon fresh lime juice (optional)

1 Heat a large saucepan over medium. Add the oil to the pan; swirl to coat. Add the onion and cook, stirring occasionally, until the onion is tender, about 4 minutes. Add the garlic and cumin and cook, stirring occasionally, for 1 minute. Add the beans, salsa, broth, and salt. Bring to a boil, stirring occasionally. Reduce the heat to low and simmer, stirring occasionally, until slightly thickened, about 10 minutes.

2 Add the pumpkin, cilantro, and, if desired, lime juice to the bean mixture, stirring to combine. Transfer half the bean mixture to a blender. Remove the center piece of the blender lid to allow the steam to escape; secure the lid on the blender. Place a clean dish towel over the opening in the lid to avoid splatters and blend until smooth. Return the pureed soup to the saucepan and cook over low until thoroughly heated.

(SERVING SIZE: 1½ CUPS): CALORIES 273; FAT 5G (SAT 1G, UNSAT 3G); PROTEIN 13G; CARB 44G; FIBER 11G; SUGARS 9G (ADDED SUGARS 0G); SODIUM 599MG; CALC 15% DV; POTASSIUM 15% DV

what toppings to add?

I love sprinkling crumbled queso fresco on top for a salty-creamy bite, but one—or a combo—of the following ingredients also adds great flavor and texture:

- Toasted sliced almonds
- Diced avocado
- Chopped fresh cilantro
- Queso fresco or feta cheese
- Chopped scallions
- Plain Greek yogurt
- Roasted pumpkin seed kernels (pepitas)

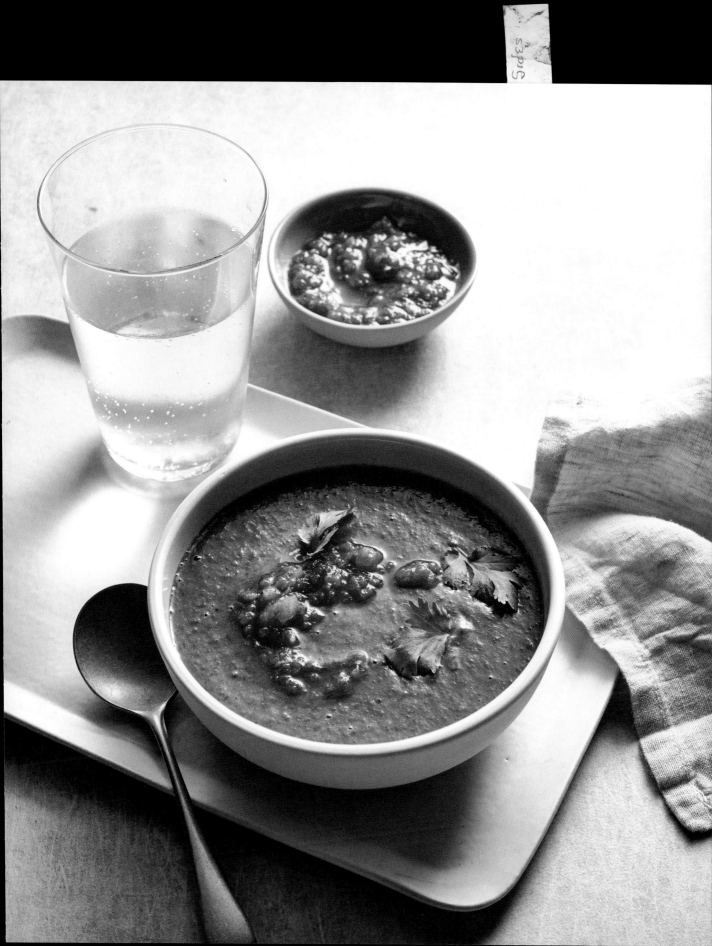

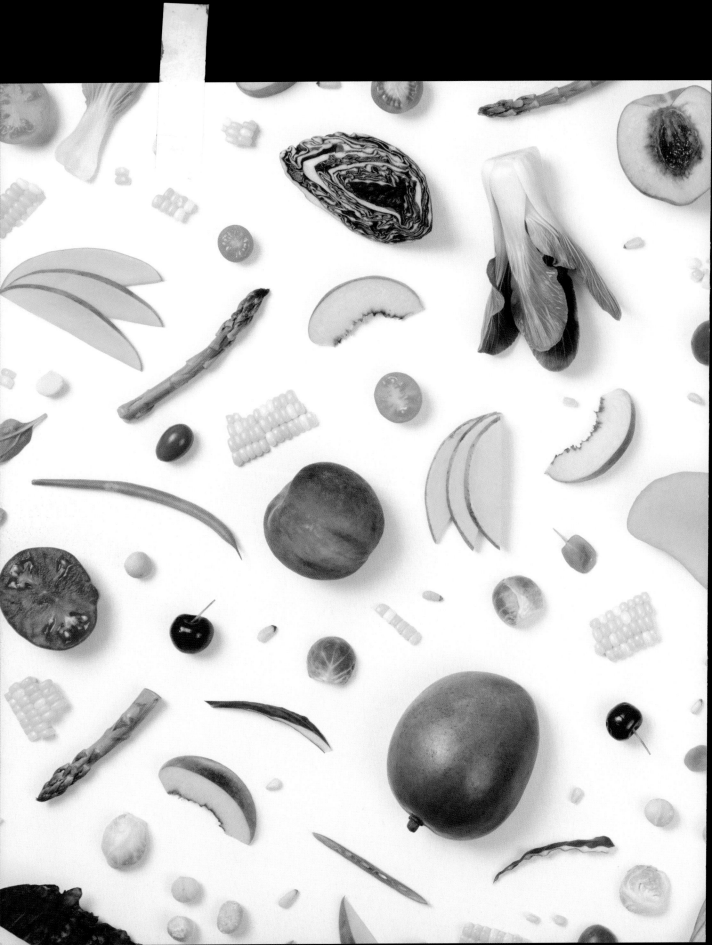

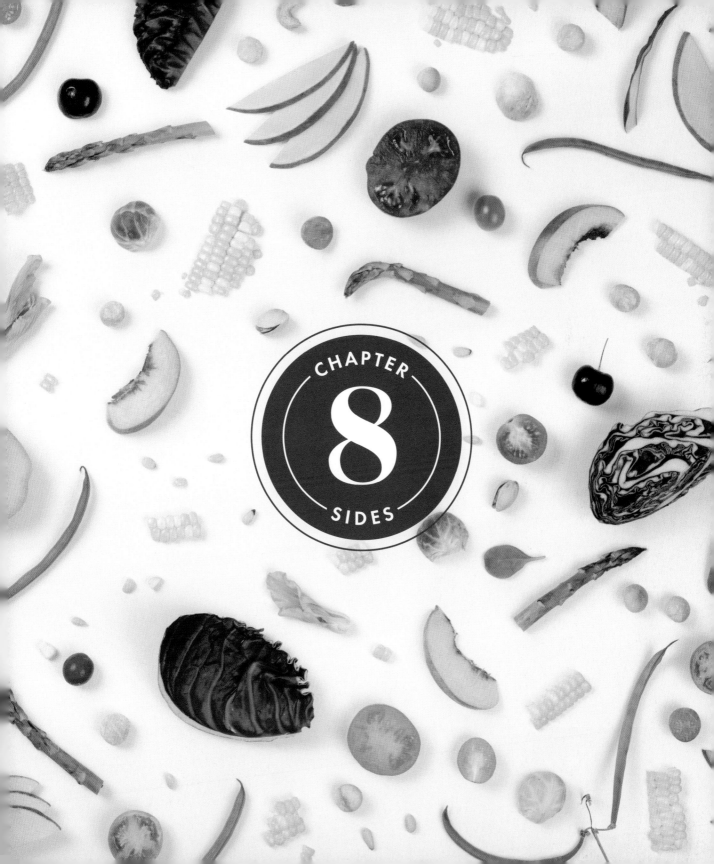

CHAPTER

8

SIDES

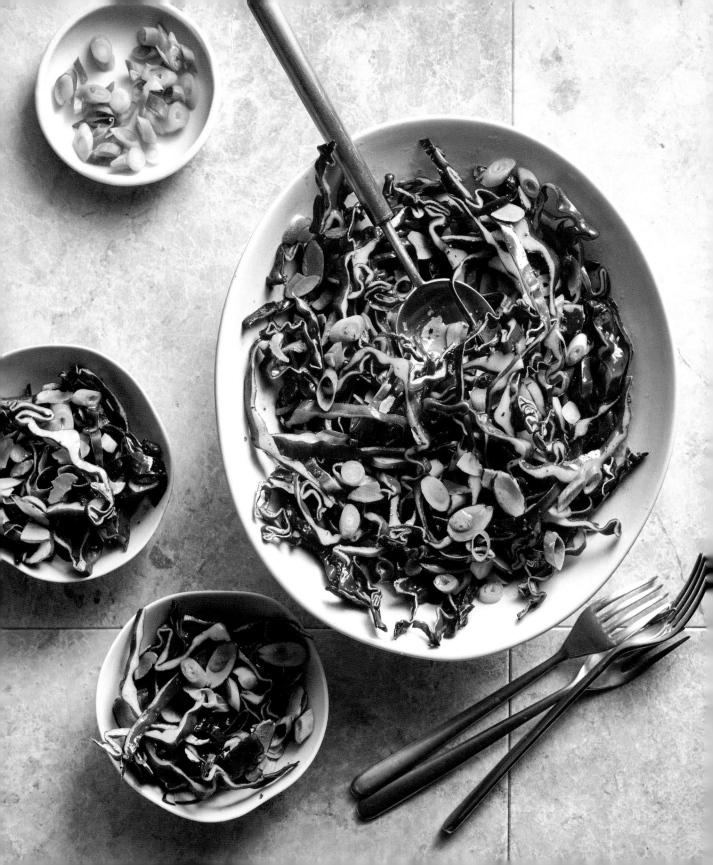

simple vinaigrette slaw

Inspired by a dish I tried at a local Mediterranean restaurant, this clean vinaigrette slaw is a refreshing change to creamy, slightly sweet mayo-based versions. It's quick to make on short notice, but also holds up well enough to make a day ahead. Serve it as a side, or use it as a bed for grilled chicken, shrimp, or fish to make a meal.

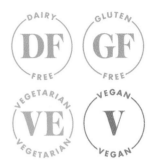

1 Place the cabbage and scallions in a large bowl or ziplock plastic bag. Whisk together the oil, vinegar, honey, mustard, Greek seasoning, garlic powder, salt, and pepper in a small bowl until blended. Pour the oil mixture over the cabbage mixture and stir well to coat the cabbage mixture.

2 Let stand for at least 20 minutes or up to overnight before serving. Sprinkle with the almonds just before serving.

(SERVING SIZE: ¾ CUP): CALORIES 103; FAT 9G (SAT 1G, UNSAT 7G); PROTEIN 2G; CARB 6G; FIBER 2G; SUGARS 3G (ADDED SUGARS 1G); SODIUM 85MG; CALC 3% DV; POTASSIUM 3% DV

SIMPLE VINAIGRETTE SLAW WITH FETA: Reduce the almonds to 3 tablespoons and add 3 tablespoons crumbled feta cheese.

SIMPLE (NUT-FREE) VINAIGRETTE SLAW WITH FETA: Omit the almonds. Add 1¼ ounces crumbled feta cheese (about ⅓ cup) to the cabbage mixture with the olive oil mixture in step 1, and proceed as directed.

- 6 cups finely shredded red or green cabbage
- ¼ cup chopped scallions
- ¼ cup extra-virgin olive oil
- 2 tablespoons red wine vinegar
- 2 teaspoons honey or brown sugar
- 1 teaspoon Dijon mustard
- 1 teaspoon salt-free Greek or Italian seasoning
- ½ teaspoon garlic powder
- ¼ teaspoon kosher salt
- ¼ teaspoon black pepper
- ⅓ cup sliced almonds, toasted

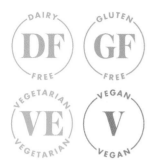

warm lemony brussels slaw

Tossing the sprouts in a skillet for just a few minutes takes the raw edge off of them, yet retains their crunch. Preshaved or shredded Brussels sprouts save time, but you can also quickly shave your own with a mandoline or by tossing them into a food processor. Use 3 tablespoons of a store-bought lemon vinaigrette like Tessemae's Lemon Garlic Dressing and Marinade instead of making your own, if desired.

3 tablespoons walnut oil or olive oil

1 pound preshaved Brussels sprouts (about 7 cups)

1½ tablespoons fresh lemon juice

½ teaspoon Dijon mustard

½ teaspoon honey or pure maple syrup

¼ teaspoon kosher salt

¼ teaspoon black pepper

¼ cup sweetened dried cranberries or cherries

3 tablespoons pine nuts, toasted

1 Heat a large skillet over medium-high. Add 2¼ teaspoons of the oil to the pan; swirl to coat. Add 3½ cups of the Brussels sprouts and cook, stirring often, until slightly wilted, about 2 minutes. Transfer to a large bowl. Wipe the skillet clean with paper towels. Repeat the procedure with 2¼ teaspoons of the oil and the remaining 3½ cups Brussels sprouts.

2 Whisk together the lemon juice, mustard, honey, salt, pepper, and remaining 1½ tablespoons oil in a small bowl until blended. Drizzle the lemon juice mixture over the Brussels sprouts and sprinkle with the cranberries and pine nuts; toss to coat. Serve warm or chilled.

(SERVING SIZE: ½ CUP): CALORIES 109; FAT 8G (SAT 1G, UNSAT 6G); PROTEIN 2G; CARB 10G; FIBER 3G; SUGARS 5G (ADDED SUGARS 0G); SODIUM 82MG; CALC 3% DV; POTASSIUM 5% DV

WARM LEMONY BRUSSELS SLAW WITH BACON: Prepare the recipe as directed, substituting 3 crumbled cooked uncured bacon slices for the pine nuts.

brussels sprouts

Who could have guessed that Brussels sprouts would become so hip? The once not-so-popular vegetable now shows up on trendy restaurant menus and in recipes shared across social media. And it's probably good we decided to give these sprouts a second look, because this veggie is good for our taste buds and our health! A serving of sprouts packs in almost a complete day's worth of vitamins C and K, plus kaempferol, a bioactive compound that appears to reduce the risk of blood clots and strokes. Kaempferol also exhibits antioxidant qualities, which reduce oxidative damage, risk of inflammatory diseases, and possibly cancer progression.

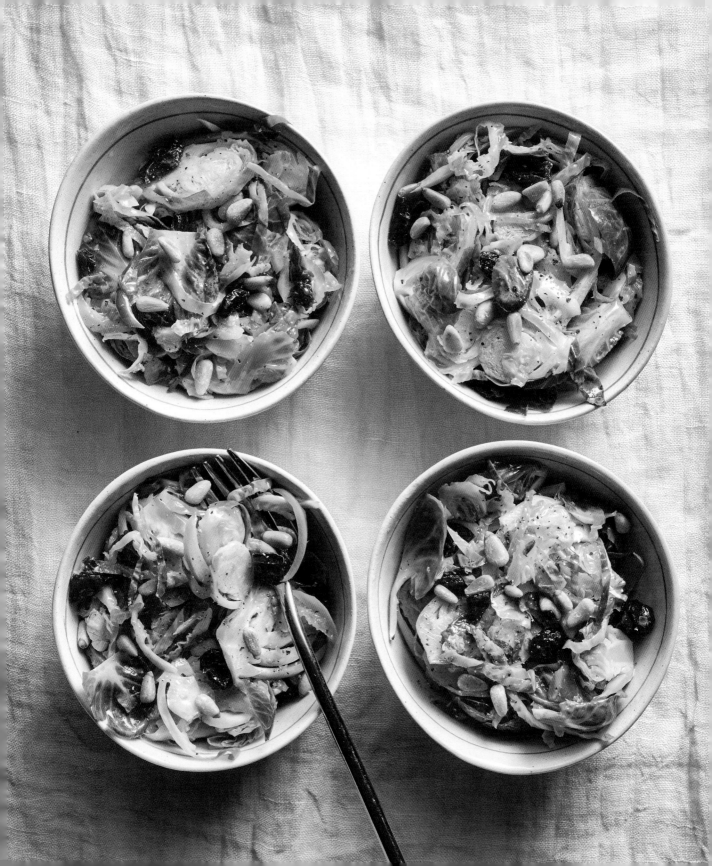

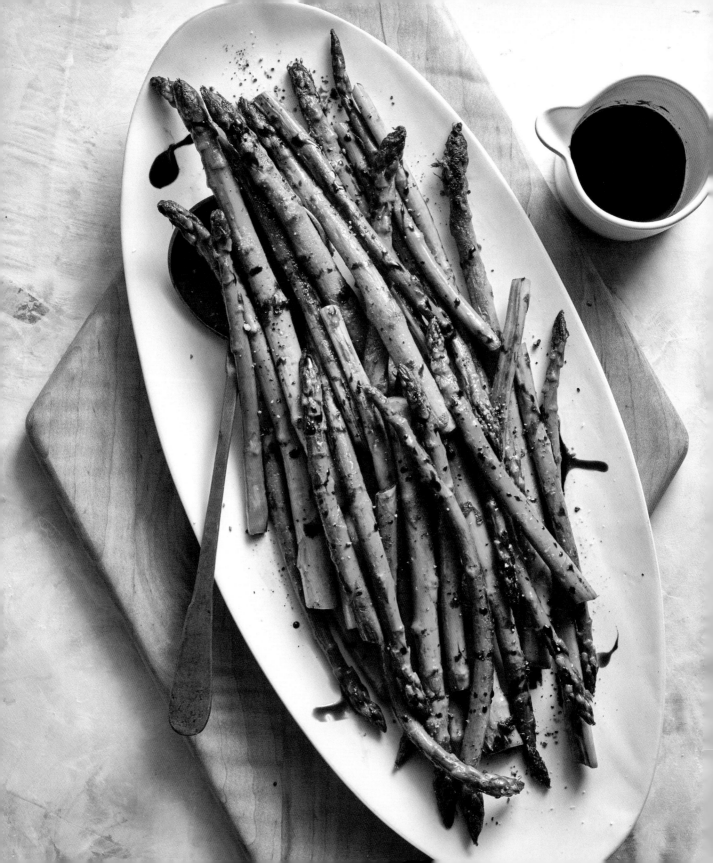

asparagus with balsamic drizzle

Simmering the vinegar tames its sharp flavor and thickens it to create a slightly sweet glaze. Drizzle it over roasted or grilled vegetables or fresh summer tomatoes. Balsamic reductions are available at most groceries, but they tend to be much pricier and may have added sugars.

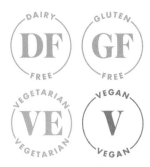

1 Preheat the oven to 400°F. Line a rimmed baking sheet with aluminum foil.

2 Arrange the asparagus on the prepared pan; toss with the oil, salt, garlic powder, and pepper. Roast for 8 to 10 minutes or until tender and beginning to brown, stirring halfway through roasting.

3 While the asparagus roasts, place the vinegar in a small saucepan over medium-high; bring to a boil. Reduce the heat to low and simmer, stirring frequently, for 5 minutes or until syrupy. Drizzle the vinegar over the asparagus.

(SERVING SIZE: ¼ OF THE ASPARAGUS AND ABOUT 1 TABLESPOON SAUCE): CALORIES 75; FAT 3G (SAT 0G, UNSAT 3G); PROTEIN 2G; CARB 9G; FIBER 2G; SUGARS 6G (ADDED SUGARS 0G); SODIUM 194MG; CALC 3% DV; POTASSIUM 4% DV

1¼ **pounds asparagus spears,** **trimmed**
1 **tablespoon olive oil**
½ **teaspoon kosher salt**
½ **teaspoon garlic powder**
¼ **teaspoon black pepper**
½ **cup balsamic vinegar**

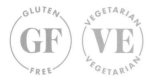

lemony garlic green beans

This recipe may use super-simple ingredients, but it's a big step up in flavor compared to plain steamed beans. Using a little of both butter and olive oil helps to coat the beans, giving them rich flavor that you couldn't get by using either fat alone.

1 (12-ounce) bag trimmed fresh green beans

2 teaspoons unsalted grass-fed butter

1 teaspoon olive oil

1 garlic clove, minced

2 teaspoons lemon zest

¼ teaspoon kosher salt

¼ teaspoon black pepper

1 Cook the green beans in the microwave for 1 minute less than directed on the package. Drain, if needed.

2 Heat the butter and oil in a large skillet over medium until the butter is melted; swirl to combine and coat the pan. Add the garlic to the pan; cook, stirring constantly, for 30 seconds. Add the cooked green beans and cook for 4 minutes or until the beans are tender. Sprinkle with the lemon zest, salt, and pepper and toss to combine.

(SERVING SIZE: ABOUT ¾ CUP): CALORIES 55; FAT 3G (SAT 1G, UNSAT 2G); PROTEIN 2G; CARB 6G; FIBER 2G; SUGARS 3G (ADDED SUGARS 0G); SODIUM 168MG; CALC 4% DV; POTASSIUM 4% DV

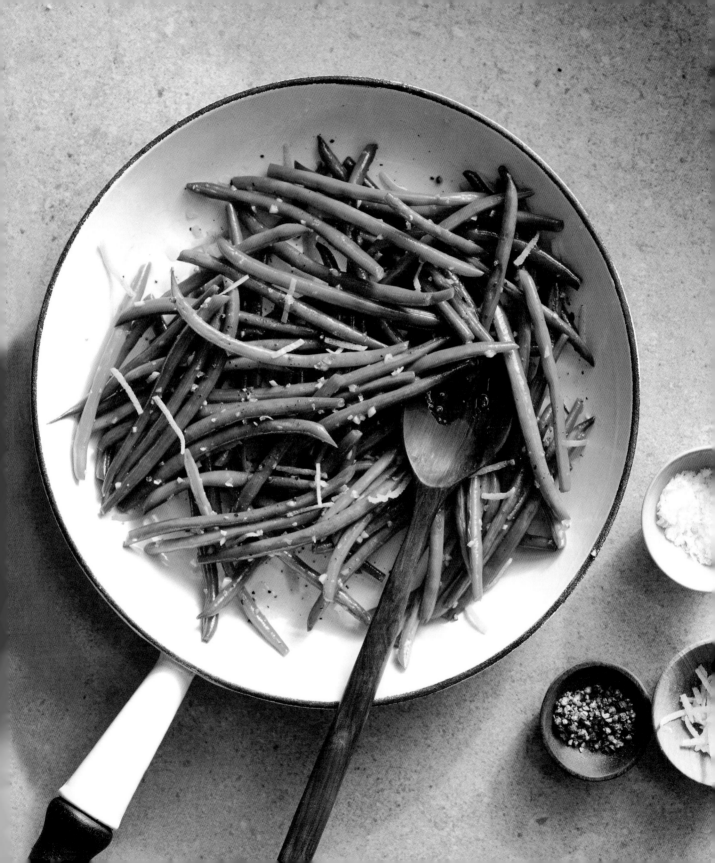

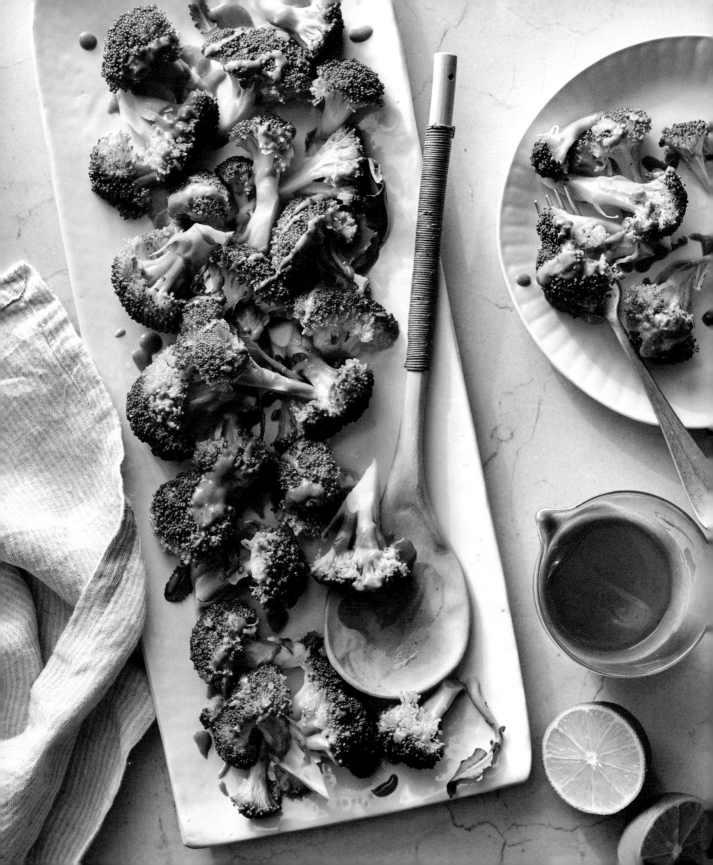

broccoli with thai almond butter sauce

Roasted broccoli is one of my favorite sides, but this broccoli dish, with a spin on peanut sauce drizzled over steamed florets, is a close runner-up. Almond butter's healthy fats give the sauce a creaminess that's able to balance some of the other ingredients' sharp flavors and create a rich drizzle. Peanut butter or another nut butter can be substituted for the almond butter.

DF DAIRY FREE **GF** GLUTEN FREE

VE VEGETARIAN **V** VEGAN

1 Cook the broccoli in the microwave according to the package instructions.

2 Whisk together the almond butter, soy sauce, lime juice, vinegar, honey, and water in a small bowl until well combined. Drizzle the almond butter mixture over the broccoli.

(SERVING SIZE: ABOUT ¾ CUP BROCCOLI AND 1½ TABLESPOONS SAUCE): CALORIES 76; FAT 5G (SAT 1G, UNSAT 4G); PROTEIN 4G; CARB 6G; FIBER 3G; SUGARS 2G (ADDED SUGARS 0G); SODIUM 185MG; CALC 7% DV; POTASSIUM 7% DV

- 1 (12-ounce) package fresh broccoli florets
- 2 tablespoons almond butter
- 1 tablespoon gluten-free lower-sodium soy sauce or tamari
- 1½ teaspoons fresh lime juice
- 1 teaspoon rice wine vinegar
- 1 teaspoon honey (optional; omit if vegan)
- 2 tablespoons warm water

cruciferous vegetables

Cruciferous vegetables have been highlighted as some of the top anti-inflammatory foods (see page 38) since all of them offer healthy doses of phytochemicals that quell inflammatory compounds. Aim for at least one daily serving of cruciferous vegetables and you should be good. Here's a list of options:

- Arugula
- Bok choy
- Broccoli
- Broccoli rabe
- Brussels sprouts
- Cabbage
- Cauliflower
- Collard greens
- Kale
- Kohlrabi
- Mustard greens
- Radishes
- Rutabaga
- Turnip greens
- Turnips
- Watercress

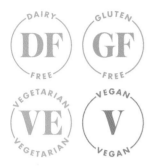

stir-fried bok choy with cashews

Thanks to its crunch and mild flavor, bok choy is a versatile vegetable that pairs well with strong or rich ingredients and can be eaten raw or cooked. If you can't find bok choy, substitute napa cabbage. A large wok is ideal for cooking this dish, but you can also cook it in two batches in a skillet like I did.

2 teaspoons sesame oil

1 garlic clove, minced

½ teaspoon minced fresh ginger (optional)

1 large head bok choy, trimmed and thinly sliced (about 6 cups)

2 tablespoons gluten-free lower-sodium soy sauce or tamari

⅛ teaspoon crushed red pepper (optional)

¼ cup chopped unsalted raw cashews

Heat a large skillet over medium-high. Add 1 teaspoon of the oil to the pan; swirl to coat. Add the garlic and, if desired, the ginger; cook, stirring constantly, until fragrant, about 1 minute. Add 3 cups of the bok choy and cook, stirring often, until just beginning to wilt, about 2 minutes. Transfer to a medium bowl. Wipe the skillet clean with paper towels. Repeat the procedure with the remaining 1 teaspoon oil and remaining 3 cups bok choy. Stir in the soy sauce and, if desired, the crushed red pepper. Sprinkle with the cashews just before serving.

(SERVING SIZE: ¾ CUP): CALORIES 89; FAT 6G (SAT 1G, UNSAT 5G); PROTEIN 3G; CARB 6G; FIBER 1G; SUGARS 2G (ADDED SUGARS 0G); SODIUM 357MG; CALC 12% DV; POTASSIUM 7% DV

vitamin k

Cruciferous vegetables, as well as leafy greens, are usually packed with vitamin K. In fact, it's not unusual for 1 cup to provide at least 50 percent of your daily vitamin K needs. This is a good thing since research suggests that vitamin K has an anti-inflammatory effect in the body, particularly for heart disease–related conditions and osteoarthritis.

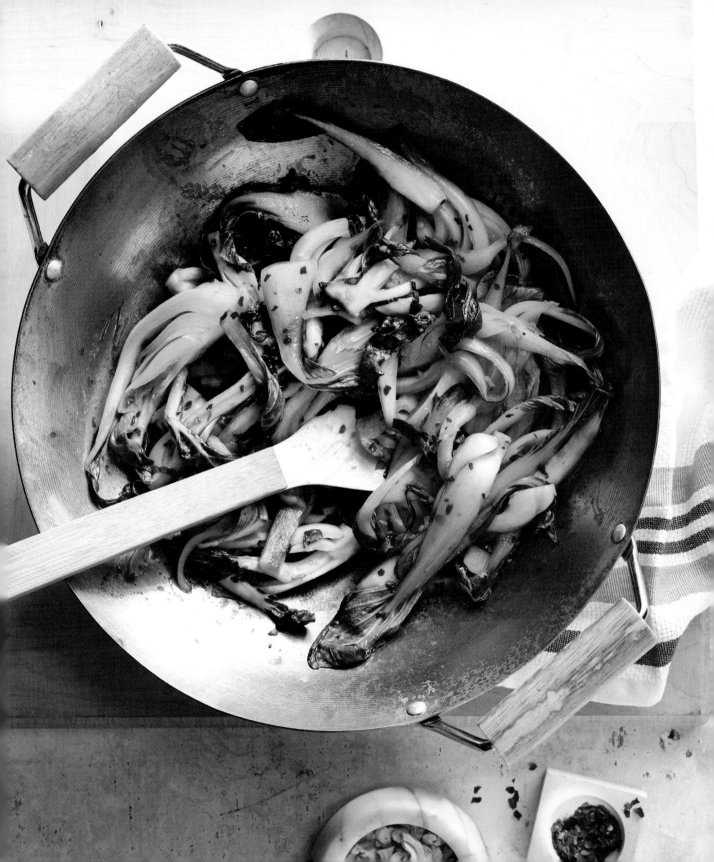

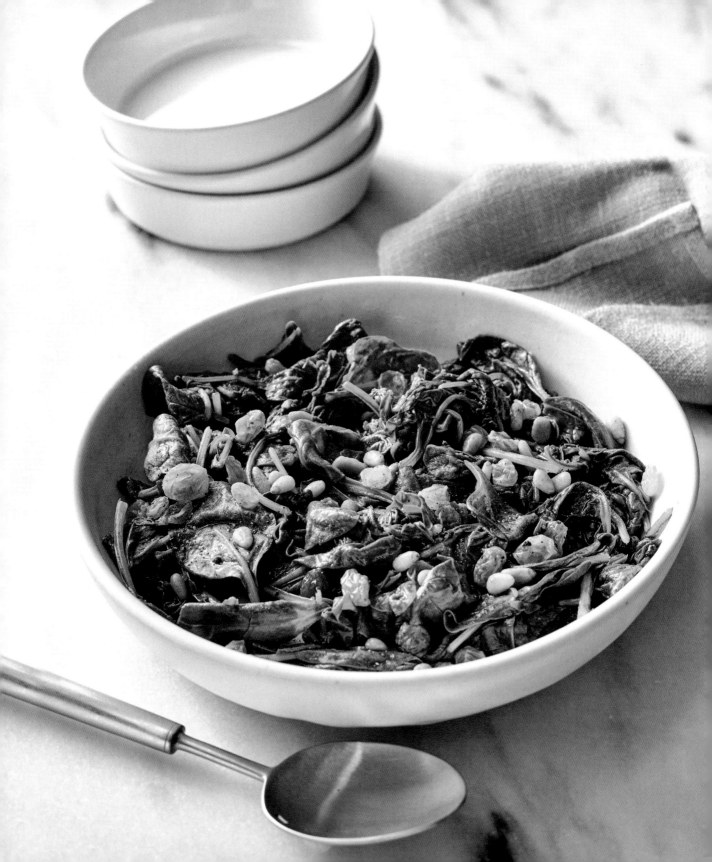

sautéed spinach with pine nuts and raisins

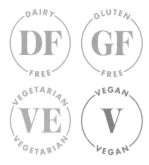

Golden raisins tend to be a little plumper, which makes them my preferred choice in this dish, and adding them to the skillet with the spinach helps this even more. If you find that your stash of raisins is a little dry, try this trick: Place the raisins in a small bowl, cover with hot water, let stand for 5 minutes or until plump, and then drain.

Heat a large saucepan over medium-high. Add the oil to the pan; swirl to coat. Add the garlic; cook for 30 seconds. Add the spinach, raisins, salt, and pepper. Cook, tossing occasionally with tongs, for 3 minutes, until the spinach wilts. Sprinkle with the pine nuts.

(SERVING SIZE: ABOUT ⅔ CUP): CALORIES 123; FAT 8G (SAT 1G, UNSAT 6G); PROTEIN 4G; CARB 11G; FIBER 3G; SUGARS 5G (ADDED SUGARS 0G); SODIUM 238MG; CALC 12% DV; POTASSIUM 16% DV.

1 tablespoon olive oil

1 garlic clove, peeled and smashed

1 (16-ounce) bag prewashed spinach

3 tablespoons golden raisins

¼ teaspoon kosher salt

⅛ teaspoon black pepper

3 tablespoons pine nuts, toasted

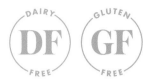

summer succotash with edamame

Limiting processed meats, as well as opting for uncured versions (see page 141 for Cured vs. Uncured Meats), is good for overall health. So when I do use a processed meat like bacon, I try to really make its flavor count. A little bit of uncured bacon goes a long way to add flavor that you can't get anywhere else.

2 uncured bacon slices

1½ teaspoons olive oil

1 cup chopped sweet onion

1⅓ cups fresh corn kernels (about 2 ears)

1 (10-ounce) bag frozen, shelled edamame, thawed

1 tablespoon red wine vinegar

½ teaspoon kosher salt

½ teaspoon black pepper

½ cup chopped summer tomatoes or halved cherry tomatoes

2 tablespoons chopped fresh basil

1 Cook the bacon in a large nonstick skillet over medium heat until crisp. Remove the bacon from the pan, reserving 2 teaspoons of the drippings in the pan; coarsely chop the bacon.

2 Increase the heat to medium-high. Add the oil to the drippings in the pan. Add the onion; sauté for 3 minutes, stirring occasionally. Add the corn kernels; sauté for 3 minutes or until lightly charred. Add the edamame and sauté for 3 minutes, stirring occasionally. Stir in the vinegar, salt, pepper, and tomatoes; cook for 30 seconds, stirring occasionally. Sprinkle with the bacon and basil.

(SERVING SIZE: ABOUT ½ CUP): CALORIES 123; FAT 5G (SAT 1G, UNSAT 3G); PROTEIN 8G; CARB 14G; FIBER 4G; SUGARS 4G (ADDED SUGARS 0G); SODIUM 251MG; CALC 4% DV; POTASSIUM 4% DV

frozen or fresh

Frozen side dishes are a quick, easy way to round out a meal, as well as incorporate grain and veggie variety and nutrients into your diet. In fact, fresh and frozen produce have been found to have similar nutrient amounts, and sometimes frozen even has slightly higher levels when flash-frozen immediately after harvest. Another plus to frozen sides is that they have a much longer shelf life with minimal nutrient loss—a big plus when comparing them to fresh produce.

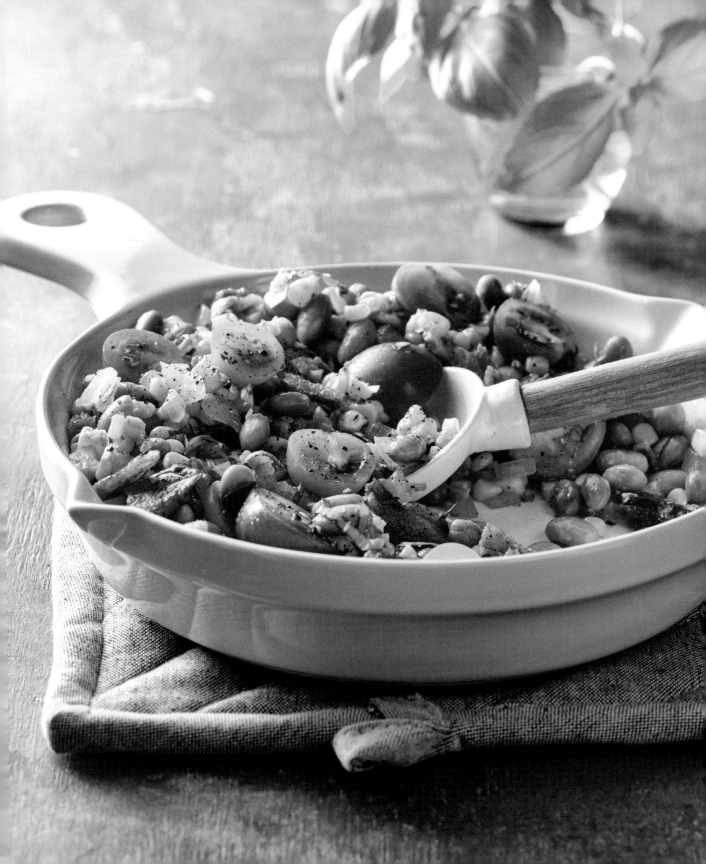

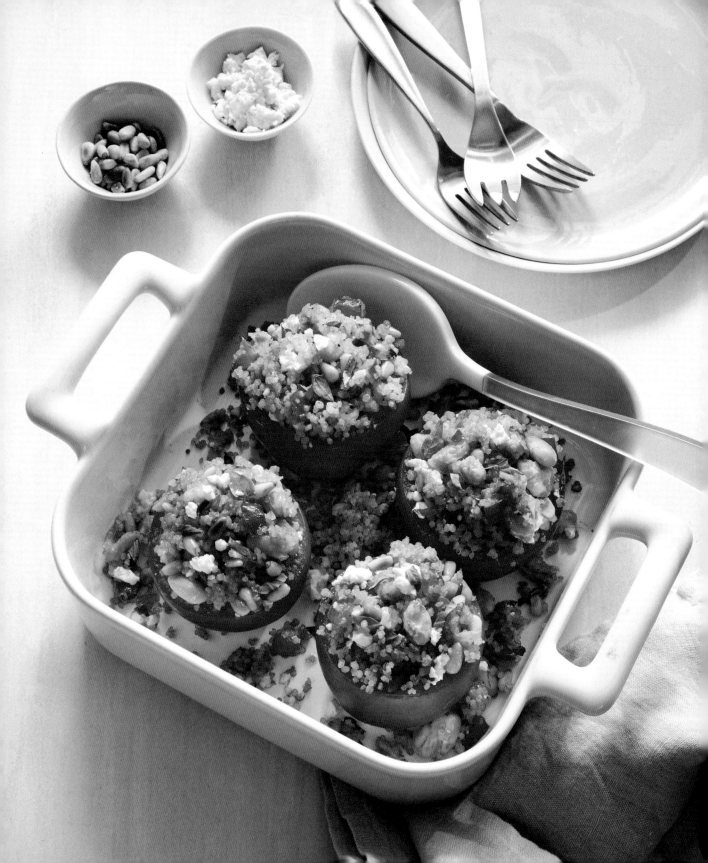

mediterranean stuffed tomatoes

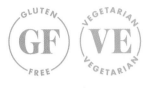

A ripe summer tomato is good by itself, but adding a little fresh basil and feta cheese makes it amazing. Use any cooked whole grain in the stuffing, but wait for a ripe tomato, or you'll be disappointed with the results.

1 Preheat the oven to 375°F.

2 Cut the tops off the tomatoes and discard. Carefully scoop out the tomato pulp, leaving the shells intact and reserving ½ cup of the pulp. Finely chop the reserved pulp. Place the tomato shells in a small square baking dish.

3 Combine the chopped tomato pulp, rice, beans, basil, feta, oil, pepper, and salt in a large bowl. Divide the mixture evenly among the tomato shells. Bake until thoroughly heated, about 12 minutes.

(SERVING SIZE: 1 TOMATO): CALORIES 132; FAT 4G (SAT 1G, UNSAT 3G); PROTEIN 5G; CARB 21G; FIBER 4G; SUGARS 4G (ADDED SUGARS 0G); SODIUM 142MG; CALC 7% DV; POTASSIUM 9% DV

DAIRY-FREE AND VEGAN OPTION: Prepare the recipe as directed, substituting ¼ cup chopped kalamata olives and 2 tablespoons toasted pine nuts for the feta cheese.

4 medium ripe tomatoes
1 cup cooked brown rice or quinoa
½ cup no-salt-added canned cannellini beans, rinsed and drained
⅓ cup torn fresh basil leaves
1 ounce feta cheese, crumbled (about ¼ cup)
1 teaspoon olive oil
¼ teaspoon black pepper
⅛ teaspoon kosher salt

tomatoes

Tomatoes are packed with potassium, folate, and vitamin C, but it's their content of the phytochemical lycopene that propels them to the next nutritional level. Studies show lycopene reduces and suppresses inflammation, lowering the risk of some cancers—particularly prostate cancer—and cardiovascular incidents. Lycopene's protection isn't limited to fresh tomatoes. Minimally processed tomato products like canned tomatoes and tomato paste provide similar levels of the compound.

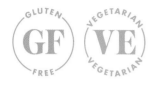

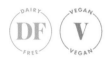

lower-carb parmesan polenta

Using a combination of polenta and cauliflower creates a creamy side dish with half the carbs and a lower glycemic impact. Extra servings make a perfect base for a polenta bowl topped with veggies and protein later in the week. For a smoother polenta, process fresh cauliflower rice in a food processor until the "grains" are significantly smaller.

2 cups unsalted vegetable broth

1 cup water

½ teaspoon kosher salt

½ cup quick-cooking polenta or grits

1 (12-ounce) package fresh or frozen riced cauliflower

⅓ cup freshly grated Parmesan cheese

1 tablespoon unsalted grass-fed butter

¼ teaspoon garlic powder

Bring the broth, water, and salt to a boil in a saucepan over high. Slowly add the polenta, stirring constantly with a whisk. Reduce the heat to low and simmer for 5 minutes. Add the cauliflower rice; cook for 5 minutes, stirring occasionally. Stir in the Parmesan, butter, and garlic powder.

(SERVING SIZE: ABOUT ⅔ CUP): CALORIES 100; FAT 3G (SAT 2G, UNSAT 1G); PROTEIN 5G; CARB 13G; FIBER 2G; SUGARS 1G (ADDED SUGARS 0G); SODIUM 322MG; CALC 5% DV; POTASSIUM 4% DV

DAIRY-FREE AND VEGAN OPTION: Use 1 tablespoon olive oil in place of the butter, and omit the cheese.

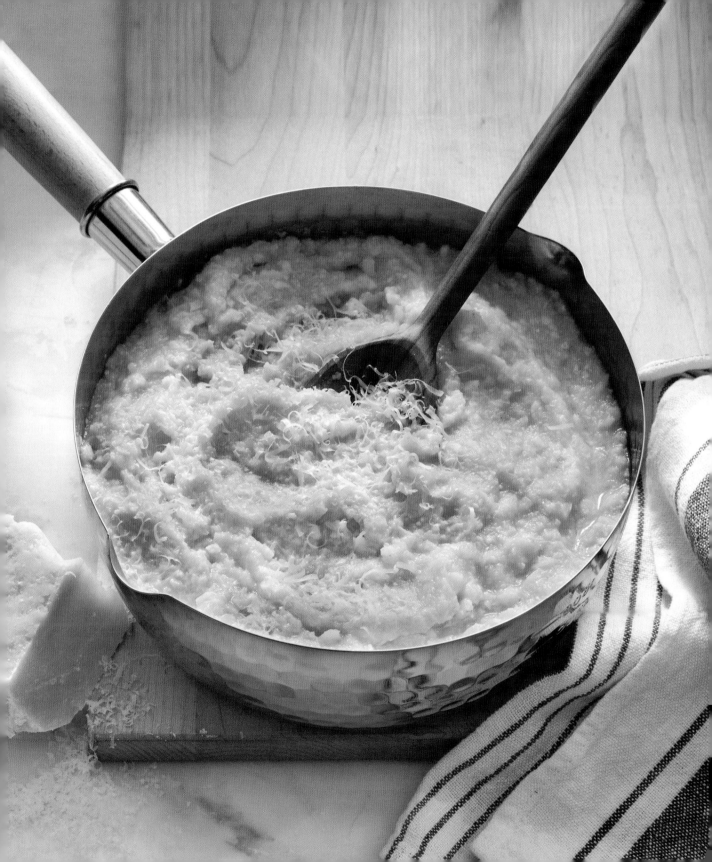

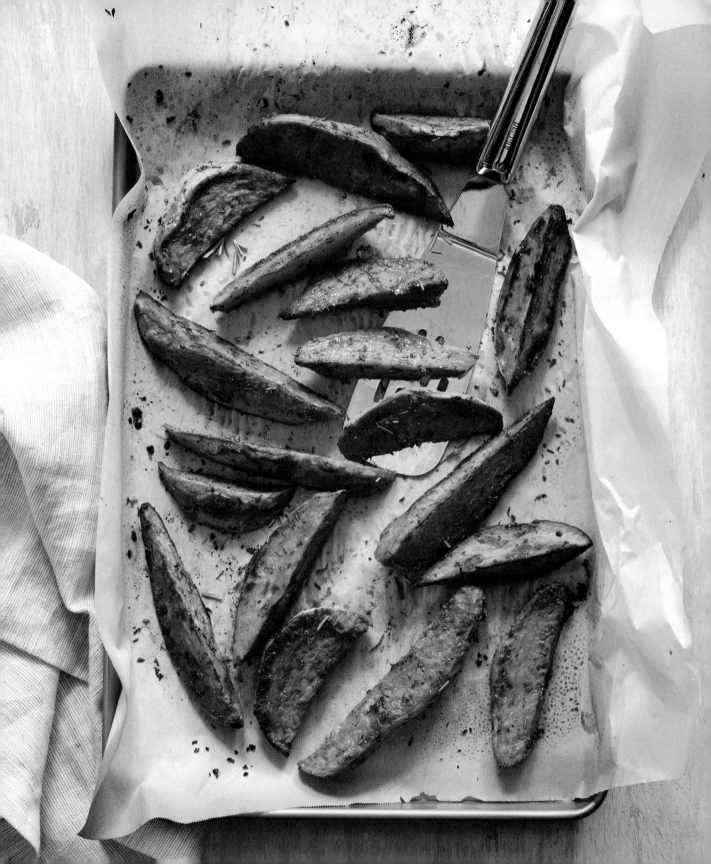

rosemary sweet potato fries

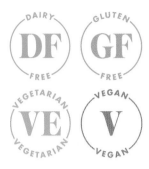

Sweetly spiced sweet potatoes are good for holidays, but I think savory is the way to go the rest of the year. The caramelization that occurs during the roasting process highlights their natural sweetness while crisping the outside—something that's complemented perfectly with just olive oil, rosemary, garlic, salt, and pepper.

1 Preheat the oven to 450°F. Line a large roasting or baking pan with aluminum foil; lightly coat with cooking spray.

2 Combine the potatoes, oil, rosemary, salt, garlic powder, and pepper in a large bowl; toss well. Arrange the potatoes in a single layer on the prepared pan.

3 Roast for 20 minutes. Gently stir the potatoes, then roast for an additional 10 minutes or until lightly browned and tender.

(SERVING SIZE: ABOUT 6 WEDGES): CALORIES 203; FAT 7G (SAT 1G, UNSAT 6G); PROTEIN 3G; CARB 33G; FIBER 5G; SUGARS 7G (ADDED SUGARS 0G); SODIUM 330MG; CALC 5% DV; POTASSIUM 12% DV

Cooking spray

3 medium sweet potatoes (about 2 pounds), each cut into 6 wedges

2 tablespoons olive oil

1½ tablespoons chopped fresh rosemary

½ teaspoon kosher salt

½ teaspoon garlic powder

¼ teaspoon black pepper

OPTIONAL

cheesy bulgur with greens

Cheese grits were the inspiration for this quick whole-grain side, which turns bulgur into a surprisingly tasty and kid-friendly dish. Short on time? Heat precooked bulgur, quinoa, or rice; then gently stir in the cheese and spinach, adding a little broth or water if needed.

2¼ cups unsalted vegetable broth

1 cup uncooked bulgur

¼ teaspoon kosher salt

2 ounces extra-sharp cheddar cheese, shredded

2 cups torn baby spinach

Combine the broth, bulgur, and salt in a small saucepan and bring to a boil. Cover, reduce the heat to low, and cook for 8 minutes. Add the cheese and gently stir until almost melted. Add the spinach; cover the pan and let sit for 2 minutes. Remove the lid, and gently toss the wilted spinach with the bulgur.

(SERVING SIZE: ABOUT ½ CUP): CALORIES 130; FAT 3G (SAT 2G, UNSAT 1G); PROTEIN 7G; CARB 19G; FIBER 3G; SUGARS 0G (ADDED SUGARS 0G); SODIUM 235MG; CALC 9% DV; POTASSIUM 2% DV

GLUTEN-FREE OPTION: Use quinoa or brown rice in place of bulgur. Adjust the broth amount and the grain cooking time based on the chart on page 63, adding salt as directed above. Follow the recipe directions above to add the cheese and spinach to the cooked grain.

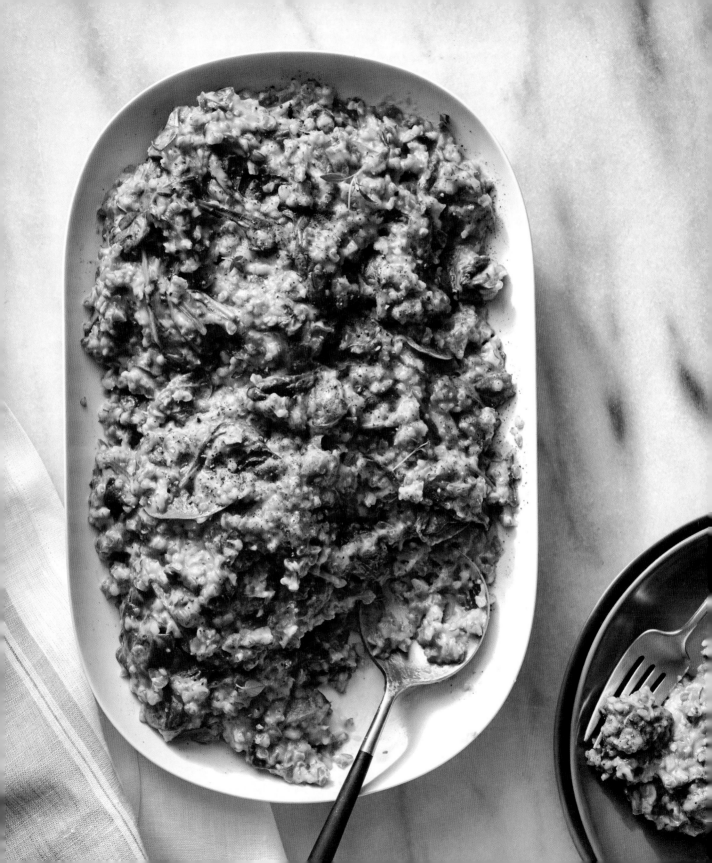

leafy green salads

Salads can be boring and tasteless—or a plate full of flavor and texture that you can't wait to dig into. I don't know about you, but I prefer the second! Here's my secret to creating crave-worthy salads: Think outside the box when it comes to what to add. I'm betting you already have several of the ingredients on hand. Combine those ingredients to create a balance of flavors using my formulas (opposite) as a guide.

fresh green options

All leafy greens are good, but consider the texture (crisp, delicate, sturdy) and flavor (mild or a little more flavorful) when deciding on greens.

- Arugula
- Cabbages (green, red, napa, or bok choy)
- Kale (baby or lacinato)
- Lettuces (butterleaf, green or red leaf, romaine)
- Spinach (baby or flat-leaf)
- Mixed greens or blends of several

kale fyi

Compared to spinach, kale is much sturdier and a little darker in color, and has a bit more flavor bite. The media has called it a superfood, largely because it was a relatively unknown green until a few years ago, and it's packed with vitamins A, C, and K, as well as potassium, fiber, iron, and calcium. Today, kale is a regular item in produce sections, and you're likely to find three common types: lacinato, curly, and baby.

- Lacinato kale (also called Tuscan kale or dinosaur kale) can be used raw in salads or cooked. It tends to have a milder flavor than curly kale, with stems that aren't as fibrous and don't necessarily have to be removed. Its leaves are a little tougher than typical salad greens, so massage them with the dressing, or toss them with dressing in advance and let them sit before adding other ingredients.
- Curly kale has large leaves that are curled on the edges. It has a little more bite and woody stems that you'll want to remove and discard. Curly is best for cooking.
- Baby kale is my favorite. It's got the mild flavor of lacinato but more tender leaves, making it ideal for quick salads.

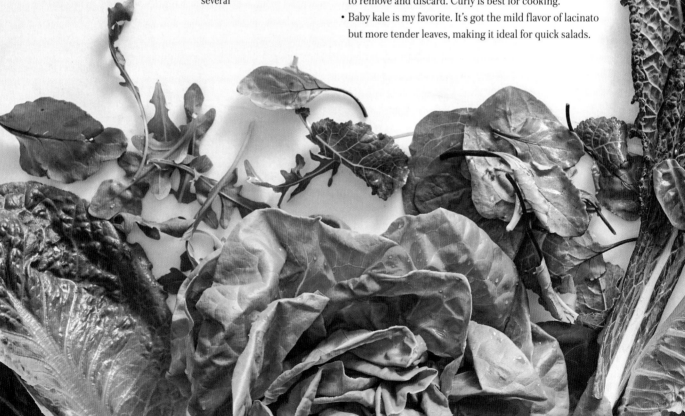

salad green blends

Containers of "salad greens" usually contain a variety of greens that you may not be as familiar with but that are just as nutrient dense. The greens vary by brand but are usually a combination of green-leaf lettuces, radicchio, escarole, red-leaf lettuces, and arugula. Most contain a mix of textures and flavors, making "mixed greens" or "salad greens" work with many toppings, including those ideas listed for spinach and kale.

SWEET

- ☐ Orange sections
- ☐ Grapefruit sections
- ☐ Sugar snap peas
- ☐ Chopped pear or apple
- ☐ Fresh peach slices
- ☐ Halved seedless grapes
- ☐ Halved cherry tomatoes
- ☐ Golden raisins
- ☐ Sliced strawberries
- ☐ Blueberries
- ☐ Pitted cherries
- ☐ Green peas
- ☐ Corn kernels
- ☐ Diced mango
- ☐ Sliced pitted dates

CRISP

- ☐ Sliced red onion
- ☐ Sliced radishes
- ☐ Chopped toasted nuts like walnuts, almonds, pecans, cashews, pine nuts, or pistachios
- ☐ Pumpkin seed kernels (pepitas) or sunflower seeds
- ☐ Shredded carrot
- ☐ Blanched asparagus pieces
- ☐ Chopped scallions
- ☐ Chopped cucumber

SAVORY

- ☐ Diced avocado
- ☐ Shelled edamame
- ☐ Freshly grated Parmesan cheese
- ☐ Cooked uncured bacon crumbles
- ☐ Hard-cooked egg
- ☐ Crumbled cheese like feta, goat, or blue
- ☐ Shredded cheese like cheddar or Monterey Jack
- ☐ Pitted kalamata olives
- ☐ Unsweetened toasted coconut

successful salad formulas

①

Lots of fresh greens
+
SWEET
+
CRISP

②

Lots of fresh greens
+
SWEET
+
SAVORY

③

Lots of fresh greens
+
CRISP
+
SAVORY

④

Lots of fresh greens
+
SWEET
+
CRISP
+
SAVORY

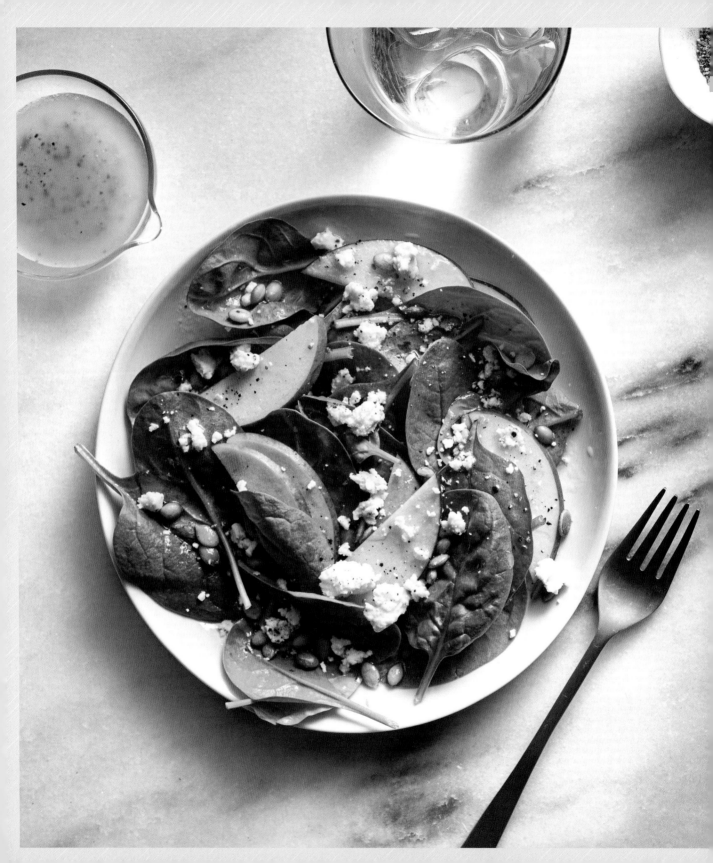

salad ideas

GREENS	SWEET	CRISP	SAVORY	DRESSING
Spinach, mixed greens, romaine, or butter	Orange sections	Pecans	Avocado	Olive oil vinaigrette
Spinach, mixed greens, or green leaf	Pear	Walnuts	Parmesan cheese	Balsamic vinaigrette
Spinach, mixed greens, or butter	Peach		Bacon	Red wine vinaigrette
Spinach, mixed greens, or green leaf	Grapefruit sections	Pecans	Blue cheese	Olive oil vinaigrette
Spinach, kale, arugula, or mixed greens	Dried cranberries	Almonds		Citrus or lemon vinaigrette
Spinach, mixed greens, romaine, or butter	Granny Smith apple and raisins	Cashews		Cider vinaigrette
Spinach, mixed greens, romaine, or butter	Jicama or apple	Pumpkin seed kernels	Queso fresco	Citrus or lemon vinaigrette
Spinach, kale, arugula, or mixed greens	Grapes			Citrus or lemon vinaigrette
Spinach, mixed greens, romaine, or butter	Tomato and corn		Bacon	Red wine vinaigrette
Romaine, kale, bok choy or napa cabbage	Sugar snap peas	Carrot or radish	Edamame	Ginger or soy vinaigrette
Spinach, kale, arugula, mixed greens, butter, or romaine	Cherry tomatoes	Cucumber	Chickpeas or feta cheese	Greek or olive oil vinaigrette
Spinach, mixed greens, or butter	Dates		Bacon	Balsamic vinaigrette
Arugula, spinach, mixed greens, or butter	Green peas	Red onion	Feta cheese	Red wine vinaigrette
Spinach, kale, arugula, mixed greens, butter, or romaine	Gala apple	Walnuts	Goat cheese	Citrus or lemon vinaigrette
Spinach, mixed greens, romaine, or butter	Strawberries			Balsamic vinaigrette
Spinach, kale, arugula, mixed greens, butter, or romaine	Mango		Avocado and coconut	Citrus or lemon vinaigrette

10-minutes-or-less sides

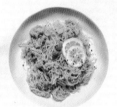

OPTIONAL

GF VE DF V

PESTO SPAGHETTI SQUASH

Toss 2 cups cooked spaghetti squash strands with 1 tablespoon pesto, 1 teaspoon fresh lemon juice, and a dash each of salt and pepper.

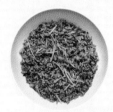

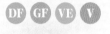
DF GF VE V

NUTTY RICE PILAF

Toast 2 tablespoons flaxseed in a skillet. Heat 1 (8.8-ounce) package ready-to-heat wild rice or brown rice according to the package directions. Place the rice, toasted flaxseed, 2 tablespoons chopped fresh parsley, 1 teaspoon lemon zest, and 1½ tablespoons fresh lemon juice or citrus vinaigrette in a bowl; toss.

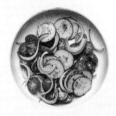

DF GF VE V

MARINATED TOMATOES AND CUCUMBERS

Place 2 cups chopped cucumbers, 2 cups halved cherry tomatoes, 1 cup sliced sweet onion, and ¼ cup extra-virgin olive oil or Greek vinaigrette in a large bowl; toss to combine. Refrigerate for at least 15 minutes before serving.

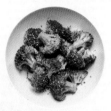

DF GF VE V

SESAME-SOY BROCCOLI

Steam 1 (12-ounce) bag fresh broccoli florets; drain. Whisk together 2 tablespoons gluten-free lower-sodium soy sauce or tamari, 2 tablespoons rice vinegar, and 1 tablespoon sesame oil until combined. Toss with the cooked broccoli. Sprinkle with 2 teaspoons toasted sesame seeds, if desired.

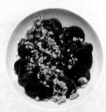

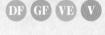
DF GF VE V

SLICED BEETS IN QUICK VINAIGRETTE

Slice 1 (8.8-ounce) package refrigerated precooked beets. Place the beets, 2 tablespoons chopped shallot, and ¼ cup red wine vinaigrette in a bowl; toss. Optional: Sprinkle with 2 tablespoons chopped toasted walnuts before serving.

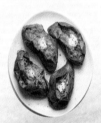

GF VE

BAKED SWEET POTATOES

Preheat the oven to 400°F. Pierce 4 medium sweet potatoes with a fork; bake for 45 minutes or until tender. Cut the potatoes in half; top each with 2 teaspoons unsalted grass-fed butter and a dash each of salt and pepper.

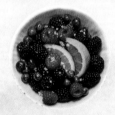

DF GF VE

GINGER-LIME BERRIES

Combine 1 tablespoon fresh lime juice, 1 teaspoon minced fresh ginger, and ½ teaspoon honey. Pour over 2 cups mixed berries (or cut-up melon, citrus sections, etc.) in a bowl and toss.

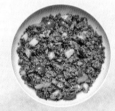

DF GF VE V

TABBOULEH QUINOA

Heat 1 (8.8-ounce) package ready-to-heat quinoa or farro according to the package directions; let cool. Place the quinoa, ½ cup each chopped tomato, cucumber, and fresh parsley, 2 tablespoons extra-virgin olive oil, 1 tablespoon fresh lemon juice, and ¼ teaspoon kosher salt in a bowl; toss. Chill until serving.

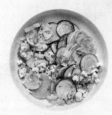

MEDITERRANEAN SQUASH SAUTÉ

Heat a large skillet over medium-high. Add 1 tablespoon olive oil to the pan; swirl to coat. Add 3 cups yellow squash or zucchini slices, 1 cup sliced leek, and ¼ teaspoon kosher salt; sauté for 5 minutes or until tender. Sprinkle with 2 tablespoons crumbled feta cheese and 1 tablespoon chopped fresh basil.

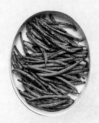

ASIAN GREEN BEANS

Cook 1 (12-ounce) package green beans according to the package directions; drain. Heat a large skillet over medium-high. Add 1 tablespoon sesame oil; swirl to coat. Add the beans, 1 tablespoon gluten-free lower-sodium soy sauce or tamari, and ½ teaspoon garlic powder. Sauté for 2 minutes.

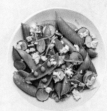

LEMONY SUGAR SNAPS WITH RADISHES

Steam 1 (8-ounce) package fresh sugar snap peas according to the package directions; drain. Place the peas, ½ cup sliced radishes, 3 tablespoons feta cheese, and 2 tablespoons each fresh lemon juice and extra-virgin olive oil in a bowl; toss.

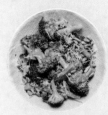

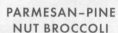

PARMESAN–PINE NUT BROCCOLI

Cook 1 (12-ounce) package fresh broccoli florets according to the package directions; drain. Place the broccoli, 1 tablespoon extra-virgin olive oil, and ¼ teaspoon each lemon zest, kosher salt, and pepper in a bowl; toss. Sprinkle with 2 tablespoons each toasted pine nuts and grated Parmesan cheese.

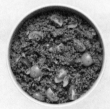

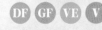

TOMATO-BASIL QUINOA

Heat 1 (8.8-ounce) package ready-to-heat quinoa according to the package directions. Let cool after cooking. Place the quinoa, 1 tablespoon extra-virgin olive oil, ¼ cup quartered cherry tomatoes, 2 tablespoons chopped fresh basil, and ¼ teaspoon kosher salt in a bowl; toss.

side dish buying guide

There are lots of side dish options to help make meals come together quickly; you just need to know how to choose those healthier ones. Since the sides category includes all types of vegetables, grains, and starches, specifics will vary, but these are the general guidelines that I follow.

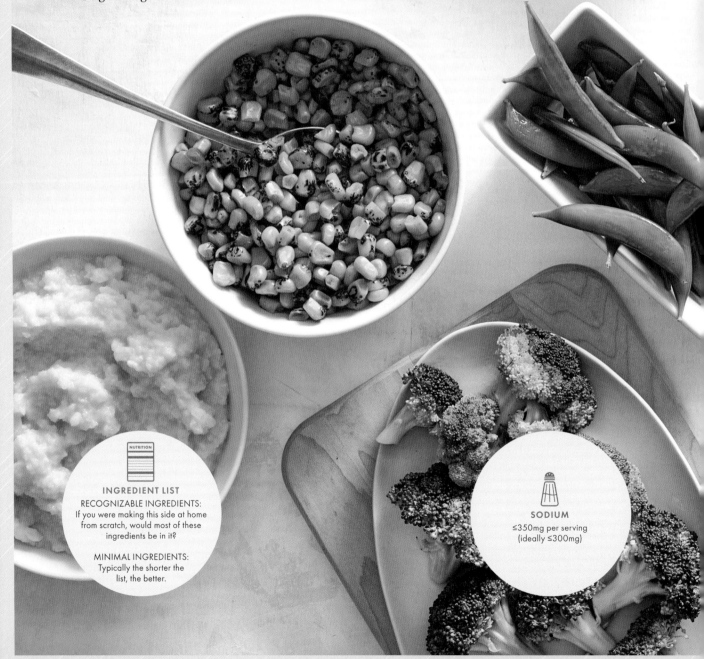

INGREDIENT LIST

RECOGNIZABLE INGREDIENTS: If you were making this side at home from scratch, would most of these ingredients be in it?

MINIMAL INGREDIENTS: Typically the shorter the list, the better.

SODIUM

≤350mg per serving (ideally ≤300mg)

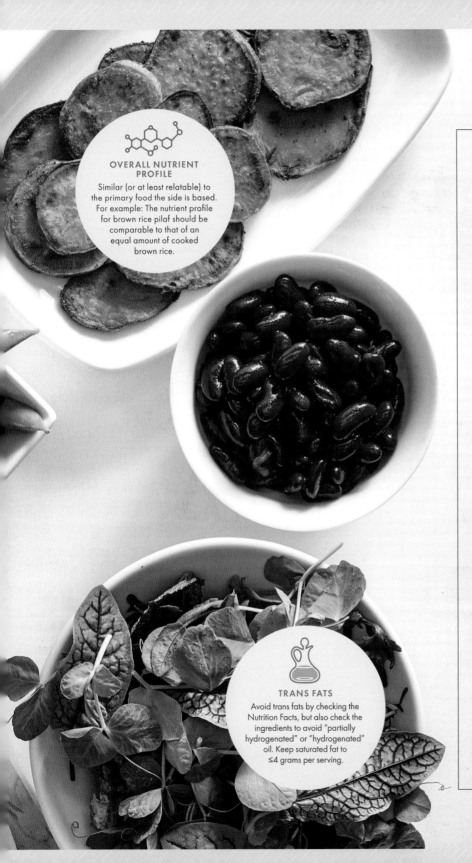

OVERALL NUTRIENT PROFILE

Similar (or at least relatable) to the primary food the side is based. For example: The nutrient profile for brown rice pilaf should be comparable to that of an equal amount of cooked brown rice.

TRANS FATS

Avoid trans fats by checking the Nutrition Facts, but also check the ingredients to avoid "partially hydrogenated" or "hydrogenated" oil. Keep saturated fat to ≤4 grams per serving.

MY REGULAR WEEKLY SIDE DISH PURCHASES

There's no way to list all the healthy options at the grocery, but these are some of my regular purchases. Use this as guidance to get started, not a definitive list of what to buy or not buy.

- Prewashed containers of leafy greens
- Ready-to-cook bags of fresh broccoli florets, green beans, and other veggies
- Steam-in-bag frozen grains, vegetables, or blends of the two
- No-salt-added canned beans
- Ready-to-heat cooked whole grains
- Chopped salad mixes

A FEW BRAND-SPECIFIC FAVORITES

- Green Giant Fresh Spaghetti Squash
- Trader Joe's Riced Cauliflower
- Veggie Noodle Co. Zucchini Spirals
- Trader Joe's Southwestern Chopped Salad
- Taylor Farms Organic Toasted Sesame Chopped Salad
- Eat Smart Broccoli Florets
- Birds Eye Veggie Made Mashed Cauliflower
- Earthbound Farms Frozen Roasted Organic Sweet Potato Slices with Olive Oil and Sea Salt
- Trader Joe's Frozen Roasted Corn
- Seapoint Farms Shelled Edamame

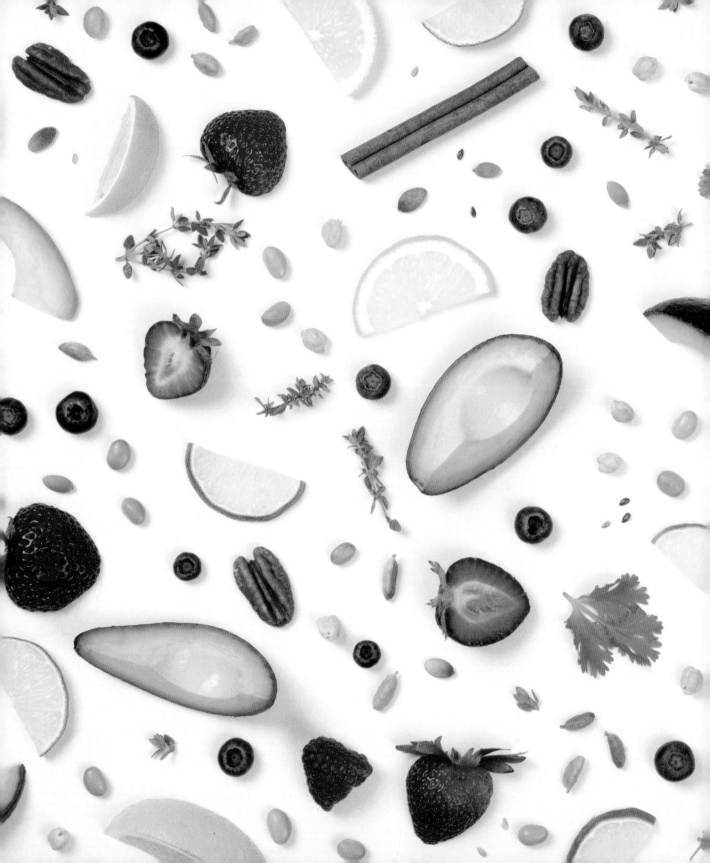

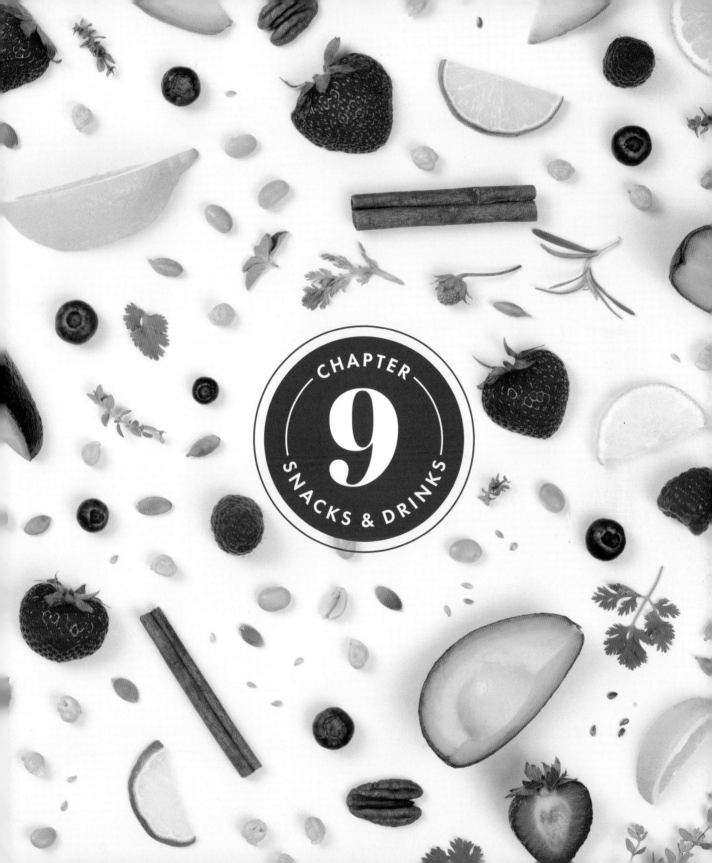

CHAPTER

9

SNACKS & DRINKS

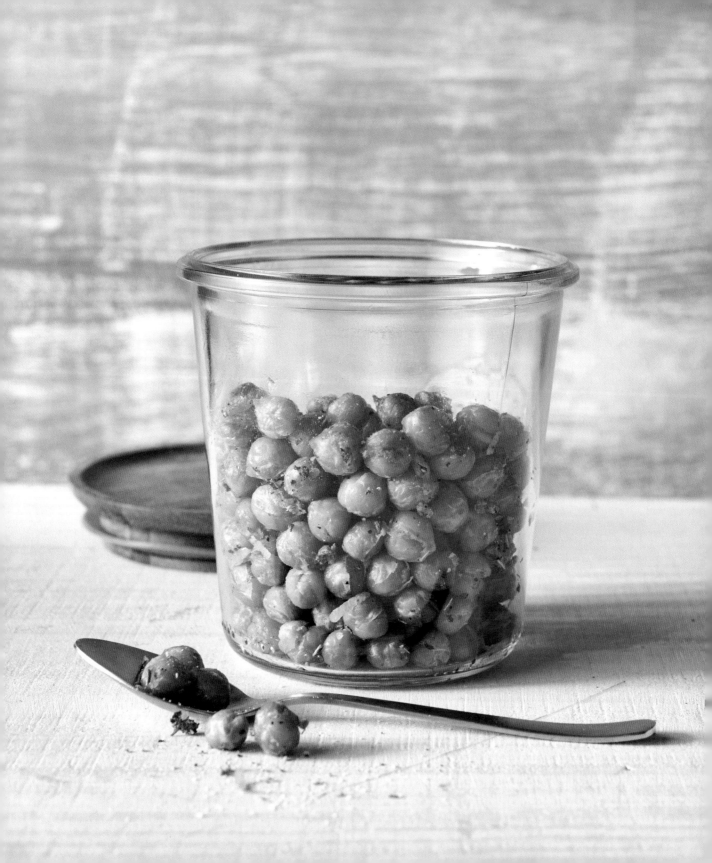

skillet-toasted chickpeas

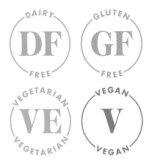

Crispy and lightly seasoned—this was how I wanted my chickpeas. But I could never find the right combination of baking time and temp—they either ended up soft or dried out—until a friend shared her trick of toasting the chickpeas in a hot skillet. The chickpeas get a crispy outside while keeping a moist inside, and in half the time it takes in the oven. Dry your chickpeas as thoroughly as possible before cooking to get a satisfyingly crisp result.

1 Pat the chickpeas dry with a paper towel. Heat a large nonstick skillet over medium-high. Add the oil to the pan; swirl to coat. Add the chickpeas; cook, stirring occasionally, for 17 minutes or until golden brown and crispy all over.

2 Transfer the chickpeas to a medium bowl. Add the garlic powder, lemon zest, oregano, salt, and pepper; toss gently. Serve immediately, or let cool in a single layer on a parchment paper–lined baking sheet before storing in an airtight container.

NOTE: For a more tender but still crispy chickpea, follow step 1 using a large ovenproof skillet. Preheat the oven to 400°F while the chickpeas are on the stovetop. Following the stovetop cooking, place the skillet in the oven and bake for 10 to 15 minutes.

(SERVING SIZE: ABOUT ¼ CUP): CALORIES 98; FAT 4G (SAT 1G, UNSAT 3G); PROTEIN 4G; CARB 11G; FIBER 3G; SUGARS 1G (ADDED SUGARS 0G); SODIUM 136MG; CALC 3% DV; POTASSIUM 3% DV

1 (19-ounce) can no-salt-added chickpeas, rinsed and drained
2 tablespoons olive oil
½ teaspoon garlic powder
½ teaspoon lemon zest
½ teaspoon dried oregano
½ teaspoon kosher salt
¼ teaspoon black pepper

add spice to cool down

Turning up the heat and flavor sounds like it might aggravate inflammation, but it actually does the opposite. In fact, incorporating fragrant spices, dried and fresh herbs, and other pungent plant foods like ginger and garlic is considered a key component to reducing inflammation, particularly when it comes to arthritis, joint pain, and swelling. Compounds in seasonings like turmeric, cinnamon, garlic, ginger, black pepper, oregano, rosemary, and cloves have been used medicinally in other cultures for thousands of years, but modern medicine in the US only recently started to use them. And the upside of using fragrant plant compounds is that there's rarely any harmful side effects associated, which means incorporating them regularly may be worth a shot for those with pain and joint issues.

Skillet-Toasted Chickpeas and Crispy Spiced Edamame (page 248) are perfect recipes to experiment with new spices and flavors. Keep the oil and salt as directed in the original recipes, and substitute one of these combinations for the other seasonings.

- ¾ teaspoon ground turmeric + ½ teaspoon ground ginger
- ½ teaspoon ground cumin + ¼ teaspoon cayenne pepper
- ½ teaspoon ground cinnamon + ¼ teaspoon ground ginger

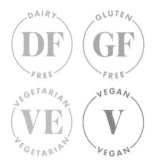

crispy spiced edamame

Cumin, paprika, and ginger are common South American spices, and in this recipe, a touch of soy sauce brings them together to give these baby soybeans a warm umami flavor with little to no heat. Feel free to add a touch of cayenne pepper, if desired.

Cooking spray

1 (16-ounce) bag frozen shelled edamame, thawed

2 tablespoons extra-virgin olive oil

2 teaspoons gluten-free lower-sodium soy sauce or tamari

¼ teaspoon ground cumin

¼ teaspoon smoked paprika

¼ teaspoon ground ginger

¼ teaspoon kosher salt

1 Preheat the oven to 300°F. Coat a large baking sheet with cooking spray.

2 Cook the edamame in the microwave according to the package directions, decreasing the cooking time by 1 minute. Spread the edamame on a clean dish towel; pat dry. Place on the prepared baking sheet. Bake for 10 minutes.

3 Whisk together the oil, soy sauce, cumin, paprika, ginger, and salt in a large bowl. Add the edamame and toss to coat. Spread the edamame on the baking sheet; bake for 30 to 40 minutes more, stirring every 20 minutes. Let cool completely before storing in airtight containers in the refrigerator for up to 3 days. You can eat them cold or reheat in the oven or toaster oven for a few minutes until warmed through.

(SERVING SIZE: ABOUT ¼ CUP): CALORIES 137; FAT 9G (SAT 1G, UNSAT 7G); PROTEIN 8G; CARB 8G; FIBER 4G; SUGARS 0G (ADDED SUGARS 0G); SODIUM 149MG; CALC 5% DV; POTASSIUM 0% DV

edamame

Edamame are young, immature soybeans that you can buy in pods or already shelled. Perfect by themselves as a snack or tossed into dishes like you would another bean, edamame are high in fiber, essential fatty acids, folate, magnesium, phosphorus, thiamin, vitamin K, and protein. In fact, soybeans are one of the few plant foods that provide all the essential amino acids, which can be key for vegetarians.

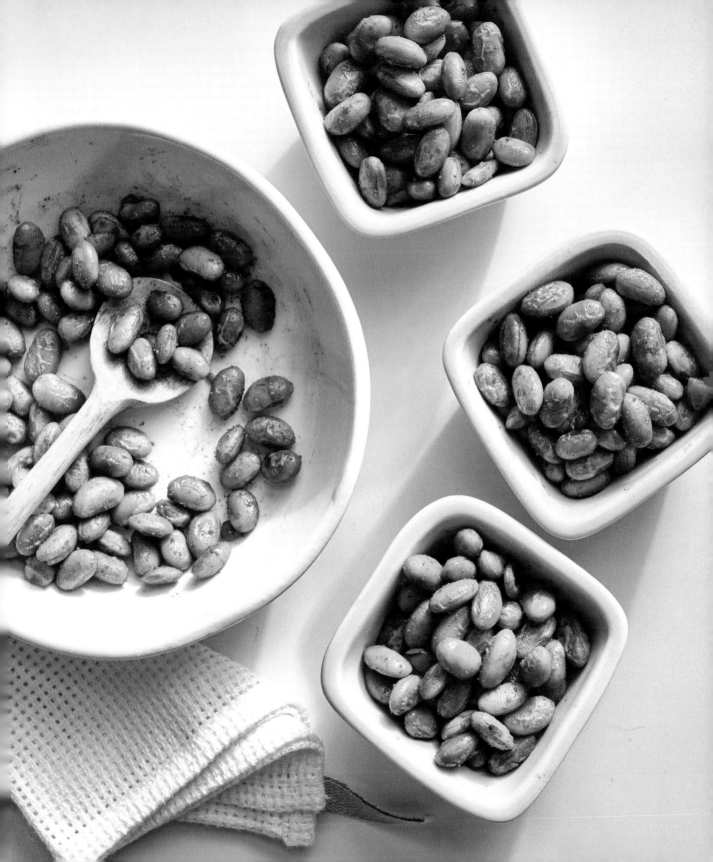

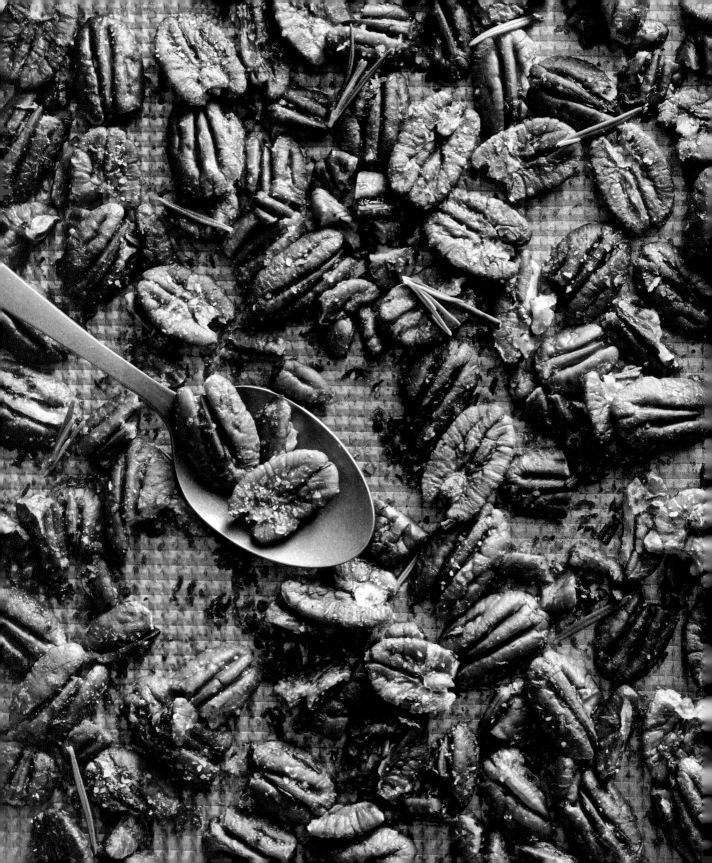

maple-rosemary pecans

Rosemary's stiff green leaves are able to stand up to extended time in the oven, making it one of my favorite herbs to incorporate into both sweet and savory baked dishes. The nuts are equally as good without the touch of sweetness, so feel free to omit the maple syrup if you're trying to avoid all added sugars.

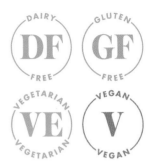

1 Preheat the oven to 325°F. Line a large baking sheet with aluminum foil and coat with cooking spray.

2 Place the rosemary, oil, and maple syrup in a small microwave-safe bowl. Microwave on high for 10 seconds or until the mixture can be whisked together and has a slightly thinner consistency. Place the pecans in a medium bowl and drizzle the rosemary mixture over the nuts; toss to coat. Arrange the coated pecans in a single layer on the prepared baking sheet. Sprinkle with the salt and cayenne; toss gently.

3 Bake for 20 minutes or until lightly toasted. Let cool completely before storing in an airtight container at room temperature for up to 1 week.

Cooking spray

1 tablespoon finely chopped fresh rosemary

1 tablespoon extra-virgin olive oil

1 tablespoon pure maple syrup

2 cups unsalted pecan halves

¾ teaspoon kosher salt

Dash of cayenne pepper

(SERVING SIZE: ABOUT 2 TABLESPOONS): CALORIES 96; FAT 10G (SAT 1G, UNSAT 9G); PROTEIN 1G; CARB 3G; FIBER 1G; SUGARS 1G (ADDED SUGARS 1G); SODIUM 90MG; CALC 1% DV; POTASSIUM 1% DV

nuts

Dry-roasted or plain, salted or unsalted, nuts pack in healthy fats along with some protein, fiber, and antioxidants like vitamin E. This combination allows just a small 1-ounce serving to satiate you for hours—something that really helps on busy days when there's little time to stop and eat. They also can impart powerful health benefits. In fact, research suggests that regularly consuming tree nuts like almonds, walnuts, pecans, hazelnuts, and pistachios may potentially have these effects:

- Reduce risk for heart disease and type 2 diabetes
- Reduce weight gain and likelihood of becoming overweight or obese
- Reduce loss of brain function associated with aging
- Reduce inflammatory markers in the blood

Regular intake is defined in many studies as approximately five 1-ounce servings a week or most days of the week, but even small increases in nut consumption appear to have positive effects.

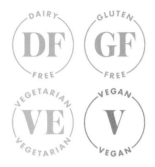

cilantro-avocado hummus

How do you improve on guacamole? Add a little creaminess and protein with the help of chickpeas to turn the dip into more of a hummus-type treat. Use it as a dip for raw veggies, pita chips, or tortilla chips, or spread it on a tortilla to add flavor to a wrap.

1 (15-ounce) can no-salt-added chickpeas, rinsed and drained

2 tablespoons extra-virgin olive oil

1 ripe small avocado, pitted and peeled

¼ cup chopped fresh cilantro

3 tablespoons fresh lime juice

1 teaspoon minced garlic

½ teaspoon ground cumin

¼ teaspoon kosher salt

½ teaspoon cayenne pepper (optional)

3 tablespoons water

Place the chickpeas, oil, avocado, cilantro, lime juice, garlic, cumin, salt, cayenne (if using), and the water in a food processor; process for 1 to 2 minutes or until smooth, stopping once to scrape down the sides. Add additional water, 1 tablespoon at a time, if needed to reach a smooth or desired consistency. Transfer to a medium bowl. Cover and chill until serving.

(SERVING SIZE: ABOUT 2 TABLESPOONS): CALORIES 72; FAT 4G (SAT 1G, UNSAT 3G); PROTEIN 2G; CARB 7G; FIBER 2G; SUGARS 0G (ADDED SUGARS 0G); SODIUM 43MG; CALC 2% DV; POTASSIUM 3% DV

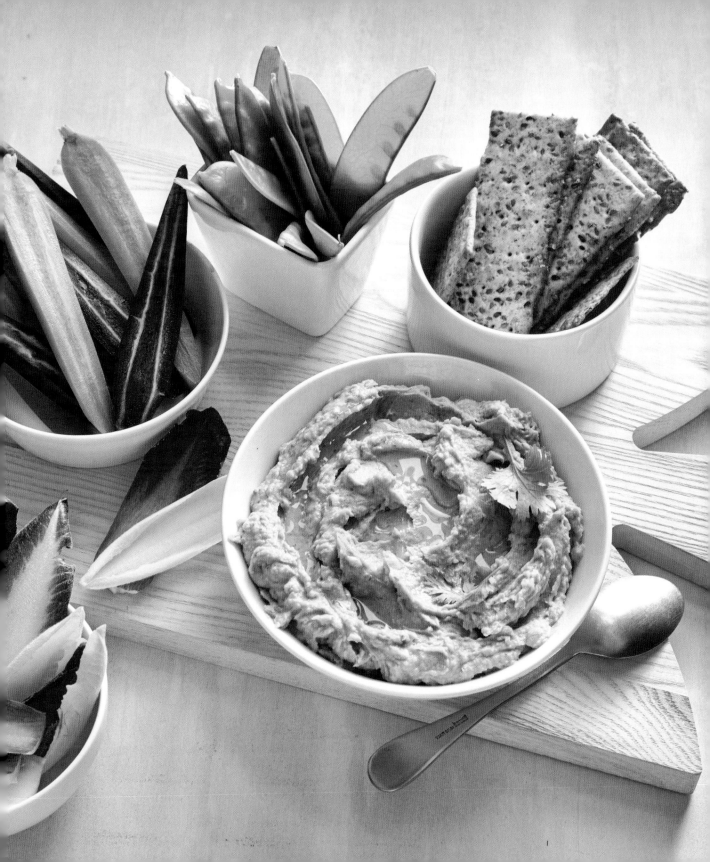

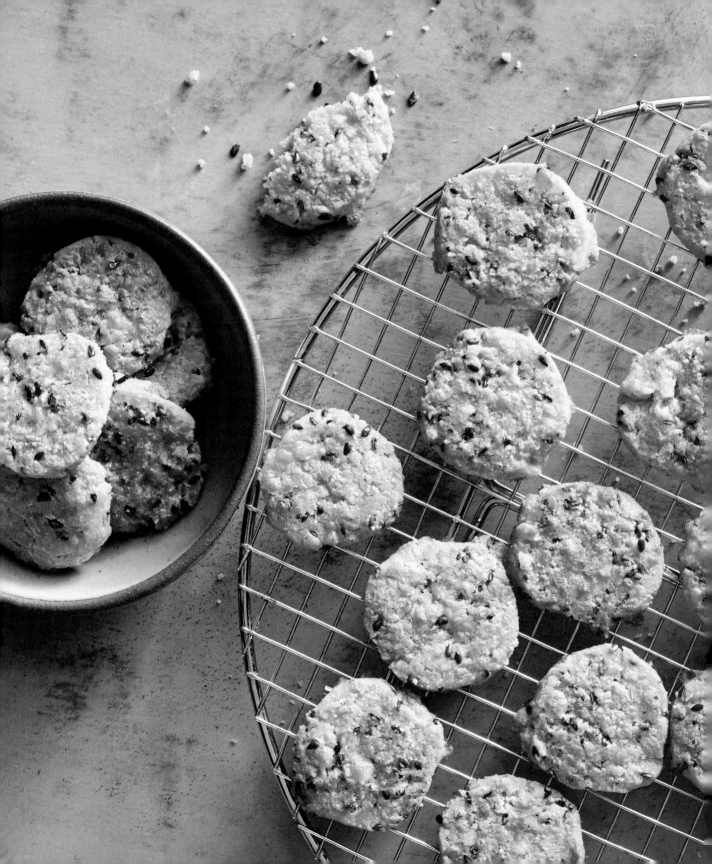

nutty cheese wafers

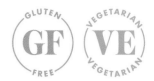

I knew these crispy cracker bites were a keeper when I heard the professionals in the publisher's test kitchen describing them as tasting "just like a Cheez-It." And they've been a hit for all ages: for my kids when served as a cheesy snack and for my friends when served as a bite to go with a glass of wine. It only takes a few minutes to combine the dough and roll it into a log. Slice and bake immediately, or freeze the unbaked log, then cut slices and bake as needed.

1 Preheat the oven to 350°F. Line a large baking sheet with parchment paper.

2 Whisk together the almond flour, flaxseed, salt, and cayenne in a large bowl until well blended. Add the cheese to the flour mixture; toss or stir until combined. Whisk together the egg and oil in a small bowl until blended. Add to the flour mixture and stir until incorporated. Knead the dough until thoroughly combined, and roll it into a 9-inch log (2 inches in diameter). Cut the dough into ¼-inch-thick slices and arrange them on the prepared baking sheet. (Freeze or refrigerate any unbaked dough.)

3 Bake until golden and set, 12 to 14 minutes. Let the wafers cool on the baking sheet for about 20 minutes. Store in an airtight container for up to 1 week.

(SERVING SIZE: 1 WAFER): CALORIES 73; FAT 6G (SAT 2G, UNSAT 4G); PROTEIN 3G; CARB 2G; FIBER 1G; SUGARS 0G (ADDED SUGARS 0G); SODIUM 91MG; CALC 6% DV; POTASSIUM 0% DV

1 cup blanched almond flour (about 3½ ounces)

2 tablespoons ground flaxseed

½ teaspoon kosher salt

¼ teaspoon cayenne pepper

6 ounces sharp cheddar cheese, grated (about 1½ cups)

1 large egg

2 tablespoons olive oil

almond flours

Alternative flours are taking over the baking aisle, and it's likely you'll see "almond flour" and "almond meal," as well as the words "blanched" and "unblanched," on packaging, making buying a simple flour slightly confusing. Here's the difference and benefits to each:

- **ALMOND FLOUR** is made by grinding almonds to a flour-like texture. Superfine almond flour is the closest in texture to white flour. Sold both ways, blanched almond flour is the more common type.
- **ALMOND MEAL** is made by grinding almonds to a slightly coarser texture or larger size than finely ground almond flour. You'll usually find almond meal made with unblanched almonds.
- **BLANCHED** means the outer skin on the almonds was removed. Small amounts of some nutrients are lost, but removing the skins allows for a finer grind.
- **UNBLANCHED** means the nut was ground with the outer skin intact. This can give the ground almonds a slightly darker tint and nuttier flavor, but also makes it a little more nutrient dense.

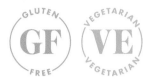

almond butter–yogurt–dipped fruit

Serve as a dip for fresh fruit, or try it the way I love it: frozen, so the dip creates a shell similar to dark chocolate–dipped fruit. The creamy almond butter coating is really all you need, but a sprinkle of a topping like cacao nibs, shredded coconut, or finely chopped nuts can add a little crunch and variety.

1 tablespoon honey

1 cup plain 2% Greek yogurt

3 tablespoons creamy almond butter, warmed in the microwave

1 pint fresh strawberries

Mix the honey, yogurt, and almond butter in a small bowl, stirring well. Dip the strawberries in the yogurt mixture. Eat immediately, or place on a small baking sheet covered with parchment paper and freeze for 20 minutes.

(SERVING SIZE: ABOUT 3 DIPPED STRAWBERRIES): CALORIES 76; FAT 4G (SAT 1G, UNSAT 3G); PROTEIN 3G; CARB 8G; FIBER 1G; SUGARS 6G (ADDED SUGARS 2G); SODIUM 36MG; CALC 8% DV; POTASSIUM 4% DV

how to eat sugar

Sugar will always be in the pantry, and giving up dessert forever isn't realistic. So how do we create a healthy relationship with it?

- **STOP COMPLACENT SUGAR:** The prevalence of added sugars in today's food supply has made us complacent and often unaware of them. It's estimated that the average person consumes around 20 teaspoons (82 grams) of sugar each day—a large majority of which may be from hidden added sugars. So eliminate added sugars that are mindlessly consumed in everyday food and drink by looking more closely at labels. Making slight changes to what you buy usually decreases some added sugars. Also, take a close look at drinks, which often are loaded with sugars.

- **FOLLOW THE 80/20 RULE:** My daily goal is to limit added sugars to 3 teaspoons (12 grams) or less. This allows a touch of added sugar in things like salad dressings or a small piece of dark chocolate. On those occasions that I do indulge, my goal is to stay around 6 teaspoons (25 grams) or less or as close to that as possible.

- **MAKE DESSERT COUNT:** Once you've cut out sugars hidden in products that you use daily, then this allows you the freedom to indulge in an occasional dessert or sugary treat. And when you do, anticipate, savor, and appreciate that sweet sugary taste.

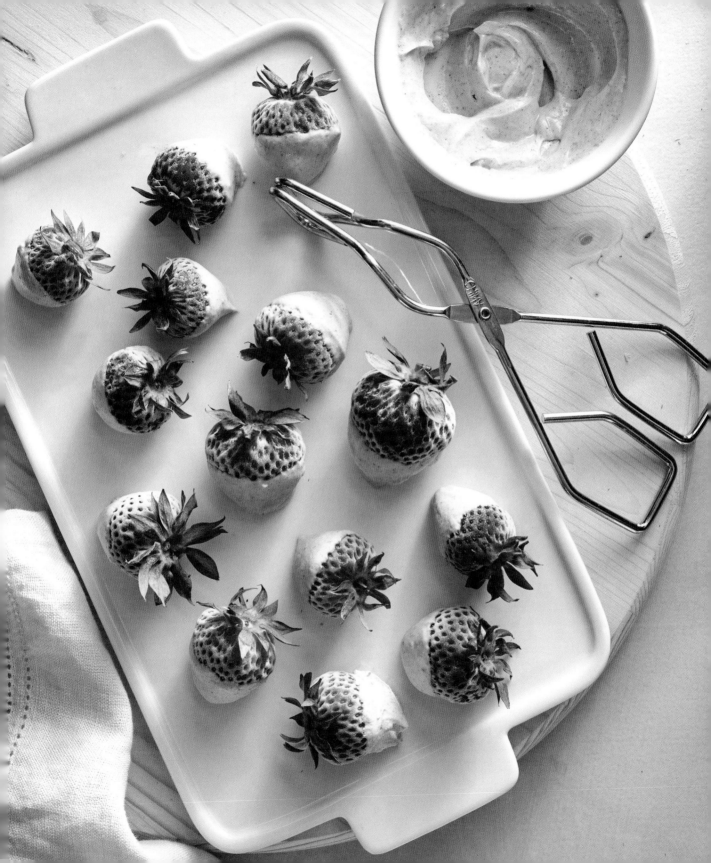

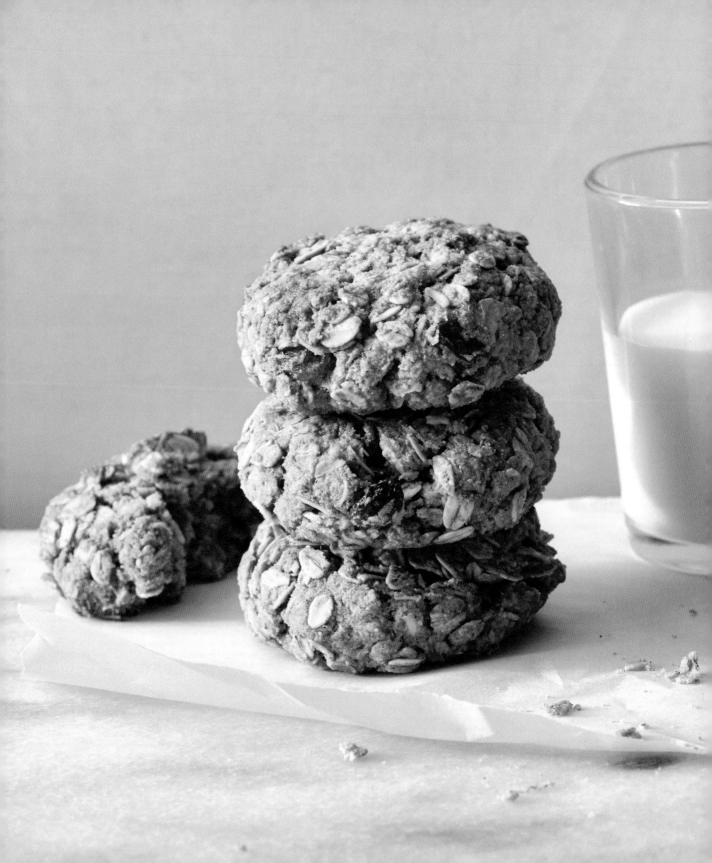

HANDS-ON: 5 MIN. // TOTAL: 50 MIN. // MAKES 9

oatmeal-raisin snack cookies

A filling snack that tastes more like a dessert? Yes, please! Pairing brown sugar with ripe banana provides enough sweetness for these to taste like a treat, but keeps added sugars in check, making them a decent-for-you snack option. This is also a great recipe to help get the kids involved in the kitchen.

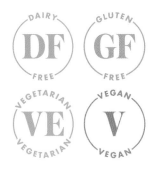

1 Preheat the oven to 350°F. Line a large rimmed baking sheet with parchment paper.

2 Place the banana, brown sugar, oil, and vanilla in a large bowl; stir well until creamy and most of the lumps are gone. In a small bowl, whisk together the flours, salt, baking soda, and cinnamon. Gently fold the flour mixture into the banana mixture until a thick dough forms. Add the oats and raisins and stir to distribute them evenly throughout the dough.

3 Divide the dough into 3-tablespoon portions and roll each portion into a ball. Place on the prepared baking sheet and flatten each ball slightly. Bake until the cookies are beginning to brown on the edges, about 13 minutes. Let cool completely on the baking sheet, about 30 minutes. Store in an airtight container at room temperature for up to 1 week.

(SERVING SIZE: 1 COOKIE): CALORIES 176; FAT 6G (SAT 1G, UNSAT 4G); PROTEIN 3G; CARB 29G; FIBER 3G; SUGARS 11G (ADDED SUGARS 6G); SODIUM 146MG; CALC 2% DV; POTASSIUM 2% DV

½ cup mashed ripe banana (about 1 small)

¼ cup packed light brown sugar

2 tablespoons olive oil

1 teaspoon vanilla extract

½ cup brown rice flour (about 2½ ounces)

¼ cup blanched almond flour (about ⅞ ounces)

½ teaspoon kosher salt

¼ teaspoon baking soda

¼ teaspoon ground cinnamon

1½ cups uncooked old-fashioned rolled oats

¼ cup golden raisins or other dried fruit (such as unsweetened cranberries)

cinnamon

A spice that's already in many kitchens, cinnamon is full of antioxidants and is being researched as a possible treatment for neurological diseases such as Alzheimer's, bacterial and fungal infections, and fat loss. While there's little evidence that cinnamon speeds fat loss, there is research suggesting that cinnamon can help lower blood sugar in type 2 diabetics, as well as healthy individuals. Consuming as little as ¼ teaspoon per day has been shown to have positive results, so sprinkle some on yogurt, stir it into oatmeal, or add it to a smoothie.

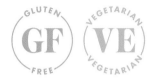

dark chocolate with cranberries and pepitas

This recipe is super easy to make and is a big upgrade from any chocolate candy you can find at the grocery store. A touch of salt plays up the cranberries' sweetness when paired with dark chocolate. Use this as a base and substitute other nuts and dried fruits like dried cherries and slivered almonds, or peanuts and raisins. The recipe directions give you the option to make chocolate cups in mini-muffin pans, bark, or granola crumbles.

5 ounces bittersweet chocolate chips (about ¾ cup)

½ teaspoon ground cinnamon

¼ cup sweetened dried cranberries or other chopped dried fruit

3 tablespoons raw unsalted pumpkin seed kernels (pepitas)

Cooking spray (optional)

⅛ teaspoon flaky sea salt or kosher salt

1 Microwave the chocolate in a microwave-safe bowl on high until melted, about 1½ minutes, stopping to stir the chocolate every 30 seconds. Stir in the cinnamon, cranberries, and pumpkin seed kernels.

2 Lightly coat 9 baking cups of a mini-muffin pan with cooking spray, or line a 15 x 10-inch rimmed baking sheet with aluminum foil. Spoon the chocolate mixture by tablespoons into the prepared muffin cups, or spread it over the prepared baking sheet to ¼-inch thickness. Sprinkle the salt over the chocolate mixture. Freeze for 30 minutes. Remove the pieces from the muffin pan, or break the chocolate sheet into 9 equal pieces. Transfer to an airtight container; store in the freezer for up to 2 months or in the refrigerator for up to 1 week.

(SERVING SIZE: 1 CHOCOLATE CUP OR 1 PIECE OF BARK): CALORIES 122; FAT 8G (SAT 4G, UNSAT 3G); PROTEIN 2G; CARB 12G; FIBER 2G; SUGARS 9G (ADDED SUGARS 6G); SODIUM 32MG; CALC 1% DV; POTASSIUM 2% DV

DARK CHOCOLATE GRANOLA CLUSTERS: Prepare the recipe as directed in step 1, and stir 3 cups whole-grain, gluten-free granola (such as KIND Maple Quinoa Clusters with Chia Seeds) into the chocolate mixture. Spread the mixture evenly over a foil-lined baking sheet. Freeze for 30 minutes. Break the larger clusters apart. Store in an airtight container in the refrigerator for up to 1 week. Eat like trail mix or use as a yogurt topping. Makes about 6 cups (serving size: ⅓ cup).

dark chocolate

The satisfying bittersweet bite is rich in flavonoids, which have been shown to improve cognitive function and possibly reduce blood pressure and the risk of blood clots. It also encourages the release of endorphins, which elevate your mood. For maximum flavonoid benefit, choose a dark chocolate that contains 60% cacao or higher, and avoid those made with alkalized or Dutch-processed cocoa.

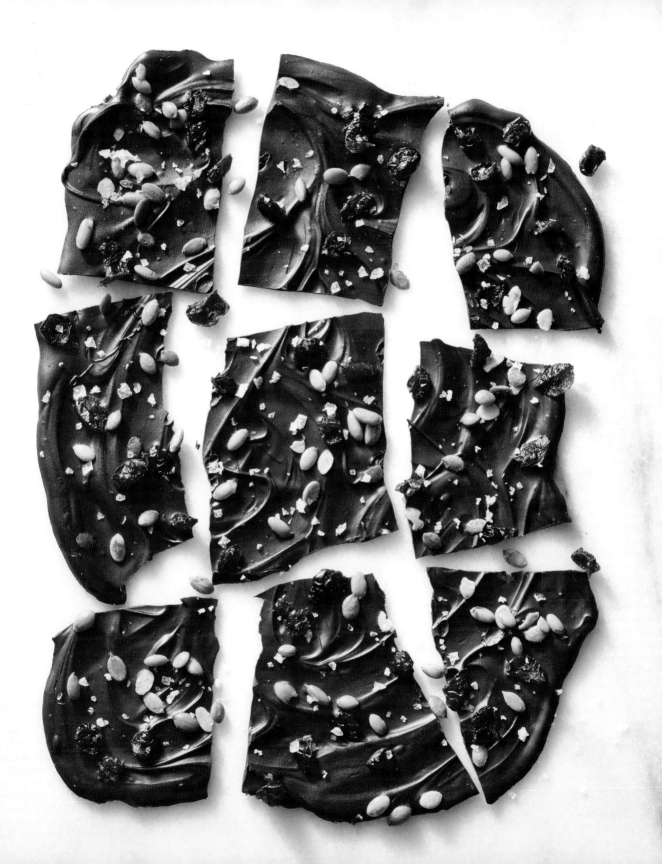

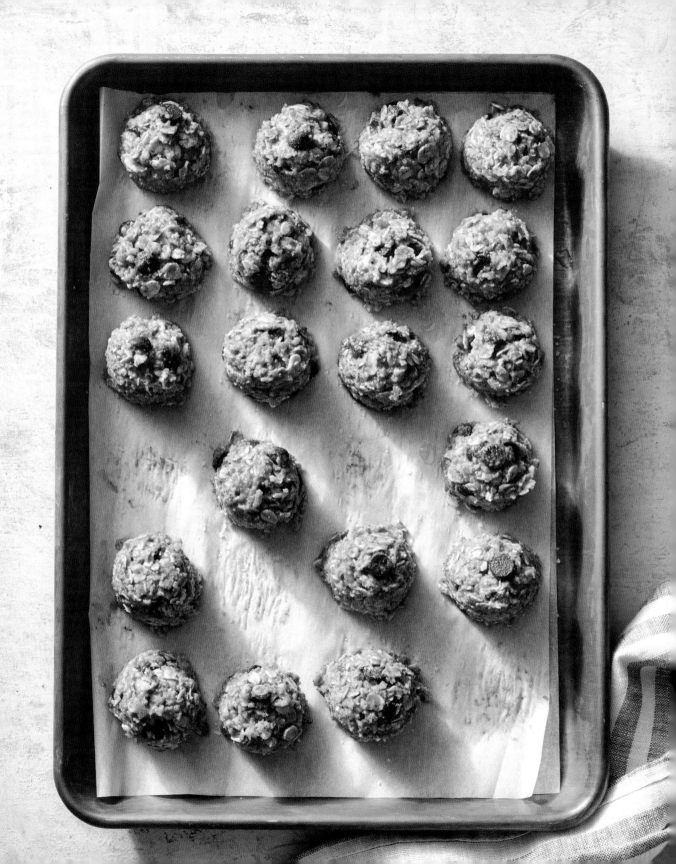

peanut butter–chocolate chip "cookie dough" bites

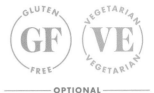

OPTIONAL

Possibly my favorite recipe in the book, this "cookie dough" is seriously good and a bit addictive. A spoonful gives you a sweet, chocolaty, creamy, slightly salty fix all in one. You'll never know the base is chickpeas—trust me on this one. I promise they won't hang around long in your house!

1 Place the chickpeas, peanut butter, brown sugar, almond milk, vanilla, and salt in a food processor; process until smooth, 1 to 2 minutes, stopping to scrape the sides of the bowl as needed.

2 Add 1 cup of the oats and pulse until the oats are blended into the dough, four or five times. Transfer the dough to a large bowl; stir in the chocolate chips and the remaining ½ cup oats.

3 Cover and chill for at least 1 hour or until ready to serve, and serve by the spoonful. Or roll the dough into 1-tablespoon balls. Place the balls on a parchment paper–lined rimmed baking sheet or in an airtight container. Cover and freeze until ready to serve. Let stand at room temperature for 10 minutes before serving.

(SERVING SIZE: 1 BALL): CALORIES 124; FAT 6G (SAT 2G, UNSAT 3G); PROTEIN 4G; CARB 16G; FIBER 2G; SUGARS 8G (ADDED SUGARS 6G); SODIUM 120MG; CALC 1% DV; POTASSIUM 1% DV

DAIRY-FREE AND VEGAN OPTION: Substitute 100% cacao or vegan dark chocolate morsels (such as the Enjoy Life brand) for the dark chocolate chips.

canned chickpeas

I've found that the quality of canned chickpeas varies greatly among brands. The texture of some lower-quality ones tends to be a little drier and crumbly, neither of which is desirable when pureeing chickpeas for hummus or "dough" or roasting them whole. Two brands that seem to consistently provide good-quality chickpeas are Bush's Best and Goya, so stock up when you see those on sale.

- 1 (15-ounce) can no-salt-added chickpeas, rinsed and drained
- ½ cup natural peanut butter or almond butter
- 6 tablespoons light brown sugar
- 3 tablespoons unsweetened almond milk
- 1 tablespoon vanilla extract
- ¾ teaspoon kosher salt
- 1½ cups uncooked old-fashioned rolled oats
- ⅔ cup dark chocolate chips (70% to 85% cacao)

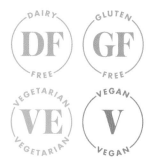

strawberry-basil "nice" cream

Coconut and almond milks create a creamy, dairy-free way to satisfy your sweet tooth and ice cream cravings. I like adding a touch of lemon juice to enhance sweetness and fresh basil to highlight the berries' ripe flavors. Using an ice cream maker incorporates air into the mixture to give the frozen treat a lighter, smoother consistency, but there are also directions to freeze it without one.

3 cups unsweetened vanilla almond milk

1 (13.5-ounce) can coconut milk

1 (16-ounce) package unsweetened frozen whole strawberries (about 3 cups)

½ cup pure maple syrup or honey

3 tablespoons fresh lemon juice

¼ cup packed fresh basil leaves

⅛ teaspoon kosher salt

1 Place the almond milk, coconut milk, strawberries, maple syrup, lemon juice, basil, and salt in a blender; blend until smooth, about 2 minutes.

2 Transfer the mixture to a 1½-quart electric ice cream maker and churn according to the manufacturer's instructions. Transfer to an airtight container; freeze until firm, about 3 hours.

NOTE: If you don't have an ice cream maker, prepare the recipe as directed in step 1, then pour the mixture into a shallow airtight container. Cover and freeze until firm, about 3 hours.

(SERVING SIZE: 1 CUP): CALORIES 141; FAT 9G (SAT 7G, UNSAT 2G); PROTEIN 1G; CARB 16G; FIBER 1G; SUGARS 12G (ADDED SUGARS 10G); SODIUM 79MG; CALC 16% DV; POTASSIUM 3% DV

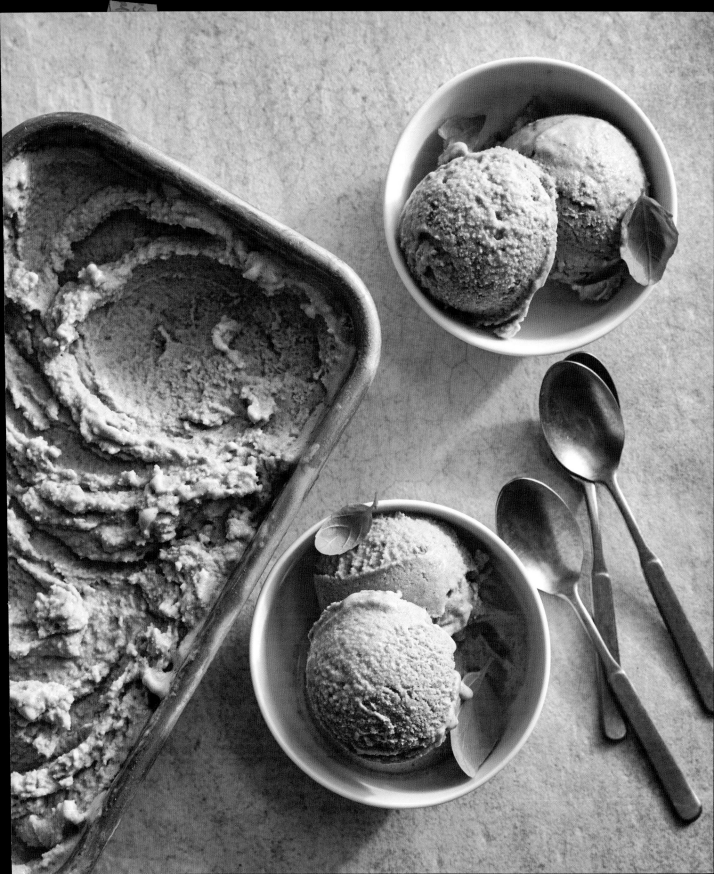

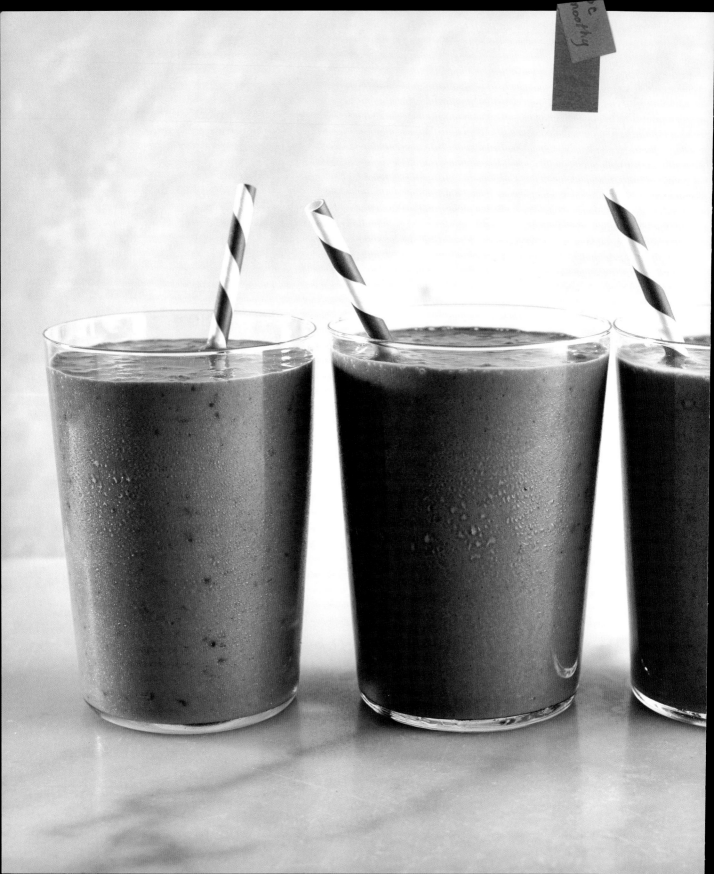

rich dark chocolate smoothie

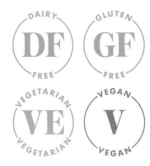

This super-chocolaty smoothie is a tasty nondairy option with no added sugars thanks to dates, which offer up lots of natural richness and a caramel-like sweetness. I originally designed this smoothie as a complete breakfast meal or snack for days when I'm hungrier. When you just need a little boost to tide you over, split the smoothie into two servings.

1 Place the dates in a small bowl; cover with hot water. Let stand for 3 minutes or until softened; drain.

2 Place the milk and dates in a blender; blend for 30 seconds or until pureed. Add the ice, cocoa powder, yogurt, banana, and coffee (if using); blend for 30 seconds or until smooth.

(SERVING SIZE: ABOUT 2⅓ CUPS): CALORIES 302; FAT 7G (SAT 1G, UNSAT 5G); PROTEIN 9G; CARB 58G; FIBER 7G; SUGARS 37G (ADDED SUGARS 13G); SODIUM 200MG; CALC 48% DV; POTASSIUM 14% DV

3 pitted dates

1 cup unsweetened chocolate almond milk

1 cup ice

1 tablespoon unsweetened cocoa powder

1 (5.3-ounce) container vanilla soy yogurt

½ banana, sliced and frozen

Dash of instant coffee or espresso granules (optional)

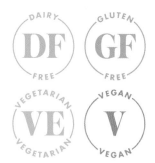

DAIRY FREE DF

GLUTEN FREE GF

VEGETARIAN VE

VEGAN V

cold-brew iced green tea

I remember making sun tea with my mom when I was little, and this process is similar—but you don't have to wait for warm summer weather. To sweeten it, I like to add a touch of stevia or stir in a little honey thinned with warm water.

6 cups water, at room
   temperature
4 green tea bags
2 or 3 lemon slices

Combine the water, tea bags, and lemon slices in a pitcher or a large container with a lid. Refrigerate for at least 8 hours. Remove the tea bags, straining the liquid. Return the tea to a pitcher. Discard the tea bags and lemon slices. Sweeten as desired, stirring well. Chill until ready to serve. Serve over ice.

(SERVING SIZE: 1 CUP): CALORIES 0; FAT 0G (SAT 0G, UNSAT 0G); PROTEIN 0G; CARB 0G; FIBER 0G; SUGARS 0G (ADDED SUGARS 0G); SODIUM 0MG; CALC 0% DV; POTASSIUM 0% DV

STRAWBERRY-CITRUS ICED GREEN TEA: Omit the lemon slices, and replace with 1 small (thin-skinned) orange, peeled and sliced, and 6 to 10 large strawberries, hulled and halved. Chill and strain as directed, reserving the orange sections; squeeze the juice from the orange sections into the pitcher. Sweeten as desired, stirring well. Chill until ready to serve. Serve over ice.

GINGER-MINT ICED GREEN TEA: Omit the lemon slices, and replace with 1 (1-inch) piece peeled fresh ginger and 4 to 6 fresh mint sprigs. Chill and strain as directed above. Sweeten as desired, stirring well. Chill until ready to serve. Serve over ice.

green tea

This antioxidant-rich beverage appears to be one of the best ways to keep the brain hydrated thanks to compounds called catechins. Not only do catechins appear to be some of the most effective antioxidants in preventing free radical damage, but some research suggests they can help block amyloid plaque formation associated with Alzheimer's disease. Green tea is also associated with reducing heart disease risk and preventing cancer. Most research points to drinking a cup, hot or cold, one to three times per day, but remember that even green tea has a small amount of caffeine, so balance your intake with other caffeine consumed or if you have sensitivities to caffeine.

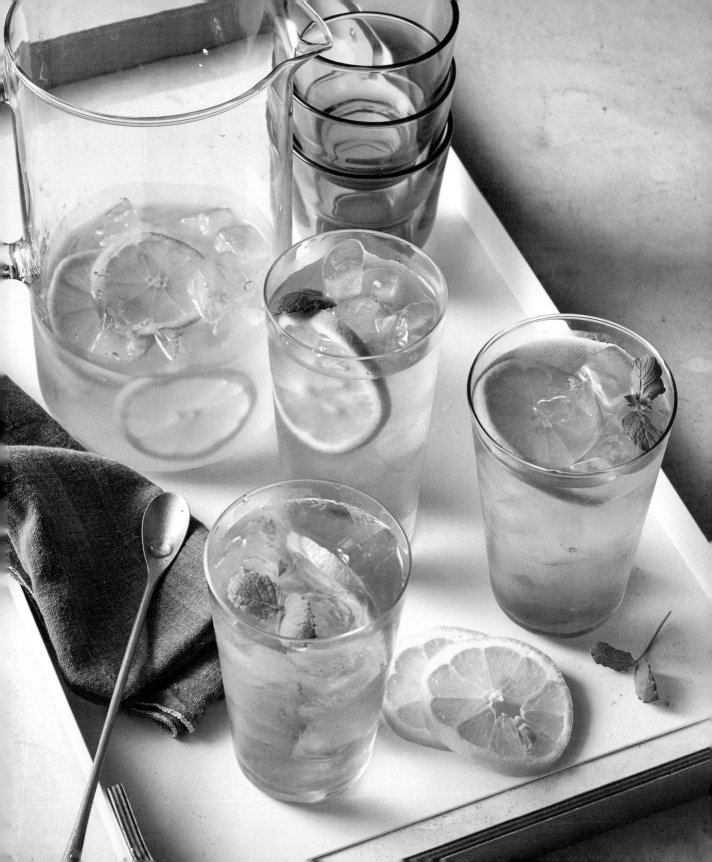

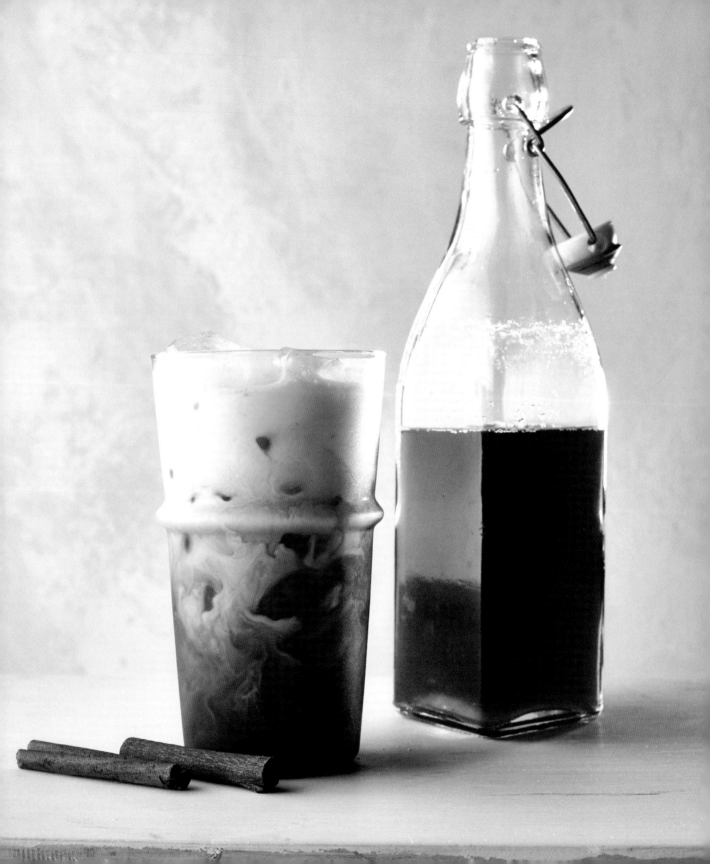

chai concentrate

Warm, fragrant spices transform an ordinary tea into something special while also soothing inflammation. Toasting the spices in a saucepan helps to bring out their flavors before steeping the tea bags. Adjust the syrup for sweetness, or substitute for stevia, if desired.

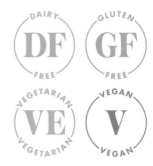

1 Place the peppercorns, cardamom, cloves, and cinnamon in a medium saucepan and cook over medium, stirring frequently, for 3 to 4 minutes until fragrant and lightly golden. Add the water and ginger, and bring to a boil. Reduce the heat to medium-low; simmer, partially covered, for 10 minutes. Remove from the heat; add the tea bags and steep for 5 minutes. Remove the tea bags, gently squeezing them to release excess water; discard the bags.

2 Add the maple syrup and vanilla and stir to combine. Let stand for 1 hour; strain and discard the solids. Store the concentrate in an airtight container in the refrigerator for up to 1 week. To prepare, combine ½ to ¾ cup milk with 1 cup concentrate. Serve hot or cold over ice.

(SERVING SIZE: ¾ CUP CONCENTRATE): CALORIES 29; FAT 0G (SAT 0G, UNSAT 0G); PROTEIN 0G; CARB 7G; FIBER 0G; SUGARS 6G (ADDED SUGARS 6G); SODIUM 8MG; CALC 1% DV; POTASSIUM 2% DV

- 20 black peppercorns
- 8 cardamom pods
- 10 cloves
- 2 cinnamon sticks
- 4 cups water
- 1 (2-inch) piece fresh ginger, sliced
- 4 black tea bags (such as English Breakfast)
- 2 tablespoons maple syrup or honey
- ¼ teaspoon pure vanilla extract
- Dairy or nondairy milk for serving

coffee or tea?

Looks like you may not have to pick, because coffee (in moderate amounts) appears to offer health perks, too. Harvard researchers found that people who drink 3 to 5 cups of coffee (caffeinated or decaf) a day may have a lower risk of developing neurological diseases and type 2 diabetes. Coffee lovers can thank chlorogenic acid, a compound in coffee that acts as an anti-inflammatory and decreases cells' insulin resistance. Caffeine also blocks adenosine, a chemical that inhibits the activity of nerve cells; several studies correlate caffeine intake with higher scores on memory tests.

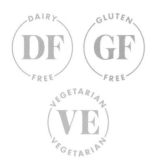

simple honey syrup

Try a simple syrup made with honey instead of granulated sugar to cut the added sugar content in cocktail mixers while still getting a touch of needed sweetness. Making the Simple Honey Syrup in the microwave is quick and easy, but you can also heat it on the stovetop. Store in the refrigerator, and shake before using.

3 tablespoons local honey
1 cup warm water

Place the honey in a microwave-safe bowl or jar. Microwave on high until warm, 10 to 15 seconds. Add the water and whisk until blended. (If using a jar, cover with the lid and shake well.) Store in an airtight container in the refrigerator for up to 1 month.

(SERVING SIZE: 2 TABLESPOONS): CALORIES 22; FAT 0G (SAT 0G, UNSAT 0G); PROTEIN 0G; CARB 6G; FIBER 0G; SUGARS 6G (ADDED SUGARS 6G); SODIUM 0MG; CALC 0% DV; POTASSIUM 0% DV

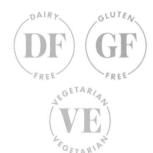

classic margarita

Fresh juices and my easy Simple Honey Syrup create a margarita with all the tart, slightly sweet flavor that I love. But the calories and sugar are drastically lower when compared to a margarita of similar size made with a standard syrup or mixer. Add a little bit of club soda if you like to sip on your drink a bit longer.

¼ cup Simple Honey Syrup
2 tablespoons fresh lime juice
1 tablespoon fresh orange
   juice
6 tablespoons (3 ounces)
   blanco tequila
Ice
½ cup club soda (optional)

1 Combine the honey syrup, lime juice, orange juice, and tequila in a cocktail shaker, and add enough ice to fill the shaker. Cover with the lid and shake vigorously until chilled, about 30 seconds.

2 Fill two glasses with ice, and strain the tequila mixture evenly into the glasses. Top each with club soda for a taller drink, if desired.

(SERVING SIZE: 1 DRINK): CALORIES 139; FAT 0G (SAT 0G, UNSAT 0G); PROTEIN 0G; CARB 8G; FIBER 0G; SUGARS 7G (ADDED SUGARS 6G); SODIUM 1MG; CALC 0% DV; POTASSIUM 1% DV

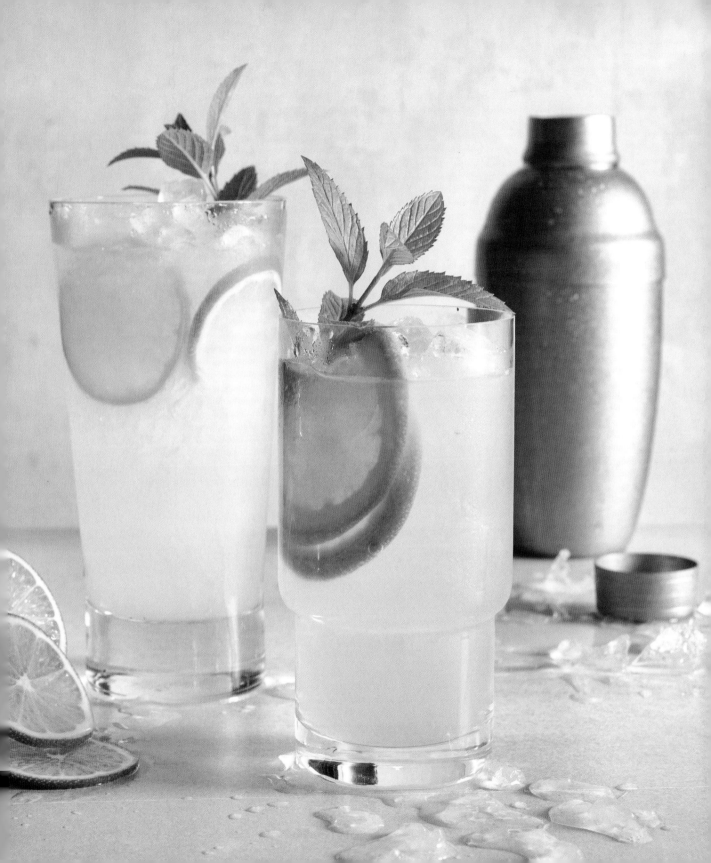

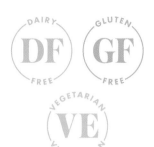

DAIRY FREE **DF**

GLUTEN FREE **GF**

VEGETARIAN **VE** VEGETARIAN

kombucha margarita

It's important to buy a kombucha that will work well with the other flavors in this drink. If you can't find a plain citrus Kombucha, opt for one labeled "original."

3 tablespoons Simple Honey Syrup (page 272)

2 tablespoons fresh lime juice

6 tablespoons (3 ounces) blanco tequila

Ice

1 cup citrus kombucha (such as GT's Enlightened Organic Raw Citrus Kombucha)

1 Combine the honey syrup, lime juice, and tequila in a cocktail shaker, and add enough ice to fill the shaker. Cover with the lid and shake vigorously until chilled, about 30 seconds.

2 Fill two glasses with ice and strain the tequila mixture evenly into the glasses. Top evenly with the kombucha, and stir.

(SERVING SIZE: 1 DRINK): CALORIES 144; FAT 0G (SAT 0G, UNSAT 0G); PROTEIN 0G; CARB 9G; FIBER 0G; SUGARS 6G (ADDED SUGARS 5G); SODIUM 6MG; CALC 0% DV; POTASSIUM 0% DV

kombucha

Kombucha is made by fermenting tea, usually black tea, to create a fizzy beverage that's tart and slightly sweet. Variations may be flavored with fruit, herbs, spices, or a combination. Drinking kombucha has become a mainstream craze that touts some pretty good health benefits. The fermentation process used to make it means the beverage has live cultures—which you may hear more commonly referred to as probiotics—that promote good gut health. Two tips for when you try:

• Don't be tempted to shake the bottle. Similar to soda, the fizzy drink will expand and overflow once opened if shaken.

• Choose one with 4g or less of sugar per 1-cup serving (8 fluid ounces). All kombuchas require a little sugar to initiate fermentation, but some have sugar added post-fermentation to sweeten them.

pomegranate cape cod

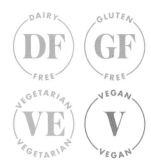

Pomegranate juice packs a powerful punch of heart-healthy polyphenols. For an added touch, muddle a few pomegranate seeds (also known as arils) with the ginger and lime. The more the arils break down, the more color and flavor they release into the drink.

Muddle the ginger and lime wedge in a cocktail shaker. Add the cranberry juice, pomegranate juice, vodka, and 3 ice cubes; cover, and shake well for 15 seconds. Fill two highball glasses with ice and strain the mixture evenly into the glasses. Top each glass evenly with the club soda.

(SERVING SIZE: 1 DRINK): CALORIES 154; FAT 0G (SAT 0G, UNSAT 0G); PROTEIN 0G; CARB 14G; FIBER 0G; SUGARS 14G (ADDED SUGARS 0G); SODIUM 21MG; CALC 2% DV; POTASSIUM 3% DV

2 teaspoons thinly sliced
   fresh ginger
1 (1-inch) lime wedge
¾ cup cranberry juice
¼ cup pomegranate juice
6 tablespoons (3 ounces)
   silver vodka
Ice
½ cup club soda

alcohol and inflammation

Getting health professionals to talk about the benefits associated with drinking alcohol is tough, and understandably so since it's so easy to cross the line from beneficial to harmful. And most doctors still don't think the benefits are great enough to suggest you start drinking if you don't already drink. But for those who do occasionally consume a glass of wine or a beer, moderate alcohol intake is associated with a lower cardiovascular risk and possibly reduced severity of rheumatoid arthritis. Both of these benefits are attributed to the slight anti-inflammatory effect seen with moderate alcohol intake. Here are a few things to consider before pouring your next drink.

- Moderate consumption is the key to reaping any potential benefits from drinking alcohol. The definition of "moderate" varies among researchers, but it is commonly understood to be no more than 1 drink per day for women and no more than 2 drinks per day for men.
- A "drink" is generally considered a 5-ounce glass of wine, a 12-ounce beer, or a 1½-ounce serving of hard liquor.
- The type of alcohol appears to have little impact on potential health benefits. Studies have found similar cardiovascular risk reduction in those who drank moderate amounts of wine, and those who drank moderate amounts of beer or liquor.
- Alcohol isn't a nutrient, but it still has calories. Those calories can contribute to obesity, which is an inflammatory risk factor. Minimize calories from alcohol by choosing a glass of wine, a light beer, or a serving of liquor mixed with a low- or no-calorie mixer.

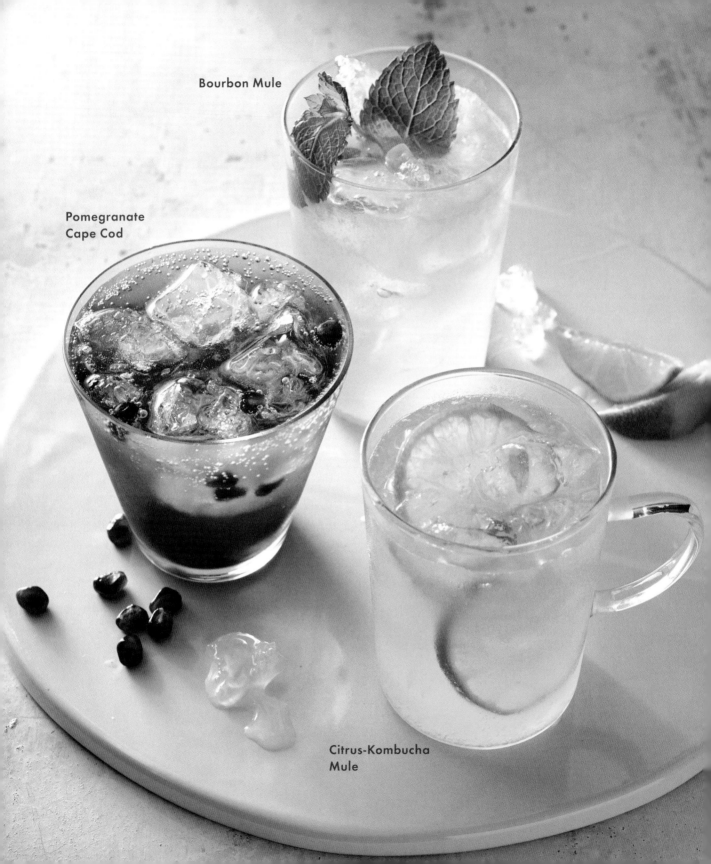

Bourbon Mule

Pomegranate
Cape Cod

Citrus-Kombucha
Mule

HANDS-ON: 4 MIN. // TOTAL: 4 MIN. // SERVES 2

bourbon mule

Ginger beers are available in both alcoholic and nonalcoholic varieties, so check the label depending on preference. Ginger beer has a spicier kick than ginger ale, which you can substitute, if desired.

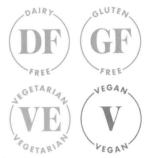

- Ice
- 6 tablespoons (3 ounces) bourbon
- 2 tablespoons fresh lime juice
- 1 cup (8 ounces) ginger beer
- 2 fresh mint sprigs
- 2 lime slices

Fill two copper mule mugs with ice. Divide the bourbon, lime juice, and ginger beer evenly between the mugs; stir to combine. Serve garnished with the mint and lime slices.

(SERVING SIZE: 1 DRINK): CALORIES 166; FAT 0G (SAT 0G, UNSAT 0G); PROTEIN 0G; CARB 18G; FIBER 0G; SUGARS 0G (ADDED SUGARS 0G); SODIUM 1MG; CALC 0% DV; POTASSIUM 0% DV

HANDS-ON: 5 MIN. // TOTAL: 5 MIN. // SERVES 2

citrus-kombucha mule

Kombucha and orange juice are a fun variation to the classic mule cocktail, which is traditionally made with ginger beer, lime juice, and vodka. Orange, grapefruit, tangerine, blood orange—use any freshly squeezed citrus juice that you have on hand. Then serve over ice, and garnish with fresh lime slices or wedges.

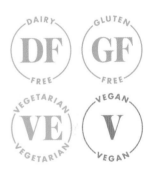

- Ice
- ¾ cup (6 ounces) ginger beer
- ½ cup citrus or ginger kombucha
- ½ cup fresh orange or grapefruit juice
- 6 tablespoons (3 ounces) vodka
- 2 tablespoons fresh lime juice

Fill two copper mule mugs with ice. Divide the ginger beer, kombucha, orange juice, vodka, and lime juice evenly between the mugs; stir to combine.

(SERVING SIZE: 1 DRINK): CALORIES 185; FAT 0G (SAT 0G, UNSAT 0G); PROTEIN 0G; CARB 22G; FIBER 0G; SUGARS 6G (ADDED SUGARS 1G); SODIUM 4MG; CALC 1% DV; POTASSIUM 3% DV

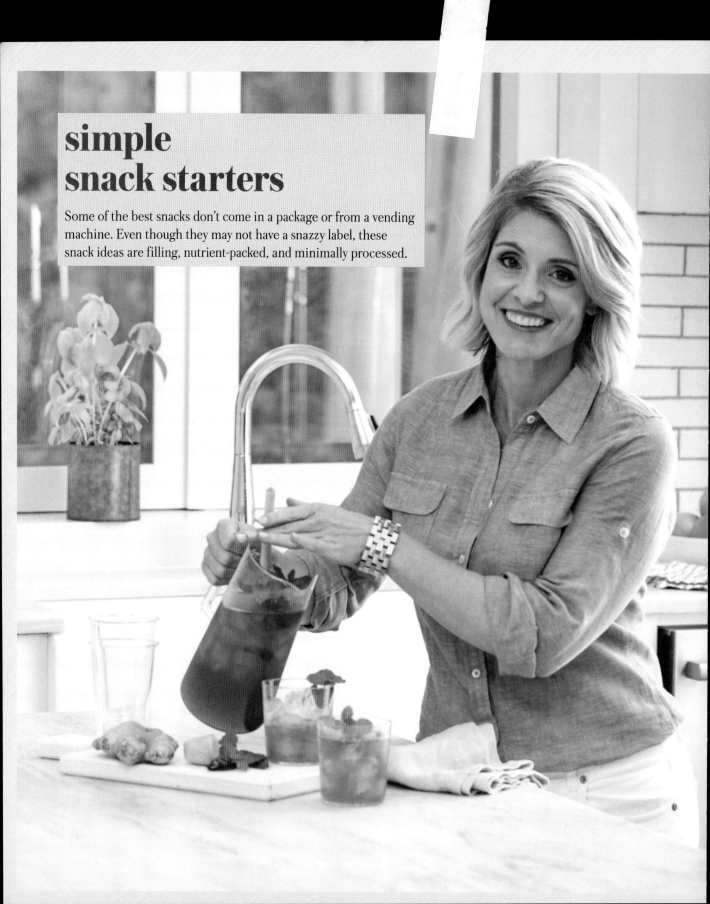

simple snack starters

Some of the best snacks don't come in a package or from a vending machine. Even though they may not have a snazzy label, these snack ideas are filling, nutrient-packed, and minimally processed.

proteins and carbs

Hard-boiled egg · Roasted chickpeas · Edamame · Yogurt · Cheese slices or stick · Cottage cheese · Whole-grain or legume-based crackers

Popcorn · Corn or whole-grain tortilla · Tortilla chips · Whole-grain pita bread · Kale chips or sweet potato chips

veggies and fruit

Cucumber slices · Carrots · Cherry tomatoes · Sugar snap peas · Celery sticks · Apple slices · Peach, nectarine

Berries · Fruit salad · Citrus sections · Melon cubes · Pineapple chunks · Grapes · Clementine

nuts, dips, spreads, and extras

Walnuts, almonds, cashews, pistachios, etc. · Hummus · Avocado · Guacamole · Salsa · Goat cheese · Tzatziki sauce

Peanut butter or other nut butter · Piece of dark chocolate · Chocolate-covered nuts · Chocolate milk or nondairy milk with protein

easy snack combinations

Mixed berries + cheese stick

Whole-grain bread slice + avocado

Roasted chickpeas + an orange

Whole corn tortilla chips + guacamole + salsa

Hard-boiled egg + watermelon cubes

Cucumber + hummus

Dark chocolate square + peanut butter

Plain yogurt + sliced almonds + drizzle of honey

Pear + almond butter

Steamed or roasted edamame

Sugar snap peas + tzatziki sauce + grapes

snack buying guide

Snack foods range widely in nutrient composition and food type, which makes it difficult to define parameters. Here are some general guidelines to use when shopping:

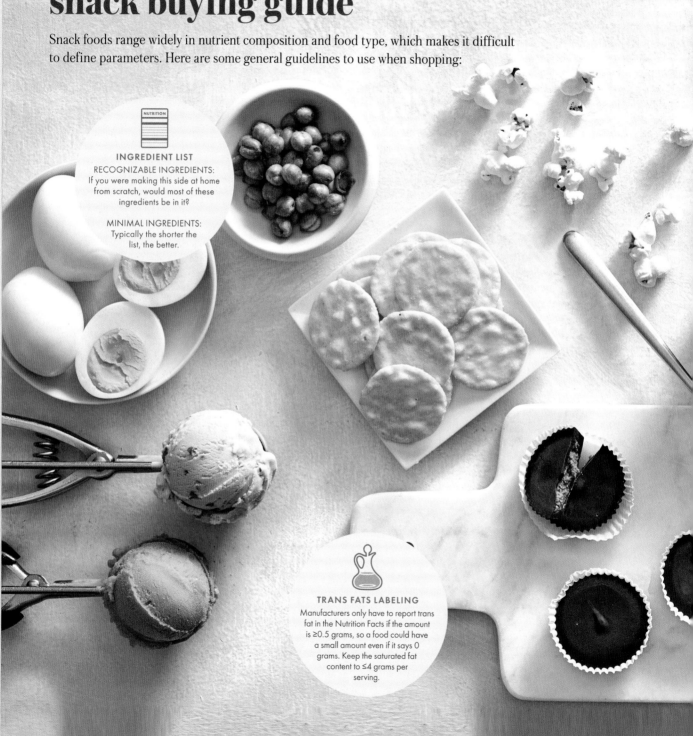

INGREDIENT LIST

RECOGNIZABLE INGREDIENTS:
If you were making this side at home from scratch, would most of these ingredients be in it?

MINIMAL INGREDIENTS:
Typically the shorter the list, the better.

TRANS FATS LABELING

Manufacturers only have to report trans fat in the Nutrition Facts if the amount is ≥0.5 grams, so a food could have a small amount even if it says 0 grams. Keep the saturated fat content to ≤4 grams per serving.

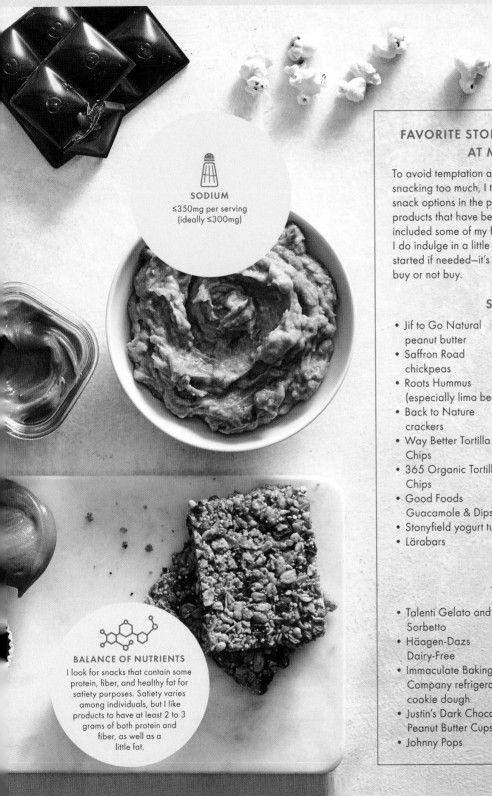

SODIUM

≤350mg per serving
(ideally ≤300mg)

BALANCE OF NUTRIENTS

I look for snacks that contain some
protein, fiber, and healthy fat for
satiety purposes. Satiety varies
among individuals, but I like
products to have at least 2 to 3
grams of both protein and
fiber, as well as a
little fat.

FAVORITE STORE-BOUGHT SNACKS AT MY HOUSE

To avoid temptation and to keep my kids from
snacking too much, I try not to keep too many
snack options in the pantry. These are some newer
products that have been hits at my house. I've also
included some of my favorite sweet treats when
I do indulge in a little sugar. Use this list to get
started if needed—it's not a definitive list of what to
buy or not buy.

SNACKS

- Jif to Go Natural peanut butter
- Saffron Road chickpeas
- Roots Hummus (especially lima bean)
- Back to Nature crackers
- Way Better Tortilla Chips
- 365 Organic Tortilla Chips
- Good Foods Guacamole & Dips
- Stonyfield yogurt tubes
- Lärabars
- Chobani Greek Yogurt tubes
- Hope Foods Hummus
- Cedar's Foods Hommus Snack Packs
- Angie's Boom Chicka popcorn
- Planters NUT-trition Packs
- KIND Protein Crunchy Peanut Butter Bar (also good for breakfast)
- Eggland's Best Hard-Cooked Eggs
- Justin's Classic Almond Butter

TREATS

- Talenti Gelato and Sorbetto
- Häagen-Dazs Dairy-Free
- Immaculate Baking Company refrigerated cookie dough
- Justin's Dark Chocolate Peanut Butter Cups
- Johnny Pops
- BarkTHINS Snacking Chocolate
- Ghiradelli Chocolate Sea Salt Soiree squares
- Green & Black's Pure Dark Chocolate with Salted Caramel 70% Cacao

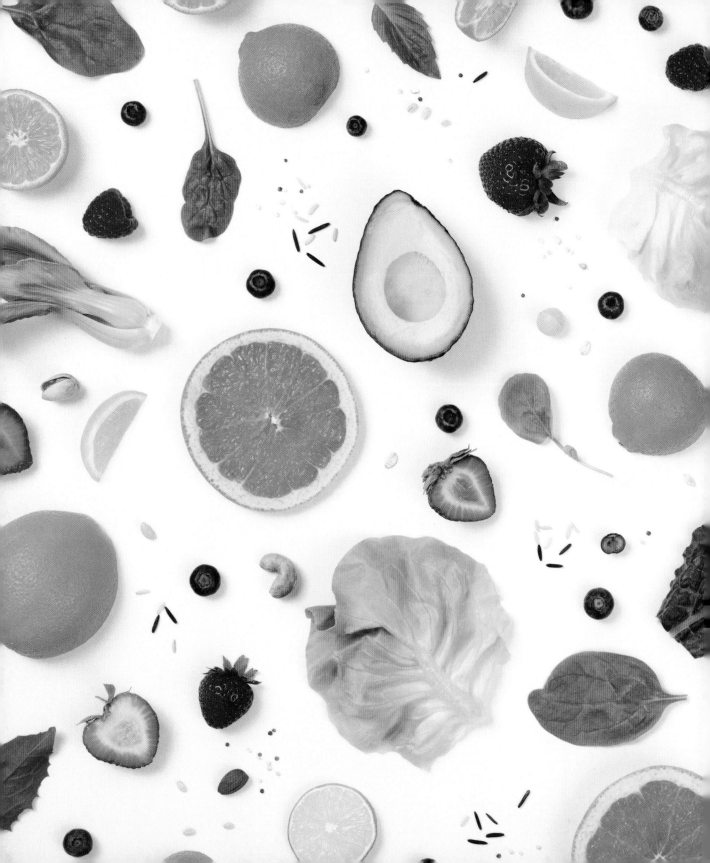

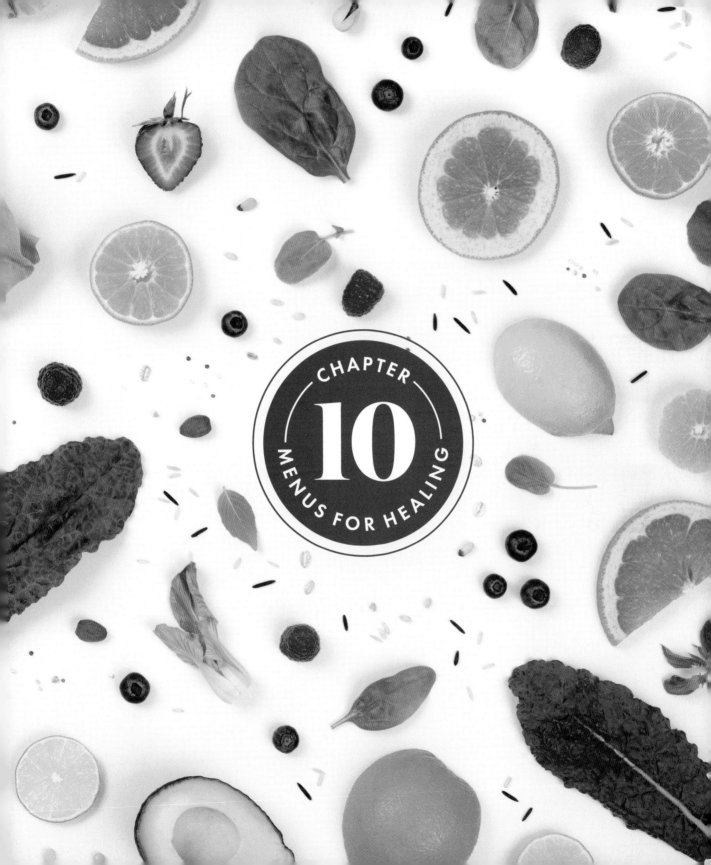

CHAPTER

10

MENUS FOR HEALING

Ready to see how *quick*, easy, and delicious anti-inflammatory eating can really be? Let me walk you through the process to begin healing your body and then target your specific health concerns.

———

Before you know it, making and eating anti-inflammatory food choices will be second nature—I promise!

how this chapter is designed

One thing I've learned while trying to incorporate anti-inflammatory eating at my house, as well as teaching others how to do it, is that most people *get* the guidelines and research. They also love the recipes. The trouble comes when they try to pull the guidelines and recipes together to create a weekly menu. Because of this, I've created weekly menus using recipes in the book and other simple food items for you to use as guides. The Menu Plan to Detox and Restore can be used by all individuals for the first couple of weeks. Weekly menu-planning guides are then provided for the most common inflammatory disease conditions.

These menus incorporate the key nutrients and diet aspects that current research has associated with risk prevention or easing of symptoms.

1 // DETOX AND RESTORE
2 // PREVENT OR MANAGE TYPE 2 DIABETES
3 // CANCER PREVENTION
4 // HEART HEALTH
5 // BRAIN HEALTH
6 // JOINT HEALTH AND PAIN RELIEF
7 // AUTOIMMUNE CONDITIONS

how to incorporate these guides

STEP #1: ASSESS. Use the assessment on page 41 to determine where your initial focus should be.

STEP #2: DETOX AND RESTORE. Start the healing process by using the Menu Plan to Detox and Restore (page 288) to immediately begin calming inflammation and replenishing the body and gut. Follow this plan for at least two weeks.

STEP #3: TARGET OR REASSESS. When you want to target certain health issues, choose the eating guidelines and menus for your specific health concerns. They are designed to prevent, soothe, or ease related symptoms. If you feel like you need to target additional eating habits before focusing on specific concerns, then reassess and continue the Detox and Restore process (see "Defining Your Own Plan" on page 42).

STEP #4: EAT AND FEEL GOOD!

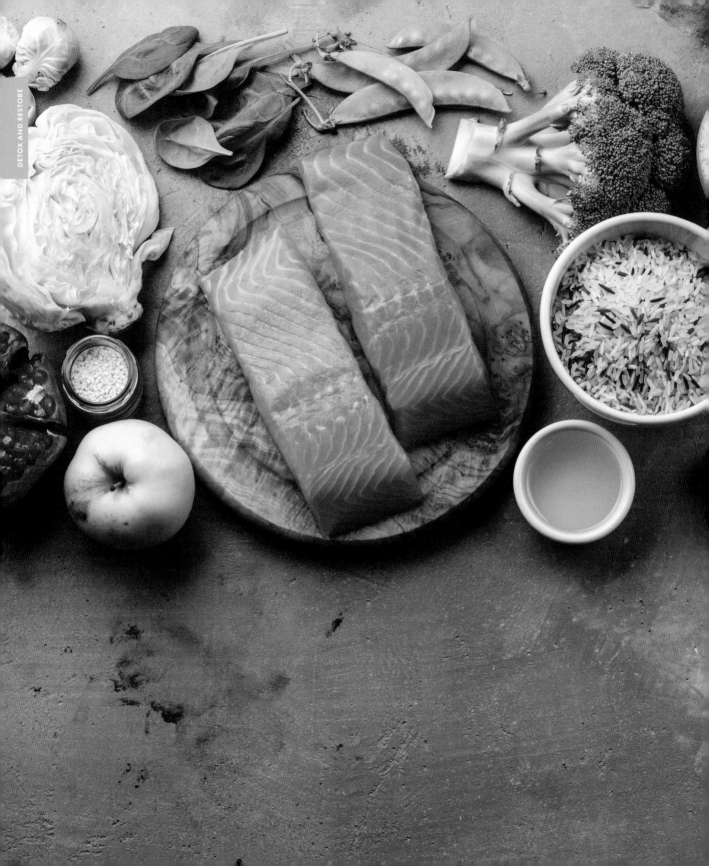

EATING TO
detox and restore the body

Add additional vegetables, fruits, dairy or nondairy yogurt, and healthy fat sources as desired to supplement breakfast, lunch, and snack suggestions.

essential focus areas

- **USE** the Anti-inflammatory Eating Recommendations on page 38 as a guide for food sources and amounts.
- **EMPHASIZE** variety in vegetable intake, and regularly incorporate cruciferous vegetables and leafy greens.
- **FOCUS** on vibrant colors when choosing fruits, and regularly incorporate berries and citrus.
- **CHOOSE** starchy vegetables, beans, lentils, peas, and whole grains as complex carbohydrate sources. Avoid all refined grains and highly processed starch sources.
- **CONSUME** only whole or minimally processed foods when possible to eliminate any unnecessary additives like colorings, artificial sweeteners, chemicals, and pesticides.
- **INCREASE** intake of probiotic and prebiotic foods (see page 18 for a list).
- **INCREASE** the proportion of plant-based proteins to animal-based proteins in your meals.
- **HYDRATE** the body daily with adequate water intake (a minimum of 64 fluid ounces and increasing based on thirst, environment, and physical activity demands).

additional considerations

- Eliminate all potential irritants like gluten, added sugars, alcohol, excessive caffeine, etc. (Don't worry—most of these are temporary unless a specific condition suggests continued elimination.)
- Keep coffee and/or tea consumption to less than 3 cups or 300mg caffeine daily.

- Focus on incorporating more omega-3-rich fats into your diet in place of or in addition to omega-6 fats (see page 30 for a list).
- If you have reason to think you may have a sensitivity to dairy foods, I encourage you to eliminate these as well during this period so you can later determine if your symptoms are being caused by dairy or other irritants.

REMEMBER, DETOX DOES _NOT_ MEAN:

- Eliminating food group(s) unless you have specific allergies or sensitivities
- Consuming only liquids, juices, or odd food combinations
- Severely restricting calories
- Cutting out flavor, taste, salt, or fat

GOALS

①	②	③
Allow the body to calm existing inflammation by eliminating potential irritants.	Consume nutrient-dense foods to replenish nutrient stores and to support the liver's natural detoxification process.	Begin to restore, balance, and nourish gut bacteria.

start here: menu plan to detox and restore

DETOX AND RESTORE

DAY 1 MEALS

BREAKFAST

Grain- or greens-based savory breakfast bowl (page 97)

LUNCH

Avocado-Chicken Salad (page 105)

DINNER

Grilled Salmon with Quick Romesco (page 159)

Sautéed spaghetti squash (page 53)

Sautéed Spinach with Pine Nuts and Raisins (page 225)

DAY 2 MEALS

BREAKFAST

Super Green Frittata Bites (page 89)

LUNCH

Build-your-own Spaghetti Squash Bowl (page 53)

DINNER

Chicken Fried Quinoa (page 138)

Steamed green beans

DAY 3 MEALS

BREAKFAST

Berry Green Smoothie (page 82)

LUNCH

Tuna, White Bean, and Arugula Salad (page 109) or tuna salad with greens

DINNER

Lemony Black Bean–Quinoa Salad (page 191)

Yogurt and mixed berries

DAY 4 MEALS

BREAKFAST

Sweet Potato Home Fries with Eggs (page 90)

LUNCH

Leftover Chicken Fried Quinoa (page 138) from Day 2 Dinner

DINNER

Sea Bass with Strawberry-Citrus Salsa (page 163)

Brown rice

Mixed greens with vinaigrette

DAY 5 MEALS

BREAKFAST

Warm Spinach Breakfast Bowl
(page 93)

LUNCH

Chicken Salad with Apple,
Cashews, and Basil (page 106)
or other chicken salad over
greens

DINNER

Seared Tofu with Gingered
Vegetables (page 187)

Sesame-Soy Broccoli (page
240)

DAY 6 MEALS

BREAKFAST

Berry Green Smoothie
(page 82)

LUNCH

Pack-and-Go Lunch Bowl
(page 124)

DINNER

Salmon over Kale-Quinoa Salad
(page 172)

Roasted carrots

DAY 7 MEALS

BREAKFAST

Grain- or sweet potato–based
breakfast bowl (page 97)

LUNCH

Chopped Greek Salad Bowls
with Chicken (page 114) or
mixed greens with chicken

DINNER

Creamy Tomato Soup with
Spinach (page 207)

Warm Lemony Brussels Slaw
(page 214)

breakfast and lunch supplements

Apple or pear with nut butter

Hummus and baby carrots
or other raw vegetable

Toasted chickpeas or edamame

Mixed greens with vinaigrette

Yogurt with berries

Black coffee, green tea, water
(including flavored seltzer)

snack ideas

Skillet-Toasted Chickpeas
(page 247)

Crispy Spiced Edamame
(page 248)

Cilantro-Avocado
Hummus (page 252)

Cold-Brew Iced Green
Tea (page 268)

Nuts and nut butters

Legume-based
crackers or chips

Hummus

Yogurt or nondairy yogurt
with live cultures

Fruit

Raw vegetables

Guacamole

Salsa

Hard-boiled
omega-3–rich eggs

EATING TO
prevent or manage type 2 diabetes

Inflammation triggers insulin resistance, the key issue that ultimately leads to prediabetes and type 2 diabetes. This inflammation is caused by irritants in the body like high blood glucose levels, excess body fat, a lack of physical activity, and food choices.

If not stopped, inflammation progresses to slowly deteriorate the body's insulin sensitivity and blood glucose management. This can lead to type 2 diabetes as well as associated complications such as heart disease.

The goal of this targeted anti-inflammatory approach is to maintain or achieve healthy blood glucose management by combining guidelines from the American Diabetes Association and research that has demonstrated a direct correlation to improved glucose regulation, decreased insulin resistance, reduced risk of developing type 2 diabetes, and reduced risk of obesity.

essential focus areas

- INCORPORATE beans and legumes into meals at least 3 times per week. Choose high-fiber, low-GI carbohydrate foods (see Best Carb Choices on page 26) for additional complex carb sources.
- CONSUME a minimum of 5 servings of produce each day (approx. 2 ½ cups).
- CONSUME nuts (approx. a 1-ounce serving) 5 days per week.
- CHOOSE whole foods or minimally processed foods (see page 72) over processed to increase daily fiber intake and to minimize refined grain, added sugar, and sodium intake.
- EAT fish rich in omega-3 fats at least once per week, and increase intake of other omega-3-rich foods.
- MINIMIZE saturated fat intake by choosing lean animal proteins and increasing the proportion of plant- to animal-based proteins.
- GREATLY LIMIT processed foods, trans fats, fried foods, processed and refined sweets, pastries, and foods with high amounts of added sugars.

additional considerations

The following recommendations are not as substantiated by research as the Essential Focus Areas; they are more lifestyle-related approaches. They are additional factors to consider incorporating once the Essential Focus Areas are being actively met.

- The ideal proportion of daily calories from carbohydrates, protein, and fat is specific to each individual. However, research suggests many individuals respond well to a lower to moderate carbohydrate intake (30 to 45 percent calories from carbohydrate). These menus reflect an emphasis on this approach.
- Regular physical activity is an essential component to improve insulin sensitivity and to reduce the production of inflammatory compounds in the body.
- Maintain or work toward achieving a healthy body weight.

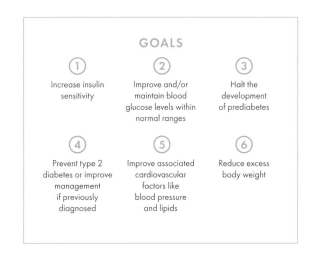

GOALS

① Increase insulin sensitivity

② Improve and/or maintain blood glucose levels within normal ranges

③ Halt the development of prediabetes

④ Prevent type 2 diabetes or improve management if previously diagnosed

⑤ Improve associated cardiovascular factors like blood pressure and lipids

⑥ Reduce excess body weight

breakfast ideas

Super Green Frittata Bites
(page 89)

Sweet Potato Home Fries
with Eggs (page 90)

Warm Spinach
Breakfast Bowl (page 93)

Yogurt or nondairy yogurt
with live cultures

Bowls made with greens

Nuts and nut butters

Omega-3–rich eggs

lunch ideas

Avocado-Chicken Salad
(page 105)

Chicken Salad with Apple,
Cashews, and Basil (page 106)

Tuna, White Bean, and
Arugula Salad (page 109)

Citrus-Balsamic Steak Salad
(page 113)

Chopped Greek Salad Bowls
with Chicken (page 114)

Chopped Southwestern Salad
(page 117)

dinners

Zucchini Taco Skillet (page 142)

Mixed salad greens with
vinaigrette

Personal Pepperoni
Cauliflower Pizzas (page 141)

Roasted broccoli

Fish Tacos with Cilantro Slaw
(page 167)

Marinated Tomatoes and
Cucumbers (page 240)

Greek Spaghetti Squash Toss
(page 204)

Asparagus with Balsamic Drizzle
(page 217)

Seared Scallops with Roasted
Tomatoes (page 179)

Pesto Spaghetti Squash
(page 240)

Chicken Tostadas with
Avocado Salsa (page 133)

Citrus sections

Pork Scaloppine with White
Beans (page 150)

Lemony Garlic Green Beans
(page 218)

snack ideas

Skillet-
Toasted
Chickpeas
(page 247)

Cilantro-
Avocado
Hummus
(page 252)

Nuts and
nut butters

Guacamole
or hummus
with raw
vegetables

Yogurt or
nondairy
yogurt with
live cultures

Hard-boiled
omega-3-rich
eggs

EATING FOR
cancer prevention

Research suggests that cancer risk largely comes down to how our genetics interact with the environment, and our environment includes what we eat and drink.

While we can't change the genetic hand we were dealt, we can limit exposure to carcinogenic food, and we can flood the body with protective antioxidants and phytochemicals to minimize risks and potential cancerous cell mutations by free radicals. This targeted anti-inflammatory approach is based on guidelines advised by the American Cancer Society and the American Institute for Cancer Research, as well as research that has demonstrated a direct correlation to reducing cancer risk and/or development.

essential focus areas

- AIM to consume 6 to 9 servings (3 to 5 cups) of vegetables and fruits each day, if possible, and a minimum of 5 servings each day (approx. 2 ½ cups).
- EMPHASIZE variety in vegetable intake, and regularly incorporate cruciferous vegetables and leafy greens. Focus on vibrant colors when choosing fruits, and regularly incorporate berries and citrus.
- CHOOSE starchy vegetables, beans, lentils, peas, and whole grains. Greatly limit refined grains and highly processed starch sources.
- INCREASE the proportion of plant-based proteins compared to animal-based proteins.
- SLOWLY increase your total daily fiber intake, working up to approximately 25 grams daily for females and 38 grams daily for males.
- AVOID processed meats, fast foods, highly processed foods, and sugary beverages.
- DECREASE added sugar intake, and if consuming alcohol, drink in moderation (see page 275).

additional considerations

These recommendations are not as substantiated by research as the Essential Focus Areas; they are more lifestyle-related approaches. They are additional factors to consider incorporating once the Essential Focus Areas are being actively met.

- Incorporate green tea into daily or weekly intake.
- Consider buying local and/or organic product to limit intake of chemicals and synthetic compounds.
- Step up flavor with fragrant spices, herbs, garlic, and onions.
- Incorporate soy foods unless your doctor advises against it.
- Choose uncured or nitrate-free variations when consuming minimally processed meats.
- Incorporate daily stress management tools or exercise.

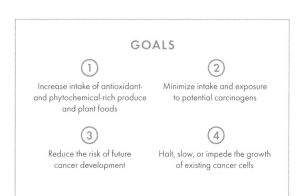

GOALS

① Increase intake of antioxidant- and phytochemical-rich produce and plant foods

② Minimize intake and exposure to potential carcinogens

③ Reduce the risk of future cancer development

④ Halt, slow, or impede the growth of existing cancer cells

breakfast ideas

Berry Green Smoothie
(page 82)

Sweet Potato Home Fries
with Eggs (page 90)

Cherry Power Smoothie
(page 85)

Fruit with nut butter

Bowls made with whole grains
and/or greens

Yogurt or nondairy yogurt
with live cultures and berries

lunch ideas

Tuna, White Bean, and Arugula
Salad (page 109)

Black Bean and Spinach
Quesadillas (page 110)

Chopped Southwestern Salad
(page 117)

Spinach-Quinoa Bowls with
Chicken and Berries (page 121)

Chopped Greek Salad Bowls
with Chicken (Vegetarian
Option; page 114)

dinners

Quick Roasted Tomato Pasta
(page 200)

Spinach salad with vinaigrette

Pesto Spring Grain Bowl
(page 199)

Ginger-Lime Berries (page 240)
or mixed berries

Sea Bass with Strawberry-
Citrus Salsa (page 163)

Nutty Rice Pilaf (page 240)
or cooked whole grain

Lemony Garlic Green Beans
(page 218)

Seared Tofu with Gingered
Vegetables (page 187)

Stir-Fried Bok Choy
with Cashews (page 222)

Salmon over Kale-Quinoa Salad
(page 172)

Rosemary Sweet Potato Fries
(page 233)

Creamy Black Bean and
Cilantro Soup (page 208)

Warm Lemony Brussels Slaw
(page 214)

Lemony Shrimp and Spinach
with Feta (page 176)

Mediterranean Stuffed Tomatoes
(page 229)

snack ideas

Skillet-
Toasted
Chickpeas
(page 247)

Crispy
Spiced
Edamame
(page 248)

Cilantro-
Avocado
Hummus (page
252)

Cold-Brew
Iced Green
Tea (page
268)

Guacamole
and salsa

Berries and
yogurt

Nuts and
nut butters

Legume-
based
crackers or
chips

EATING FOR
heart health

Sure, genetics and body weight increase risks, but every individual is susceptible to lifestyle-related cardiovascular issues such as atherosclerosis, high blood pressure, stroke, and heart attack.

All of these are directly correlated to underlying chronic inflammation typically triggered by a poor diet and a sedentary lifestyle. These factors lead to circulating LDL (aka "bad" cholesterol) that slowly forms deposits within the lining of blood vessels, triggering additional inflammation and creating narrower passageways that require increased pressure to circulate blood.

This targeted anti-inflammatory approach incorporates guidelines from the American Heart Association and research that has demonstrated a direct correlation to either decrease inflammatory factors and increase those associated with reducing inflammation within the cardiovascular system.

essential focus areas

- AIM to consume 100% of the DV for potassium (4,700mg) and to slowly increase total daily fiber intake to approximately 25 grams daily for females and 38 grams daily for males.
- CONSUME a *minimum* of 5 servings of fruits and vegetables each day (approx. 2 ½ cups). Emphasize variety in vegetable and fruit intake, and regularly incorporate leafy greens.
- CHOOSE starchy vegetables, beans, lentils, peas, and whole grains as complex carbohydrate food sources, making sure to incorporate beans and legumes several times per week.
- MINIMIZE saturated fat intake by choosing lean animal proteins and increasing the proportion of plant- to animal-based proteins.
- EAT fish rich in omega-3 fats two to three times a week.
- SUBSTITUTE omega-3-rich foods when possible to improve omega-3 to omega-6 intake ratio.
- CONSUME nuts (approx. a 1-ounce serving) 5 to 7 days per week.

- CONSUME no more than 2,300mg sodium daily.
- GREATLY LIMIT processed foods, trans fats, fried foods, refined grains, highly processed starch sources, and foods with high amounts of added sugars. Limit added sugar content in foods to less than 2 grams per serving.

additional considerations

These recommendations are not as substantiated by research as the Essential Focus Areas; they are more lifestyle-related approaches. They are additional factors to consider incorporating once the Essential Focus Areas are being actively met.

- Regular physical activity is considered an essential component—for all individuals regardless of body weight and age—to reduce the production of inflammatory compounds in the body.
- Excess body weight is associated with increased inflammation in the body. To reduce inflammation, maintaining a healthy body weight or slowly reducing excess body weight is strongly recommended.

GOALS

1. Improve blood lipid numbers
2. Maintain blood pressure within normal range or gradually reduce it to within healthy parameters
3. Prevent, halt, and/or reverse the development of atherosclerosis and hypertension
4. Reduce the risk of major cardiovascular events and conditions

breakfast ideas

Cherry Power Smoothie
(page 85)

Yogurt or nondairy yogurt
with live cultures

Warm Spinach Breakfast Bowl
(page 93)

Bowls made with whole grains
and/or greens

Fruit with nut butter

Berries

lunch ideas

Avocado-Chicken Salad
(page 105)

Chopped Southwestern Salad
(Dairy-Free Option; page 117)

Tuna, White Bean, and Arugula
Salad (page 109)

Chopped Greek Salad Bowls
with Chicken (Vegetarian
Option; page 114)

dinners

Chicken Fried Quinoa (page 138)

Stir-Fried Bok Choy with Cashews
(page 222)

Lemony Black Bean–Quinoa
Salad (page 191)

Roasted carrots

Southwestern Grilled Shrimp
Salad (page 175)

Mixed berries and citrus sections

Thai Zoodle Bowls (page 188)

Steamed green beans

Creamy Black Bean and
Cilantro Soup (page 208)

Mixed salad greens with
vinaigrette

Grilled Salmon with Quick
Romesco (page 159)

Mediterranean Squash Sauté
(page 241)

Quick Roasted Tomato Pasta
(page 200)

Parmesan–Pine Nut Broccoli
(page 241)

snack ideas

Skillet-Toasted Chickpeas (page 247)

Crispy Spiced Edamame (page 248)

Almond Butter–Yogurt-Dipped Fruit (page 256)

Cold-Brew Iced Green Tea (page 268)

Nuts and nut butters

Guacamole or hummus with raw vegetables

Yogurt or nondairy yogurt with live cultures

Hard-boiled omega-3-rich eggs

EATING FOR
brain health

Sure, some slow mental decline is expected as we age, but inflammation in the brain due to lifestyle choices drastically increases the rate and progression of this natural process.

It also appears to be the driving force behind development and progression of brain-deteriorating diseases like Alzheimer's and Parkinson's. The anti-inflammatory eating approach below emphasizes guidelines from the MIND diet, which was developed by researchers at Rush University and emphasizes eating key therapeutic brain foods while avoiding certain inflammatory diet components. Research suggests this protocol has a profound impact on brain functioning by slowing mental decline and memory loss associated with aging and reducing risk and progression of Alzheimer's disease.

essential focus areas

• **AIM** to consume 6 to 9 servings (3 to 5 cups) of vegetables and fruits each day if possible, and a minimum of 5 servings each day (approx. 2 ½ cups).
• **INCLUDE** approximately 1 cup of leafy greens (spinach, kale, cooked greens, salad greens) daily.
• **MAKE** berries your predominant fruit choice, and include them several times a week.
• **EAT** fish rich in omega-3 fats at least once per week.
• **CONSUME** nuts (approx. a 1-ounce serving) 5 to 7 days per week.
• **USE** extra-virgin olive oil as your primary oil in food preparation.
• **INCORPORATE** beans and legumes into meals at least 4 times per week. Choose whole grains and starchy vegetables for additional complex carb sources.
• **_LIMIT_** alcohol consumption to no more than one glass daily, cheese intake to 1 to 2 times per week, and red meats to fewer than 3 times per week.
• **_GREATLY LIMIT_** processed foods, trans fats, fried foods, processed and refined sweets, pastries, and foods with high amounts of added sugars.

additional considerations

These recommendations are not as substantiated by research as the Essential Focus Areas; they are more lifestyle-related approaches. They are additional factors to consider incorporating once the Essential Focus Areas are being actively met.

• Incorporate soy foods such as edamame, soy milk, miso, tofu, and tempeh.
• Consume coffee and/or tea (staying below 3 cups or 300mg caffeine daily).
• Consume eggs rich in omega-3 fats and choline.
• Stay active mentally by regularly reading, doing puzzles or strategy games such as crosswords or sudoku, and getting physical activity that incorporates balance and coordination.

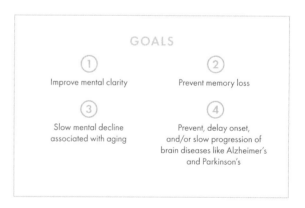

GOALS

① Improve mental clarity

② Prevent memory loss

③ Slow mental decline associated with aging

④ Prevent, delay onset, and/or slow progression of brain diseases like Alzheimer's and Parkinson's

breakfast ideas

Berry Green Smoothie
(page 82)

Cherry Power Smoothie
(page 85)

Sweet Potato Home Fries
with Eggs (page 90)

Warm Spinach Breakfast Bowl
(page 93)

Bowls made with whole grains
and/or greens

Yogurt or nondairy yogurt
with live cultures and berries

lunch ideas

Tuna, White Bean, and Arugula
Salad (page 109)

Chopped Southwestern Salad
(page 117)

Spinach-Quinoa Bowls with
Chicken and Berries (page 121)

Thai Salmon-Brown Rice Bowl
(page 118)

dinners

Salmon over Kale-Quinoa Salad
(page 172)

Rosemary Sweet Potato Fries
(page 233)

Huevos Rancheros Tostadas
(page 195)

Ginger-Lime Berries (page 240)
or mixed berries

Pan-Seared Chicken with Basil–
Pine Nut Gremolata (page 130)

Brown rice or quinoa

Roasted carrots

Lemony Shrimp and Spinach
with Feta (page 176)

Steamed green beans

Creamy Tomato Soup with
Spinach (page 207)

Warm Lemony Brussels Slaw
(page 214)

Sea Bass with Strawberry-
Citrus Salsa (page 163)

Brown rice or quinoa

Spinach salad with vinaigrette

Greek Spaghetti Squash Toss
(page 204)

Roasted broccoli

snack ideas

Skillet-
Toasted
Chickpeas
(page 247)

Crispy
Spiced
Edamame
(page 248)

Almond
Butter–
Yogurt-Dipped
Fruit (page
256)

Cold-Brew
Iced Green
Tea (page
268)

Chai
Concentrate
(page 271)

Nuts and
nut butters

Berries with
yogurt

Hard-boiled
omega-3-rich
eggs

TARGET OR REASSESS

joint health and pain relief

No matter if it's caused by natural wear-and-tear, a previous injury, or an autoimmune reaction, inflammation is at the root of most stiffness, pain, swelling, and deterioration of joints and cartilage.

Choosing foods with an anti-inflammatory effect can ease symptoms to provide mild to significant pain relief and halt further deterioration. The anti-inflammatory eating approach below emphasizes recommendations from the Arthritis Foundation and research that has demonstrated a direct correlation to decreased inflammation within joints, potential pain relief, and long-term joint health.

essential focus areas

- **CONSUME** a minimum of 5 servings of produce each day (approx. 2½ cups).
- **EMPHASIZE** variety in vegetable and fruit intake.
- **CHOOSE** starchy vegetables, beans, lentils, peas, and whole grains as complex carbohydrate food sources, making sure to incorporate beans and legumes several times per week.
- **EAT** fish rich in omega-3 fats two to three times a week.
- **SUBSTITUTE** omega-3-rich foods when possible to improve omega-3 to omega-6 intake ratio (see page 32 for a list).
- **CONSUME** nuts (approx. a 1-ounce serving) 5 to 7 days per week.
- **GREATLY LIMIT** processed foods, trans fats, fried foods, refined grains, highly processed starch sources, and foods with high amounts of added sugars.
- **LIMIT** added sugar content in foods to less than 2 grams per serving.
- **STEP UP** flavor with fragrant spices, herbs, garlic, and onions.

additional considerations

- Consider eliminating nightshade vegetables for 2 to 4 weeks; then reintroduce them one at a time to determine possible effects on arthritis and/or joint pain.
- Eliminate or greatly reduce artificial sweeteners for 2 to 4 weeks to determine if these are affecting arthritis and joint inflammation.
- Take an omega-3 supplement if you're unable to meet the fish or omega-3 food intake recommendations.
- Consider taking a vitamin D and/or calcium supplement if unable to meet daily needs.
- To ease symptoms, consume green tea, cherries or cherry juice, turmeric or curries with turmeric, ginger, pomegranate or pomegranate juice, glucosamine, and/or chondroitin.
- Incorporate daily stress management tools or exercise.

autoimmune joint conditions

Following an anti-inflammatory eating plan appears to be particularly important if you have been diagnosed with an autoimmune condition that affects joints and mobility such as rheumatoid arthritis or systemic lupus. Individuals with one of these conditions can try this guide or may take a slightly more aggressive approach by using the Menu Planning Guide for Autoimmune Conditions (page 300).

GOALS

① Improve or maintain joint health and mobility

② Ease and reduce musculoskeletal stiffness, pain, swelling, and tenderness

③ Prevent or halt joint deterioration caused by inflammation

breakfast ideas

Cherry Power Smoothie (page 85)

Super Green Frittata Bites (page 89)

Sweet Potato Home Fries with Eggs (page 90)

Fruit with nut butter

Cherries and berries

Yogurt or nondairy yogurt with live cultures

Whole grains and/or greens bowls

lunch ideas

Avocado-Chicken Salad (page 105)

Tuna, White Bean, and Arugula Salad (page 109)

Black Bean and Spinach Quesadillas (page 110)

Chopped Southwestern Salad (page 117)

Spinach-Quinoa Bowls with Chicken and Berries (page 121)

dinners

Sheet Pan Honey-Soy Salmon, Sweet Potatoes, and Green Beans (page 160)

Gluten-Free Chicken Tenders (page 129)

Lower-Carb Parmesan Polenta (page 230)

Roasted broccoli

Zucchini Frittata with Goat Cheese (page 203)

Cherries

Green Curry with Halibut (page 164)

Gluten-Free Margherita Flatbread (page 192)

Lemony Sugar Snaps with Radishes (page 241)

Grilled Salmon with Quick Romesco (page 159)

Brown rice or quinoa

Spinach salad with vinaigrette

Thai Zoodle Bowls (page 188)

Roasted baby carrots

snack ideas

Cilantro-Avocado Hummus (page 252)

Cold-Brew Iced Green Tea (page 268)

Nuts and nut butters

Guacamole or hummus with raw vegetables

Yogurt or nondairy yogurt with live cultures

Fruit

Hard-boiled omega-3-rich eggs

autoimmune conditions

An autoimmune condition is a dysfunctional state where the body is inflamed, confused, and attacking the structure or proper functioning within itself. Basically, the system that is responsible for inflammation is itself inflamed.

This creates a very delicate, self-debilitating state that is very susceptible to further irritation and inflammation, causing a cascade of effects. Unlike some inflammatory conditions that progress slower—like diabetes or heart disease—autoimmune conditions are either exacerbated or calmed by food and lifestyle habits; individuals with these conditions can usually feel the impact immediately.

The anti-inflammatory protocol will be specific to each autoimmune condition, and it's important to identify the key diet and lifestyle factors that both negatively and positively impact symptoms. Once identified, then inflammation in the body can be reduced to help manage the disease and ease symptoms and side effects.

essential focus areas

- CONSUME a minimum of 5 servings of produce each day (approx. 2 ½ cups).
- CONSUME only whole or minimally processed foods when possible to eliminate any unnecessary additives like colorings, artificial sweeteners, chemicals, and pesticides.
- ELIMINATE gluten for several weeks before reintroducing, and avoid if potential sensitivity is identified.
- EAT fish rich in omega-3 fats two to three times a week.
- SUBSTITUTE omega-3-rich foods when possible to improve omega-6 to omega-3 intake ratio (see page 32 for a list).
- CONSUME nuts (approx. a 1-ounce serving) 5 to 7 days per week.
- GREATLY LIMIT processed foods, trans fats, fried foods, refined grains, highly processed starch sources, and foods with high amounts of added sugars.

- LIMIT added sugar content in foods to less than 2 grams per serving.
- INCREASE intake of probiotic and prebiotic foods (see page 18 for a list).
- INCREASE the proportion of plant-based proteins compared to animal-based proteins.
- STEP UP flavor with fragrant spices, herbs, garlic, and onions.

additional considerations

- Increase your intake of produce during periods of physical or emotional stress to increase antioxidant intake.
- Consider taking an omega-3 supplement if unable to meet the fish or omega-3 food intake recommendations.
- Discuss the need for possible supplementation of vitamin D, calcium, probiotics, and/or vitamin B_{12} with your doctor.
- Avoid excessive caffeine intake.
- Consider trying a grain-free diet if eliminating gluten does not ease symptoms.
- Consider eliminating nightshade vegetables for 2 to 4 weeks; then reintroduce them one at a time to determine the possible effects on arthritis and/or joint pain.
- Consider eliminating dairy for 2 to 4 weeks; then slowly reintroduce it to determine if dairy is an irritant that exacerbates symptoms.
- Curcumin may slightly ease symptoms. Obtain curcumin through supplements and/or turmeric or curries with turmeric, and/or ginger.
- Incorporate daily stress management tools or exercise.
- Get adequate sleep.
- Consider following an elimination protocol under the supervision of a registered dietitian if you're unable to effectively identify food sensitivities.

diet and autoimmune conditions

The prevalence of autoimmune dysfunction and disease is notably higher in wealthier, industrialized societies, something researchers suggest is largely due to the excess calories, fat, salt, sugar, and processed food components in the Western diet. The combination of diet, a lack of diverse and balanced gut bacteria, and other lifestyle practices appears to lead to systemic inflammation, which triggers alterations in proper immune system functioning, particularly in those with a genetic predisposition. Individuals in the eastern hemisphere and less-developed countries do not have less genetic susceptibility to autoimmune conditions, but they likely have less exposure to inflammatory conditions to trigger a disease state.

top diet components related to autoimmune conditions

Autoimmune conditions differ in onset and symptoms, but there are four things that research suggests play the biggest role when it comes to management and easing of autoimmune symptoms.

GLUTEN-FREE DIET: One of the first recommendations is to eliminate gluten to determine if it is exacerbating inflammation. While it may not appear to have an effect during symptom-free periods, it may become an irritant during flare-ups.

ADEQUATE OMEGA-3 INTAKE: EPA and DHA are key fatty acids found in fish oil and appear to play a key role in managing autoimmune conditions and easing flare-ups and symptoms. Daily recommendations range from 250 to 1,000mg of omega-3 fatty acids (from DHA and EPA), which can be accomplished by eating fatty fish regularly and/or taking a supplement.

ADEQUATE VITAMIN D: Low levels of vitamin D are associated with increased likelihood of being diagnosed with an autoimmune condition. Adequate intake appears to reduce or minimize risks of flare-ups. Daily requirements are 600 to 800 IUs for adults. Many have a hard time achieving this, particularly those who do not consume dairy or who are vegetarian.

HEALTHY GUT: It's when foreign compounds and irritants leak through the intestinal wall into the bloodstream that inflammation occurs, and consuming a diet with adequate probiotic and prebiotic foods to strengthen gut health decreases permeability of the intestinal walls.

GOALS

(1) Calm inflammation to ease symptoms related to autoimmune diseases such as lupus, multiple sclerosis, irritable bowel diseases, arthritis, and thyroid conditions.

(2) Identify specific diet and lifestyle habits.

(3) Reduce flare-ups by targeting specific diet and lifestyle habits.

(4) Halt progression of disease and/or insidious development of additional conditions.

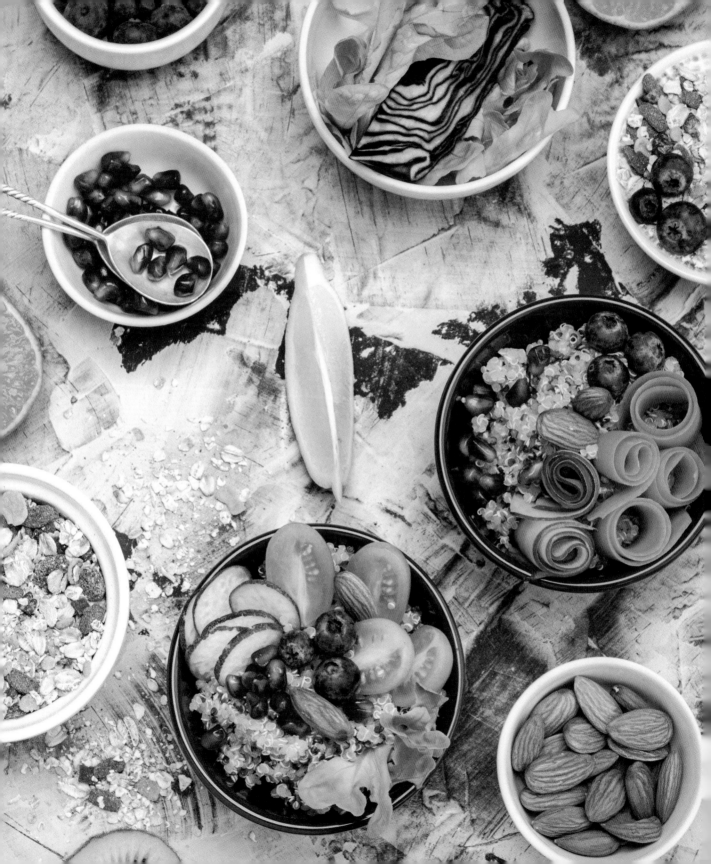

breakfast ideas

Easy Make-Ahead Granola
(Grain-Free Option; page 81)

Cherry Power Smoothie
(page 85)

Super Green Frittata Bites
(page 89)

Sweet Potato Home Fries with Eggs
(page 90)

Bowls made with whole grains
and/or greens

Yogurt or nondairy yogurt with live
cultures and berries

lunch ideas

Chicken Salad with Apple,
Cashews, and Basil (page 106)

Tuna, White Bean, and Arugula
Salad (page 109)

Chopped Southwestern Salad
(Dairy-Free Option; page 117)

Chopped Greek Salad Bowls
with Chicken (Dairy-Free
Option; page 114)

Spinach-Quinoa Bowls
with Chicken and Berries
(Dairy-Free Option; page 121)

dinners

Seared Tofu with Gingered
Vegetables (page 187)

Broccoli with Thai Almond Butter
Sauce (page 221)

Thai Chicken Noodle Soup
(page 134)

Ginger-Lime Berries (page 240)
or mixed berries

Greek Lamb Lettuce Wraps
(page 149)

Baked Sweet Potatoes
(page 240)

Green Curry with Halibut
(page 164)

Gluten-Free Margherita
Flatbread (page 192)

Warm Lemony Brussels Slaw
(page 214)

Sheet Pan Honey-Soy
Salmon, Sweet Potatoes, and
Green Beans (page 160)

Thai Zoodle Bowls (page 188)

Stir-Fried Bok Choy with
Cashews (page 222)

snack ideas

Skillet-
Toasted
Chickpeas
(page 247)

Crispy
Spiced
Edamame
(page 248)

Cold-Brew
Iced Green
Tea (page
268)

Chai
Concentrate
(page 271)

Nuts and
nut butters

Guacamole
or hummus
with raw
vegetables

Yogurt or
nondairy
yogurt with
live cultures

Fruit

seasonal produce guide

When you use fresh fruits, vegetables, and herbs, you don't have to do much to make them taste great. Although many fruits, vegetables, and herbs are available year-round, you'll get better flavor and prices when you buy what's in season. This guide helps you choose the best produce so you can create tasty meals all year long.

spring

FRUITS
Bananas
Blood oranges
Coconuts
Grapefruit
Kiwifruit
Lemons
Limes
Mangoes
Navel oranges
Papayas
Passion fruit
Pineapples
Strawberries
Tangerines
Valencia
  oranges

VEGETABLES
Artichokes
Arugula
Asparagus
Avocados
Baby leeks
Beets
Belgian endive
Broccoli
Cauliflower
Dandelion
  greens
Fava beans
Green peas
Kale
Lettuce
Mushrooms
Radishes
Red potatoes
Rhubarb
Scallions
Snap beans
Snow peas
Spinach
Sugar snap peas
Sweet onions
Swiss chard

HERBS
Chives
Dill
Garlic chives
Lemongrass
Mint
Parsley
Thyme

summer

FRUITS
Apricots
Blackberries
Blueberries
Boysenberries
Cantaloupes
Casaba melons
Cherries
Crenshaw
  melons
Figs
Grapes
Guava
Honeydew
  melons
Mangoes
Nectarines
Papayas
Peaches
Plums
Raspberries
Strawberries
Watermelons

VEGETABLES
Avocados
Beans: snap,
  pole, and shell
Beets
Bell peppers
Cabbage
Carrots
Celery
Chile peppers
Collards
Corn
Cucumbers
Eggplant
Green beans
Jicama
Lima beans
Okra
Pattypan squash
Peas
Radicchio
Radishes
Summer squash
Tomatoes

HERBS
Basil
Bay leaves
Borage
Chives
Cilantro
Dill
Lavender
Lemon balm
Marjoram
Mint
Oregano
Rosemary
Sage
Summer savory
Tarragon
Thyme

fall

FRUITS
Apples
Cranberries
Figs
Grapes
Pears
Persimmons
Pomegranates
Quinces

VEGETABLES
Belgian endive
Bell peppers
Broccoli
Brussels sprouts
Cabbage
Cauliflower
Eggplant
Escarole
Fennel
Frisée
Leeks
Mushrooms
Parsnips
Pumpkins
Red potatoes
Rutabagas
Shallots
Sweet potatoes
Winter squash
Yukon Gold
  potatoes

HERBS
Basil
Bay leaves
Parsley
Rosemary
Sage
Tarragon
Thyme

winter

FRUITS
Apples
Blood oranges
Cranberries
Grapefruit
Kiwifruit
Kumquats
Lemons
Limes
Mandarin
  oranges
Navel oranges
Pears
Persimmons
Pomegranates
Pomelos
Tangelos
Tangerines
Quinces

VEGETABLES
Baby turnips
Beets
Belgian endive
Brussels
  sprouts
Celery root
Escarole
Fennel
Frisée
Jerusalem
  artichokes
Kale
Leeks
Mushrooms
Parsnips
Potatoes
Rutabagas
Sweet potatoes
Turnips
Watercress
Winter squash

nutritional information

Research overwhelmingly suggests that quality is the most important factor in one's diet for long-term health and disease prevention. Most health professionals define a higher-quality diet as one that focuses on choosing predominantly whole foods that are minimally processed, nutrient-dense, and with little to no added sugars or other ingredients. This means that traditional eating tools such as calorie counting, measuring portions, and tracking nutrient grams aren't effective measures to ensure overall diet quality.

Yet prioritizing diet quality doesn't mean that quantities (such as calories or macronutrients) aren't important. Research clearly demonstrates that routinely exceeding calorie and/or nutrients can lead to increases in body weight, disease risk, and inflammation. A key component of consuming a higher-quality diet is eating those healthier foods within recommended amounts for health or specific conditions, but the optimal intake and approach to meal planning will be unique to an individual's health goals.

However, many (including myself) want guidelines to ensure they are consuming a higher-quality daily diet, as well as not regularly exceeding energy intake, food group, or nutrient. Recognizing this, *Meals That Heal* provides several techniques and tools for helping you develop a balanced, higher-quality diet, in addition to recipes that emphasize the use of higher-quality foods.

TOOLS FOR BALANCING QUALITY WITH QUANTITY

• **Meal Planning and Daily Intake:** The information provided in Rethinking the Dinner Plate (page 33) is a method I use daily to plan meals and overall daily intake. It's simple with no counting, but guides you in eating close to the recommended amounts of food groups. And choosing higher-quality foods (see "best choices" for each macronutrient on pages 26–30) can provide a nutrient-dense diet. For those who need slightly more defined parameters, try planning daily food intake using the amounts in the Eating Recommendations (pages 22–23) as a starting place, adapting as needed for activity or other factors.

• **Nutritional Information:** You'll find nutrient information provided for each recipe that includes total calories, total grams of macronutrients, and amounts of a few key micronutrients. The intention in providing these values is to give a more complete picture of a recipe's nutritional qualities for each individual to support specific health goals.

• **USDA Nutrient Guidelines:** Every recipe in this book fits within the most recent Dietary Guidelines, as well as meets the specific condition-based recommendations in Chapter 10. These nutrient guidelines are provided below and should be used as a general guide.

DAILY NUTRITION GUIDE

	Women ages 25 to 50	Women over 50	Men ages 25 to 50	Men over 50
CALORIES	2,000	2,000*	2,700	2,500
PROTEIN	50g	50g	63g	60g
FAT	65g*	65g*	88g*	83g*
SATURATED FAT	20g*	20g*	27g*	25g*
CARBOHYDRATES	304g	304g	410g	375g
FIBER	25 to 35g	25 to 35g	25 to 35g	25 to 35g
ADDED SUGARS	38g	38g	38g	38g
CHOLESTEROL	300mg*	300mg*	300mg*	300mg*
IRON	18mg	8mg	8mg	8mg
SODIUM	2,300mg*	1,500mg*	2,300mg*	1,500mg*
CALCIUM	1,000mg	1,200mg	1,000mg	1,000mg

*Or less, for optimum health

Nutritional values used in our calculations either come from The Food Processor, Version 10.4 (ESHA Research), or are provided by food manufacturers.

metric equivalents

The recipes that appear in this cookbook use the standard United States method for measuring liquid and dry or solid ingredients (teaspoons, tablespoons, and cups). The information in the following charts is provided to help cooks outside the US successfully use these recipes. All equivalents are approximate.

METRIC EQUIVALENTS FOR DIFFERENT TYPES OF INGREDIENTS

A standard cup measure of a dry or solid ingredient will vary in weight depending on the type of ingredient. A standard cup of liquid is the same volume for any type of liquid. Use the following chart when converting standard cup measures to grams (weight) or milliliters (volume).

Standard Cup	Fine Powder (ex. flour)	Grain (ex. rice)	Granular (ex. sugar)	Liquid Solids (ex. butter)	Liquid (ex. milk)
1	140 g	150 g	190 g	200 g	240 ml
3/4	105 g	113 g	143 g	150 g	180 ml
2/3	93 g	100 g	125 g	133 g	160 ml
1/2	70 g	75 g	95 g	100 g	120 ml
1/3	47 g	50 g	63 g	67 g	80 ml
1/4	35 g	38 g	48 g	50 g	60 ml
1/8	18 g	19 g	24 g	25 g	30 ml

USEFUL EQUIVALENTS FOR LIQUID INGREDIENTS BY VOLUME

¼ tsp						=	1 ml	
½ tsp						=	2 ml	
1 tsp						=	5 ml	
3 tsp	=	1 Tbsp			=	½ fl oz	=	15 ml
		2 Tbsp	=	⅛ cup	=	1 fl oz	=	30 ml
		4 Tbsp	=	¼ cup	=	2 fl oz	=	60 ml
		5 ⅓ Tbsp	=	⅓ cup	=	3 fl oz	=	80 ml
		8 Tbsp	=	½ cup	=	4 fl oz	=	120 ml
		10 ⅔ Tbsp	=	⅔ cup	=	5 fl oz	=	160 ml
		12 Tbsp	=	¾ cup	=	6 fl oz	=	180 ml
		16 Tbsp	=	1 cup	=	8 fl oz	=	240 ml
		1 pt	=	2 cups	=	16 fl oz	=	480 ml
		1 qt	=	4 cups	=	32 fl oz	=	960 ml
						33 fl oz	=	1000 ml = 11

USEFUL EQUIVALENTS FOR DRY INGREDIENTS BY WEIGHT

(To convert ounces to grams, multiply the number of ounces by 30.)

1 oz	=	¹⁄₁₆ lb	=	30 g
4 oz	=	¼ lb	=	120 g
8 oz	=	½ lb	=	240 g
12 oz	=	¾ lb	=	360 g
16 oz	=	1 lb	=	480 g

USEFUL EQUIVALENTS FOR LENGTH

(To convert inches to centimeters, multiply the number of inches by 2.5.)

1 in					=	2.5 cm		
6 in	=	½ ft			=	15 cm		
12 in	=	1 ft			=	30 cm		
36 in	=	3 ft	=	1 yd	=	90 cm		
40 in					=	100 cm	=	1 m

USEFUL EQUIVALENTS FOR COOKING/OVEN TEMPERATURES

	Fahrenheit	Celsius	Gas Mark
Freeze Water	32° F	0° C	
Room Temperature	68° F	20° C	
Boil Water	212° F	100° C	
Bake	325° F	160° C	3
	350° F	180° C	4
	375° F	190° C	5
	400° F	200° C	6
	425° F	220° C	7
	450° F	230° C	8
Broil			Grill

acknowledgments

Thank you, Madeline and Griffin, for tasting endless recipes, being my toughest critics, and rolling with schedule changes when I had an inspiration and needed to get in the kitchen. And, more important, thank you for giving me this crazy, wonderful, on-the-go, hectic, fun life. It's your laughter, homework frustrations, sibling spats, messy rooms, scraped knees, soccer practices, hugs, and nightly snuggles that continuously remind me that it doesn't matter how healthy or "good" a recipe looks on paper. What really matters is that food tastes good, nourishes the body, and is simple enough so that we all end up at the table together.

Mom and Dad, the words "thank you" really don't feel adequate enough for all that you have done over the past year and a half. Without you, this cookbook wouldn't exist right now. I am grateful for your spending time with the kids while I worked, tasting recipes, editing copy, providing regular counseling, and feeding us when I was too tired to cook. Thank you also for exposing me to the culinary and restaurant world early in my life at home and in travel. It's these experiences that spurred my interest in cooking and developed an appreciation for good food—or at least that is what I tell myself when I now drag Madeline and Griffin to "fancy" restaurants!

Thank you Ann Pittman and Hunter Lewis for calling me in a pinch and opening my eyes to the concept of chronic inflammation, an area in food and nutrition that I hadn't considered exploring until then. I had no idea the caliber of the research and writing that I was stepping into for that November 2016 *Cooking Light* issue, but it was a challenge that I needed and one that has since opened doors and given me new career direction, as well as inspiration and energy in the kitchen. I am beyond grateful that I was the dietitian you chose to call.

To my editor, Rachel West, thank you for your guidance, support, encouragement, patience and candid feedback throughout this whole process. Having a friend, as well as trusted colleague and fellow dietitian, serve as editor meant more than you know. To my friend, Allison Lowery, thank you for always being my biggest cheerleader and best sounding board for work, kids, and life. To Robin Plotkin, thank you for challenging me to step outside my comfort zone. It was your coaching last summer that made me pitch cookbook ideas to Rachel. And to my amazing assistant, Amber Salmon, thank you for holding things together for me while I cooked, wrote, and edited!

To say it took a village would be an understatement, and I am so grateful for my village!

index

Page numbers in *italics* refer to recipe photos.

about the author

Carolyn Williams, PhD, RD, is a registered dietitian and culinary nutrition expert known for her ability to simplify the concept of healthy eating. She serves as a contributing editor for *Cooking Light* and *Real Simple* and won a James Beard Award for her article 2016 "Brain Health." She also develops content for a variety of media outlets and lifestyle brands such as *Real Simple*, *Parents*, Rally Health, *Eating Well*, eMeals, and *Health*. Other work includes nutrient analysis, recipe development, and writing, including her newest cookbook *Meals That Heal*, which focuses on using the healing aspects of food with a quick, easy, and practical approach. Carolyn is also a tenured faculty member at a local college teaching culinary arts and nutrition classes.

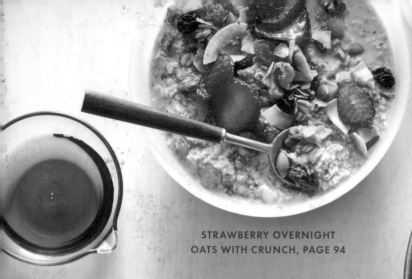

ROASTED VEGGIE-
POLENTA BOWL, PAGE 196

STRAWBERRY OVERNIGHT
OATS WITH CRUNCH, PAGE 94

Reset your microbiome with more than
100 delicious, quick, and easy anti-inflammatory recipes—all
ready in 30 minutes or less that won't break your budget! From
Sweet Potato Home Fries with Eggs for breakfast to Chopped
Greek Salad Bowls with Chicken for lunch to Personal Pepperoni
Cauliflower Pizzas or Sheet Pan Honey-Soy Salmon, Sweet
Potatoes, and Green Beans for dinner, plus Peanut Butter–
Chocolate Chip "Cookie Dough" Bites or a Classic Margarita for a
sweet treat, these are recipes for the whole family to enjoy.

Inside you'll also find:

- Recipes geared toward specific conditions like brain health, weight
  loss, cancer prevention, joint health, and autoimmune diseases.

- A complete list of anti-inflammatory foods, the top inflamers, and
  on-the-go eating guidelines.

- A menu guide to creating a personal meal and action plan
  targeting your specific health concerns.

SHEET PAN STEAK
FAJITAS, PAGE 145

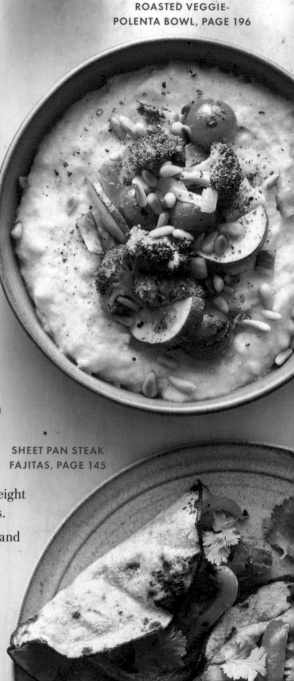

COOKING   0619

ISBN 978-1-9821-3078-7   **$22.99 U.S./**$32.00 Can.

9 781982 130787   52299

PRINTED IN THE U.S.A.

TILLER
P R E S S

SimonandSchuster.com

COVER DESIGN BY ANNAMARIA JACOB
COVER PHOTOGRAPHY BY ANTONIS ACHILLEOS

FRONT COVER: CHICKEN TOSTADAS
WITH AVOCADO SALSA, PAGE 133